Gut Microflora

Digestive Physiology and Pathology

ISBN 2-7420-0585-4

Éditions John Libbey Eurotext

127, avenue de la République, 92120 Montrouge, France

Tél : 01 46 73 06 60

E-mail : contact@john-libbey-eurotext.fr

Site internet : http://www.john-libbey-eurotext.fr

John Libbey Eurotext Limited

42-46 High Street

Esther, Surrey, KT 10 9QY

United Kingdom

© 2006, John Libbey Eurotext, Paris

Gut
Microflora

Digestive Physiology and Pathology

Edited by:
Jean-Claude Rambaud
Jean-Paul Buts
Gérard Corthier
Bernard Flourié

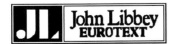

Editorial committee

Autors

Fernando Azpiroz
Servicio de Aparato Digestivo, Hospital General Vall d'Hebron,
Universidad Autónoma de Barcelona,
Barcelona, España

Annick Bernalier-Donadille
Unité de Microbiologie, INRA,
Centre de Recherches de Clermont-Ferrand / Theix,
Saint-Genès-Champanelle, France

Hervé Blottière
Institut National de la Recherche Agronomique,
Unité de Nutrition et Sécurité Alimentaire,
Domaine de Vilvert, CRJ, Jouy-en-Josas, France

Yoram Bouhnik
Service d'Hépato-Gastro-entérologie et Assistance Nutritive,
Hôpital Lariboisière, 2, rue Ambroise Paré, Paris, France

Marie-José Butel
Département de Microbiologie, Faculté de Pharmacie,
Université Paris V-René Descartes,
12, rue de l'École de Médecine, Paris, France

Jean-Paul Buts
Université Catholique de Louvain,
Cliniques Universitaires St Luc - a.s.b.l.,
Avenue Hippocrate, 10, 1200 Bruxelles, Belgique

Claire Cherbuy
Institut National de la Recherche Agronomique,
Unité de Nutrition et Sécurité Alimentaire,
Domaine de Vilvert, CRJ, Jouy-en-Josas, France

Benoît Coffin
Service d'Hépato-Gastro-entérologie, Hôpital Louis Mourier,
178, rue des Renouillers, 92000 Colombes, France

Anne Collignon
Service de Bactériologie, Hôpital Jean Verdier,
Avenue du 14 Juillet, 93140 Bondy, France

Pierre Desreumaux
Service des Maladies de l'Appareil Digestif et de la Nutrition,
EPI 0114 – CHRU de Lille, Hôpital Swynghedauw,
rue A. Verhaegh, 59037 Lille, France

Joël Doré
Unité d'Écologie et de Physiologie du Système Digestif,
INRA-CRJ, 78350 Jouy-en-Josas, France

Pierre-Henri Duée
Institut National de la Recherche Agronomique,
Unité de Nutrition et Sécurité Alimentaire,
Domaine de Vilvert, CRJ, 78350 Jouy-en-Josas, France

Philippe Marteau
Service de Gastro-entérologie, Hôpital Européen Georges Pompidou,
20, rue Leblanc, 75015, Paris, France

Marie-Christiane Moreau
Unité d'Écologie et de Physiologie du Système Digestif,
INRA, Domaine de Vilvert, 78350 Jouy-en-Josas, France

Thierry Piche
Service d'Hépato-Gastro-entérologie, CHU de Nice,
Hôpital de l'Archet 2,
151, route Saint-Antoine de Ginestière, BP 3079,
06200 Nice, France

Patrick Rampal
Service d'Hépato-Gastro-entérologie, Centre Hospitalier Princesse Grace,
avenue Pasteur, BP 48992018, 98000 Principauté de Monaco

Lionel Rigottier-Gois
Unité d'Écologie et de Physiologie du Système Digestif,
INRA-CRJ, 78350 Jouy-en-Josas, France

Christel Rousseaux
Service des Maladies de l'Appareil Digestif et de la Nutrition,
EPI 0114 – CHRU de Lille, Hôpital Swynghedauw,
rue A. Verhaegh, 59037 Lille, France

Jean-Marc Sabaté
Service d'Hépato-Gastro-entérologie, Hôpital Louis Mourier,
178 rue des Renouillers, 92000 Colombes, France

Philippe Seksik
Service de Gastro-entérologie, Hôpital Européen Georges Pompidou,
20 rue Leblanc, 75015 Paris, France

Contents

Gut Microflora

Gut Microflora
in Physiology and Pathogenesis

The Value of Administering Live Organisms

Preface

The gut microflora—which is mainly anaerobic and localized in the colon—comprises about 10^{14} microorganisms living in a symbiotic relationship with the host. For many years, its study depended on stool culture and on the skilled anaerobic culture methods, and this yielded description of the dominant, sub-dominant and transiting microflora. Despite recent technical advances, a large fraction of the dominant anaerobic microflora (i.e., 99% of the faecal microflora) cannot be grown *in vitro* in spite of its identification using molecular methods. The cloning and sequencing of 16S ribosomal DNA molecules have revealed that the majority of faecal bacteria belong to one of three major phylogenetic lineages, and that more than 80% of the molecular species observed have not hitherto been cultured. The average number of dominant species in the faecal microflora of a healthy human can be estimated at about one-hundred. Every subject carries his own range of different species and, by adulthood, this profile remains stable over time, although the microfloras of different individuals only share a small number of species. The development of 16S ribosomal RNA-recognizing probes specific for domains, groups, sub-groups and species of bacteria has made it possible to perform serial analyses—both quantitative and qualitative—of stool samples or intracolonic specimens.

The gut microflora is acquired during the first two years of life. The ability of a species to establish itself durably in the colonic ecosystem depends on complex interactions between host and bacteria as well as between the bacteria themselves. Relevant factors pertaining at birth, notably environmental conditions and hygiene, are currently a topic of great interest because of changes recently observed in intestinal colonization profiles in babies and possible links with the explosion of allergic disease in developed countries.

It is noteworthy to remember that the great majority of microbiologic investigations of the digestive system have focused on faeces, which gives an imperfect picture even of the microflora of the left colon. Although the microflora transiting the small intestine is fairly well characterized, there have been few studies of the ascending colon in which the microflora differs substantially from that in the faeces and is not as stable because of the broad variety of dietary substrates available in this segment of the gut. Similarly, the microflora which is adherent to the colonic wall—also very different from the faecal microflora—has been little studied to date. It should be noted that what is going to be described in the following pages about the functioning and malfunctioning of the microflora is the result of work conducted on either total faecal microflora or those species that can be cultured. Major progress in our view of the functioning of the microflora will result from expansion of the molecular approach to include the tools of integrative biology.

The broad diversity of the dietary and endogenous substrates metabolized by the colonic microflora largely accounts for its own diversity: anaerobic substrate breakdown is a complex process which implies the participation of different bacterial groups and various complementary metabolic activities which have been more or less comprehensively inventoried. Carbohydrate breakdown generates short-chain fatty acids (SCFA) with, in many cases, intermediate metabolites such as lactate, and gaseous end products such as carbon dioxide and hydrogen. Hydrogenotrophic bacteria, including the methanogenic archaea, play an important role by reducing the partial pressure of hydrogen. Protein fermentation results in the generation of SCFAs as well as of ammonia which is absorbed and used as a nitrogen source by many species of the microflora, thereby mitigating its toxic effects.

Imbalance between the rates of colonic gas production and consumption, and the production of malodorous gases such as hydrogen sulphide lead to the anal emission of excessive quantities of gas or unpleasantly smelling gases. Abdominal bloating—real or perceived—is a more complex topic in which increased gas production seems not involved (even when it exists). It is rather due to gas retention at the anus or to inadequate gas propulsion in the intestine. In normal subjects, the colonic motility pattern determines the establishment of the resident microflora and, in turn, the microflora influences parietal motility and colonic transit, an effect which is probably secondary to fermentation reactions.

The colonic epithelium turnover is constant. It lines the crypts where three different cell types arise, divide and differentiate, including the absorbing cells or colonocytes. It also constitutes the mucosal surface from which cells at the end of their cycle are shed, probably after apoptosis. These processes are finely regulated by molecular mechanisms, including the Wnt signal transduction pathway which plays a central role.

Butyrate, transported by MCT1 (monocarboxylate transporter 1), is the major oxidative substrate for colonocytes, in which it is also a precursor of ketogenesis. Butyrate and, to a lesser extent, other SCFAs play an important role in colonocyte division and apoptosis. Butyrate action is double-edged in that deficiency will lead to mucosal atrophy, but when energy intake is unlimited, this compound inhibits cell division both *in vivo* and *in vitro* (e.g. in transformed human colonic cell lines) by stimulating expression of the protein p21^{Cip1}.

The above-mentioned findings have been confirmed *in vivo* using animals with controlled microflora. A genuine partnership is established between the bacterial microflora and the colonic epithelium, as illustrated by the example of glycosylated glycoconjugates.

The colonic microflora certainly plays a role in the development of colon cancer, but it is a complex one. Apart from the production of protective factors like butyrate, it is possible that NH_4, H_2S and polyamines have adverse effects. Most importantly, microbial metabolism of exogenous or endogenous (bile salts) procarcinogens might be actively involved in carcinogenesis, or the microflora might produce potent mutagens like fecapentaenes. Currently, attempts are being made to prevent such effects by the administration of probiotics.

For many years, the double fonction of the mucosal immune system has been a subject of debate: this system must protect against pathogenic agents at the same time as tolerating the continuous flow of food and bacteria by suppressing cell-mediated and humoral (mainly IgE) responses to these foreign antigens in the intestine and the periphery. The gut microflora plays a key role in these processes as has been established mainly in experiments on controlled-flora animals. Bacterial components—especially lipopolysaccharide—induce maturation of the antigen-presenting cells (APC) of the innate immune system and play a particularly important role in determining the balance between Th1 and Th2 cells in children, a balance which, when inappropriate, leads to allergic disease, a pathology which is rising currently. The gut microflora also acts, through the natural immunoglobulins, on the diversity of the B cell repertoire of the humoral immune system, thereby helping to prevent autoimmune diseases.

The gut microflora plays an essential role in the development and activation of the intestinal immune system (IIS), especially in the production of secretory IgA (sIgA). Disturbance of the sequential bacterial colonization of the intestine in children affects the IIS, an effect which is probably sustained into adulthood. In acute rotaviral diarrhoea in children, specific sIgA responses are modulated by bacteria (*Bifidobacterium* and *Escherichia coli*) of the gut microflora. Oral tolerance induced by prior ingestion of a protein is also dependent on colonization (sometimes at birth) by bacterial species such as *Bifidobacterium infantis*. The mechanisms involved are as yet poorly understood but the secretion of IL-10 by Th3 cells certainly plays a major role. As far as the host tolerates its own endogenous microflora, it is believed that blocking of activation of the NFκB pathway by bacteria of the microflora inhibits synthesis of inflammatory cytokines and chemokines. One illustration of this mechanism is provided by the efficacy of probiotics in pouchitis and against the colonic lesions of ulcerative colitis, effects which are mediated through re-establishment of the disturbed balance between the microflora and the gut mucosa.

On the basis of these observations, which etiologic factors can account for the pathogenesis and chronicity of inflammatory bowel disease (IBD)? The microflora has been shown to be involved in the immune perturbations which characterize this condition by bacteriological studies in patients and in most experimental animal models of colitis. In chronic IBD, mucosal CD14 and TLR4 receptors for bacterial LPS are over-expressed and PPARγ is under-expressed, thereby perturbing the NFκB and MAPK pathways of the inflammatory response. Other molecules secreted by bacteria are also known to be involved.

Compromise of the host's tolerance of the bacteria of the microflora results in unbalanced cytokine profiles which differ between the chronic and the acute lesions of Crohn's disease. The discovery, in a sub-population of patients suffering from Crohn's disease, of mutations in the *CARD15* gene which has a central role in the control of infections of the gut mucosa and which is loop-regulated by TNFα, provides further support for the hypothesis that microbes are involved in the pathogenesis of this condition.

Disurbance of the colonic microbial ecosystem is the common denominator in antibiotic-associated diarrhoea. Curiously, this has not been studied in depth, although reduced levels of anaerobic bacteria and increased densities of aerobic bacteria in the faeces have been observed in patients with acute infectious diarrhoea, justifying preventive and curative treatment strategies based on probiotics for this type of condition. Although simple forms of antibiotic-associated diarrhoea are mainly due to reduced metabolism of a part of the colonic microflora, compromise of the barrier effect can open the way for intestinal colonization by *Clostridium difficile* sometimes leading to pseudomembranous colitis, a nosocomial problem. The epidemiology and clinical picture of this infection, how to diagnose it both endoscopically and bacteriologically (based on detection of toxins A and B whose mechanisms of actions have been elucidated), and its treatment (metronidazole and vancomycin) are all well characterized.

A more recent discovery is that the efficacy of the immune response against the bacterium is probably an essential factor in the clinical expression of *Clostridium difficile* infection and in the frequency of relapses. Probiotics, especially *Saccharomyces boulardii*, have been shown to be an effective treatment for preventing recurrence.

All the above observations justify attempts at treatment strategies based on probiotics (the utilization of which was for a long time undertaken in an empirical approach). The WHO has defined probiotics as "live microorganisms which when administered in adequate amounts confer a health benefit on the host". Since their active domains remain often unknown, our knowledge of the pharmacokinetics of probiotics are generally limited to the survival of the microorganisms during transit through the digestive tract. Probiotics mediate direct effects in the lumen or at the gut wall, notably on the immune system; they also mediate indirect effects through the endogenous microflora.

Probiotics are very safe with the rare infections due to such organisms only having been observed in very special circumstances. Probiotics can be combined with prebiotics, i.e. "indigestible dietary ingredients which, in the colon, selectively stimulate the division and activities of a limited number of bacterial groups which are capable of improving the host's health". The use of prebiotics (mainly carbohydrates) in the food processing industry is expanding but the efficacy of symbiotic combinations with probiotics remains unproven.

The prophylactic efficacy of probiotics against antibiotic-associated diarrhoea has been established for the longest time. More recently, they have been convincingly shown to prevent the recurrence of *Clostridium difficile* infection of the colon. The level of proof of their efficacy in other forms of infectious diarrhoea (notably rotaviral diarrhoea in children) is likewise high.

Application to traveller's diarrhoea (mainly due to enterotoxigenic *Escherichia coli*) was found more complex and efficacy seems to depend on travel destination. The place of certain probiotics in the treatment of symptoms of irritable bowel syndrome (especially in preventing the recurrence of pain) must be seen in the context of the vast field of research that focuses on the physiopathology of this chronic condition. The action of probiotics on the various microflora-dependent stages of colonic carcinogenesis opens the way for interventional studies in humans. In small intestinal disease, disaccharide intolerance is improved by probiotics which secrete the relevant enzyme. The efficacy of probiotics in the management of the consequences of intestinal stasis (which creates a novel ecological niche) has been investigated with contradictory findings. Beyond the digestive tract, probiotics are a very promising option in the treatment of allergic disease: the incidence of this type of pathology is inexorably rising and its development is often associated with perturbation of the infantile microflora.

Of all the probiotics, *Saccharomyces boulardii* has been the most extensively studied. In the Chapter written by J.-P. Buts, the reader will find a full description of the clinical effects of this probiotic medicinal product and, most importantly, an in-depth analysis of its pharmacodynamic properties. It can secrete on the one hand proteases which break down toxins and receptors, and on the other hand peptides which act in signal transduction pathways involved in enterocytic electrolyte transport process. It is implicated in mucosal inflammation, pathogen internalisation mechanisms, stimulation of the intestinal humoral immune responses and enhancement of the expression of enzymes in the enterocytic brush border—probably through the polyamines released into the small intestine as a result of lysis of the yeast cells.

After a long hiatus, our understanding of the gut microflora and probiotics has grown substantially over the last twenty years. However, the resultant findings have led to even more questions, and the responses to these will result is even more challenges.

Jean-Claude Rambaud

Foreward

Our colonic microflora serves important roles, digesting unabsorbed carbohydrates, but most importantly protects us! Recognition of the importance of the normal colonic microflora has expanded over the past few decades. Moreover, at some level we are what we eat since our dietary carbohydrates may influence our colonic microflora and their metabolic roles which also affects the gut's microbial balance. We take its work for granted until something goes wrong, such as acute diarrhoea due to antibiotics or acute diarrhoea due to intestinal infections or traveler's diarrhoea. World-wide, infectious diarrhoea is a significant medical problem. Millions of children die each year from infectious diarrhoea. Even adult diarrhoeas cause significant morbidity and mortality world-wide.

Understanding the pathophysiology and treatment options for gastrointestinal infections has reached world-wide importance, and this book is a welcome addition to a clinician's armamentarium. Moreover, the century old concept of probiotics has sparked increased interest. Probiotics are live microorganisms that benefit the host when taken orally. The concept arose from the Russian scientist Elie Metchnikoff's observation in the early 1900's that certain Caucasian tribes were unusually long lived—he attributed this to their ingestion of yogurt with its living microbes. There have been over thirteen hundred articles published on probiotics since 1990. With antibiotics' risks, the concept of treating illness with probiotics has much appeal, as a more "natural" remedy with fewer side effects than antibiotics. With such an increase in information it becomes important to synthesize current knowledge and to evaluate peer reviewed research.

This book provides just that excellent background to the science and the clinical significance of information in this field written by experts. In addition to the well written chapters, each has succinct key points for rapid review. I applaud its choice of topics as well as depth of inquiry. It will be invaluable for health care professionals.

Christina M. Surawicz

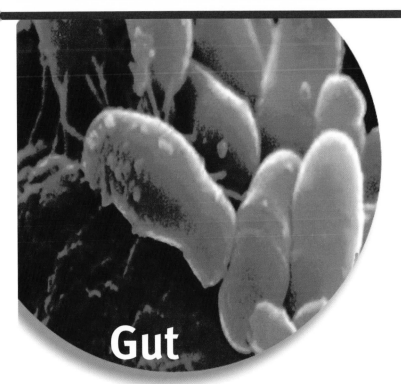

Gut
Microflora

Study Methods

**Joël Doré,
Lionel
Rigottier-Gois**

INRA. Unité d'Écologie
et de Physiologie
du Système Digestif, CRJ,
Jouy-en-Josas, France.

Microorganisms are found in all the various compartments of the digestive tract, and there are ten to one hundred times as many of them as there are cells in the human body. The highest densities are found in the intestine, especially the colon where there can be up to 10^{11} microorganisms per gram of contents. Like the vast majority of the planet's ecosystems, the digestive tract has been colonized by microbes, and long before human beings ever appeared, other animal species had already long been thus colonized (Figure 1). Because they have evolved together, there are close links between any host (or its genome) and its complex, diverse intestinal microbiota (with its multitude of different microbial genomes). In humans, these functional inter-relationships— between what could be considered as two different human genomes— ultimately have an impact on the host's state of health in the very broadest sense of the term.

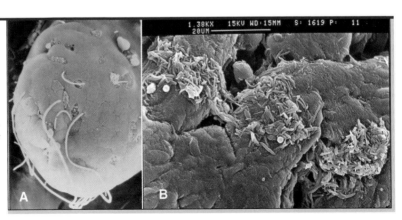

Figure 1.
A : filamentous bacteria in the murine ileum.
B : fusiform bacteria in the murine caecum (photographs: M. Bastide and F. Castex of the Pharmacy Department of Montpellier University)

This chapter deals with the methods used to investigate gut microbiota, with an emphasis on the particular insights which the various methods have brought. Our understanding of the intestinal microbiota has grown up in a chaotic fashion, highly dependent on advances in analytical methods and technology. Up until only ten years ago, our knowledge was essentially based on a few large-scale studies of faecal microbiota and characterization of those microorganisms therein which could be isolated and cultured in the laboratory. More recently, the application of molecular approaches (which do not depend on anaerobic culture techniques) is in the process of revolutionising our perception of the human digestive ecosystem, making this a particularly rich moment in the story, a time at which pre-existing ideas are being overturned as described in two recent reviews [1, 2].

Culture-based methods of studying intestinal microbiota

Since the pioneering characterization of *Bacterium coli communior* by Escherisch in 1885, regular methodological advances have led to sustained— if punctuated—progress in techniques beginning with the ability to grow intestinal microorganisms *in vitro* and later isolate pure cultures. Although it was at the very beginning of the last century that Pasteur first demonstrated that microbial life can exist in the absence of oxygen, it was not until the 1970's that the real boom in the microbiology of the human digestive tract occurred as a result of the pioneering work on anaerobiosis of Hungate and Freter [3, 4] (Figure 2).

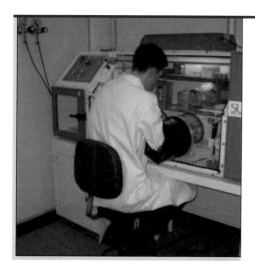

Figure 2.
An anaerobic culture chamber (photograph: BCX)

Hungate used sterile culture media under a CO_2 atmosphere in conditions designed to mimic those in the digestive tract *vis-à-vis* temperature, pH and redox potential (very low) coupled with the appropriate concentrations of minerals, trace elements, vitamins, volatile fatty acids, and ammonia (as a main nitrogen source). Although Hungate focused on the bacteria and protozoa of the rumen, his methods were subsequently applied by Moore & Holdeman to human microbiota. In parallel, Freter developed his controlled-atmosphere chamber system that is still used for preparing samples and dish cultures in the absence of oxygen. These advances made it possible to isolate and identify the dominant species found in human faeces, and these were then classified using the rules of traditional taxonomy. A small number of studies in which large numbers of faecal specimens were thus analysed gave an overview of the composition of the human faecal microbiota, at least those organisms that could be grown *in vitro* [5-8]. The main anaerobic genera thus identified were *Bacteroides, Eubacterium, Peptostreptococcus, Ruminococcus, Bifidobacterium, Fusobacterium* and *Clostridium*. Dominant genera that are amenable to culture *in vitro* are presented in Table I [7-9].

Table I. *Faecal microbiota: dominant bacterial genera that can be cultured*	Relative representation (percentage of total anaerobes)		
	Genus	Reference [7]	[8]
	Bacteroides	30	56
	Eubacterium	26	14
	Bifidobacterium	11	4
	Peptostreptococcus	9	4
	Fusobacterium	8	0.1
	Ruminococcus	4	9
	Clostridium	2	2
	Lactobacillus	2	6
	Streptococcus	2	6
	Others	3	1

By comparing the number of species detected just once with the total number of species identified, Good calculated that the faecal microbiota of humans could contain any of up to four hundred different species [10] which would make the human intestine one of the most diverse microbial ecosystems known. Ever since, this figure has always been cited without ever having been confirmed experimentally; in fact, the dominant microbiota of any individual (sometimes referred to as the indigenous or active microbiota) would only include twenty-five to forty different species [11, 12]. Dominant species correspond to those which are present at densities of between 10^8 and 10^{11} per gram of faeces, and we naturally attribute a correspondingly dominant functional role to this component. Until recently, the only way of studying these species involved a culture step which imposes the major limitation that only those species whose ecological niche can be accurately reproduced *in vitro* can be isolated and identified. Any species that is dependent on relationships with other species or which has nutritional needs that are difficult to fulfil *in vitro* is necessarily missed by culture-based methods and would have hitherto escaped culture and identification. For example, trying to isolate a microorganism in the form of a colony could deprive it of exchanges with other species on which its growth might depend. Today, we know of many examples of nutritional dependence (be it for a particular energy substrate or an essential cofactor) which are difficult to overcome: the existence of methanogenic archaea was recognized because methane could be detected in expired gases but they could not be cultured until methods based on high-pressure (2 bar) H_2/CO_2 had been developed [13]. Technical improvements in the 1970's made it possible to grow and count methanogenic archaea [14-16] and also acetogenic bacteria which are capable of using these gases as carbon and energy sources [17, 18]. Other bacterial species are still regularly being isolated from the dominant microbiota after selection for particular activities such as cellulolysis (Bernalier, personal communication) or the ability to metabolize aromatic compounds [19, 20].

Less numerous microorganisms (10^6-10^8 CFU/g) make up the sub-dominant microbiota. These can be studied using selective culture media. The presence of facultative anaerobes in the sub-dominant microbiota has meant that certain components could be studied in depth, such as *Escherichia coli*. Finally, a minor fraction consists of transient microorganisms—including some aerobic species—which only pass through the digestive tract and are present at densities of below 10^6 per gram of faeces.

The odd studies that have compared different individuals have led to the conclusion that the dominant microbiota varies from person to person [9, 21, 22].

The fact that gut microorganisms have to be cultured *in vitro* before they can be analysed has systematically led to underestimation of populations and, despite the availability of a variety of different culture media to mimic the intestinal ecosystem, investigators have consistently observed major differences—both quantitative and qualitative—between strains derived by enrichment and those sampled *in situ*. That this type of "counting error" exists has been documented in many experiments (Table II) which have shown that a large proportion of the bacterial species that make up the dominant gut microbiota in humans do not grow in anaerobic laboratory conditions. The fraction that can be cultured varies between 10% and 90% according to the study: 93% [7], 58% [23], 20-30% [24], 24% [8], 14-37% [25]—a series which reveals that the fraction estimated as "culturable" has been shrinking over the years.

Article	Year of publication	Fraction that can be cultured (%)
[7]	1974	93
[23]	1996	58
[24]	1999	20-30
[8]	1983	24
[25]	1995	14-37

Table II.
Percentage
of the faecal microbiota
that can be cultured
in vitro

Thus, for fifty years, culture-based methods provided an enormous amount of information about the intestinal ecosystem, yet only a fraction of the species actually present have been thoroughly characterized. While progress with anaerobic culture techniques can only provide more limited information, the development of phylogenetic systems based on the analysis of ribosomal nucleic acid molecules in the late 1970's [26] and subsequent application to questions of microbial ecology in the late 1980's [27-29] paved the way towards analytical methods which are not dependent on a culture step. This has opened new perspectives and led to a new wave of discovery in these matters—a wave which we are still riding. Nevertheless, for the International Systematics Committee, methods based on anaerobic culture remain the reference for the formal identification and description of new species.

Molecular techniques based on ribosomal DNA and RNA used to study the intestinal microbiota

Molecular methods based on 16S ribosomal nucleic acid molecules (16S rRNA and its corresponding rDNA gene), notably by denaturing gradient gel electrophoresis, have extensively amplified our knowledge of the ecosystem that is the human gut.

The sudden expansion and generalisation of these methods is due to properties intrinsic to RNA molecules which can be summarized in four points:
- rDNA and rRNA are found in all living cells;
- these nucleic acid molecules are not subject to lateral transfer between contemporary microorganisms;
- they contain contiguous highly conserved and variable sequences so a large and informative sequence database could be established in a very short amount of time (with more than 100,000 sequences available already);
- the primary mosaic structure provides taxonomic information from domain (Bacteria, Eukarya, Archaea) to species.

When it comes to microbial ecology, two broad types of RNA-based method can be used, and they differ from one another in terms of their resolution. The highest-resolution methods can be used to generate an inventory of dominant species whereas lower-resolution methods are applicable to the breakdown and its quantitation of the major groups of the dominant microbiota (Figure 3). We will describe the different strategies possible with these two broad approaches, the major limitation of which is that they only afford purely phylogenetic information about the specimens analysed, with limited meaning in term of functionalities.

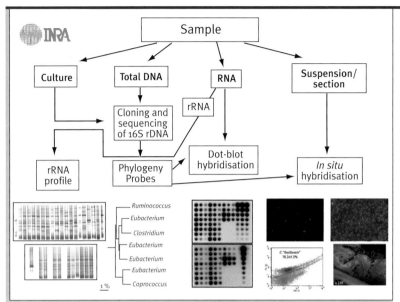

Figure 3.
Approaches to studying
the molecular ecology
of the colonic
microbiota: comparison
of ribosomal RNA
and DNA sequences

Diversity of species

Profiles of the species found in human faeces

Comparison of the sequences of 16S rDNA molecules gives an idea of the different species present and makes it possible to represent the evolutionary relationships which link organisms in a graphic form (so-called phylogenetic trees) [26]. Phylogenetic analysis was first applied to microorganisms that had been isolated and were available from culture collections. More recently, the same approach has been applied to PCR-generated 16S rDNA sequences derived from specimens isolated from natural ecosystems and separated by cloning. Following up on the pioneering work of Wilson [23] who analysed a few partial 16S rDNA sequences cloned out of a sample of human faeces, we have made an inventory of the dominant species of the faecal microbiota of a number of healthy subjects [24, 30]. To define distinct molecular species, we chose a threshold of sequence homology of 98% or over. More than one thousand cloned sequences were thus analysed, showing that:

- the faecal microbiota is composed of three principle phylogenetic lineages: the *Bacteroides-Porphyromonas-Prevotella*, *Clostridium coccoides* and *Clostridium leptum* groups;
- species which do not belong to these dominant phylogenetic groups seem to be scattered around the entire bacterial phylogeny apart from *Collinsella aerofaciens* and related species, and *Bifidobacterium* which, although not as dense as the others, are nevertheless common in the faecal microbiota of healthy adults;

- the mean number of dominant species in a healthy adult's faecal microbiota can be estimated (by mathematical inference) at about one hundred (between fifty and one hundred and eighty, depending on the individual);
- every faecal microbiota sample contains a distinct range of different species;
- gut microbiotas from different individuals only have a very limited number of species in common (one single species found in four different faecal microbiota);
- fewer than 20% of the molecularly distinct species detected are represented in current banks; therefore it is possible that fully 80% have not yet been cultured.

Recently, it has been observed that the gut microbiotas of elderly subjects contain a wider range of different species than those of younger, healthy adults. The same is true of the faecal microbiota of patients who suffer from Crohn's disease, an inflammatory bowel disease.

Comparing with similar results obtained for the digestive ecosystems of other animals [31-33], it seems that the same phylogenetic groups dominate although human faeces might harbour a relatively narrower range of microorganisms.

Molecular approaches to investigating the diversity of dominant species provide an unprecedented amount of information and they make it possible to compile comprehensive data bases of nucleic acid sequences. However, they are subject to certain methodological limitations, mainly associated with bias that can be introduced in the course of extraction or amplification. For this reason, microorganisms that are most resistant to lysis might be under-represented in today's ribosomal DNA banks. Moreover, the sensitivity of molecular methods is limited and they yield a picture of only the most common species present (accounting for about 99% of all the bacteria present). Finally, compiling an exhaustive molecular profile is an expensive process and this type of approach is not amenable for the analysis of large numbers of samples (e.g. for the purposes of dynamic or comparative studies).

Studying the dynamics of species diversity

Denaturing gradient gel electrophoresis has recently been used to compare gut microbiotas from different individuals and study dynamic aspects. The underlying principle is the separation of same-sized, PCR-generated rRNA fragments in a denaturing gel on the basis of the rate at which they become denatured—which is dependent on their sequence, notably their cytosine and guanosine content. The result is an electrophoretic fingerprint in which each band corresponds to one dominant species in the sample analysed: this technique is ideal for analysing large numbers of samples. The pioneering work of Zoetendal et al. [34] had shown that, while the diversity of dominant species in the faecal microbiota varies enormously from one person to another, it remains relatively constant in a given normal, healthy adult over a period of months; our observations have extended this time-scale to several years [35]. Thus, this method is ideal for comparative investigations and it is moreover possible to isolate and sequence any band that appears or disappears in any given nutritional or pathological conditions in order to identify the relevant species. Finally, the initial PCR step provides a means of "zooming in" on a given population and thus investigating changes in the sub-dominant microbiota at higher resolution, e.g. when applied to bifidobacteria or lactobacilli, species present at densities of the order of 10^6 per gram of faeces can be studied. Similar information can be obtained by using a sequencer to analyse single strand conformation polymorphism (SSCP) in amplified, labelled rDNA fragments. With respect to bias introduced by factors related to extraction and amplification, the limitations of these methods are the same as those for full molecular profiling [36].

Major phylogenetic groups and molecular ecology

Using a broad panel of oligonucleotide probes specific for different 16S rRNA sequences, hybridisation-based methods can be used to analyse—both quantitatively and qualitatively—the composition of gut microbiota without any dependence on culture. The pertinence of the mosaic structure of rRNA is obvious in the context of the search for nucleotide signatures: universal or domain-specific (e.g. for Bacteria, Archaea, Eucarya [37]) probes can be constructed using highly conserved regions whereas different phylogenetic groups, genera or even species can be distinguished using probes based on more variable sequences [38].

Target phylogenetic group	Sequence (5'-3')	Name (OPD system)[1]	Ref.
Universal probe	GACGGGCGGTGTGTACAA	S-*-Univ-1390-a-A-18	[53]
Bacteria domain	GCTGCCTCCCGTAGGAGT	S-D-Bact-0338-a-A-18	[54]
Archaea domain	GTGCTCCCCGCCAATTCCT	S-D-Arch-0915-a-A-20	[54]
Eucarya domain	ACCAGACTTGCCCTCC	S-D-Euca-0502-a-A-16	[54]
Bacteroides group[2]	GCACTTAAGCCGACACCT	S-*-Bacto-1080-a-A-18	[55]
Enterobacteriaceae	CTTTTGCAGCCCACT	S-G-Enter-1432-a-A-15	**
Genus *Bifidobacterium*	CCGGTTTTMAGGGATCC	S-G-Bif-1278-b-A-17	[40]
Lactobacillus group[3]	YCACCGCTACACATGRAGTTCCACT	S-G-Lacb-0722-a-A-25	[56]
C. leptum group[4]	GTTTTATCAACGGCAGTC	S-G-Clept-1089-a-A-18	[39]
C. coccoides group[4]	GCCATGRACTGATTCTTCG	S-*-Erec-0482-a-A-19	[41]

Table III.
Oligonucleotide probes used for quantitative dot-blot hybridisation

1. Oligonucleotide Probe Database [57]
2. Targets the genera *Bacteroides, Porphyromonas* and *Prevotella*
3. Targets the genera *Lactobacillus, Streptococcus, Enterococcus*
4. Targets species belonging to the genus *Clostridium* but also *Eubacterium* and *Ruminococcus* ; also *Faecalibacterium prausnitzii* in the *C. leptum* group and *Coprococcus eutactus* and *Butyrivibrio* spp. in the *C. coccoides* group
** Pochart *et al.*, unpublished results

Early applications of this type of technique to characterization of the human gut microbiota involved quantitative dot-blot hybridisation to total faecal RNA: ten different probes covering domain down to broad bacterial group were used to analyse the microbiota in frozen samples of digestive material [39]. The results are shown in Table III.

In healthy humans, Archaea and eukaryote cells make little contribution to total faecal RNA (< 3%) compared with bacteria [40]. Six of the probes specific for large bacterial groups (*Bacteroides* and its relatives, *Clostridium leptum* and relatives, *Clostridium coccoides* and relatives, Enterobacteriaceae, *Lactobacillus-Streptococcus-Enterococcus*, and the genus *Bifidobacterium*) accounted for over 70% of the faecal microbiota in young adults [39] compared with 50-70% in children and the elderly (Doré, unpublished observation) suggesting that other species are present in the latter two populations. Confirming the results of molecular profiling techniques, this method showed that in healthy adults *Bacteroides, Clostridium leptum* and *Clostridium coccoides* form a major part of the faecal microbiota, together accounting for over 50% of the total bacterial 16S rRNA found in faeces. The same method has been successfully used to follow population dynamics at the molecular level in subjects consuming dietary supplements based on fermentable compounds which are designed to promote bifidobacterial activity.

In parallel, a method based on *in situ* hybridisation on fixed faecal suspensions has been developed. In this method, faecal samples are aldehyde-fixed to preserve bacterial wall structure and then permeabilised and hybridised with fluorochrome-labelled ribosomal RNA targeted probes. When a probe binds an intracellular target sequence, the bacterial cell lights up and can be counted in a fluorescent or confocal microscope.

Bacteria thus marked can also be counted using an image analysis system or flow cytometer (which makes it possible to analyse large numbers very quickly). *In situ* hybridisation can only be used on frozen samples if they were fixed prior to freezing, and only some of the ribosomal probes available are suitable since certain regions of ribosomal RNA seem to be inaccessible in whole, fixed bacteria. Franks *et al.* [41] used a panel of six group-specific probes to investigate the dominant populations in the faecal microbiota of healthy adults, and Harmsen *et al.* [42] used the same tools to study the colonization process in children, showing that coriobacteriaceae (including the genera *Atopobium, Collinsella* and *Eggerthella*) are sometimes abundant in the faeces of very young subjects and the elderly [43]. *In situ* hybridisation has also been carried out on sections of intestinal tissue [44], a method which should eventually yield information about topographical relationships between bacteria and the host's intestinal epithelium (Figure 4).

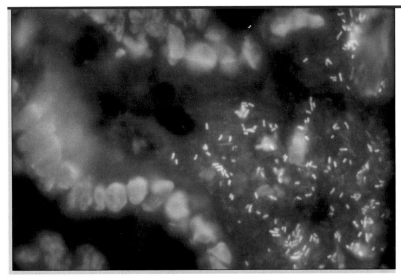

Figure 4.
DAPI-stained cells
labelled with
a fluorescent
Bif 164-Cy 3 probe
on a section
of murine caecum.
Total bacteria (blue)
and bifidobacteria
(pink)
(micrograph: V. Rochet,
INRA-UEPSD)

Using a similar set of probes targeted against six phylogenetic groups, we recently compared the techniques of *in situ* hybridisation and total rRNA dot-blotting on individual faecal specimens (Table IV).

Target phylogenetic group	[Probe]	Molecular inventory [25] (% species)	Quantitative hybridisation [39] (% rRNA)	[41] (% bacteria)
		(n = 1)	(n = 27)	(n = 10)
Bacteroides group[1]	[Bacto-1080]	23.8	36.8	
Bacteroides sub-group	[Bfra-0602] + [Bdis-]			20 .0
Enterobacteriaceae[1]	[Enter-1432]	ND	0.7	
Genus *Bifidobacterium*	[Bif-1278]	ND	0.7	3.0
Lactobacillus group[1]	[Lacb-0722]	2.4	0.6	
Strepto. sub-group	[Str-]			< 0.3
C. leptum group[1]	[Clept-1089]	23.8	16.3	
C. leptum sub-group	[LowGC2P]			12.0
C. coccoides group[1]	[Erec-0482]	36.9	14.5	29.0
C. histolyticum group	[Chis-]			< 0.3
C. lituseburense group	[Clit-]			< 0.3
Others		13.0	30.0	

Table IV.
Faecal microbial
distributions
as determined
by different
molecular methods

1. See Table III for details on the genera recognized by the various target groups.
ND : not detected

Whichever method was used, the same proportions of certain groups were observed, namely *Clostridium coccoides*, *Faecalibacterium prausnitzii* (related to *Clostridium leptum*), *Bifidobacterium* and enteric bacteria. In contrast, the proportions of *Bacteroides* and *Atopobium* were significantly different ($p < 0.05$): the discrepancy between the relative quantities of rRNA detected and the numbers of bacterial cells counted [45] is due to differential levels of metabolic activity in the colon.

The number and quality of probes available for *in situ* hybridisation is constantly increasing. In the course of work on detecting five species belonging to the *Bacteroides* in the faeces, we defined a protocol for the validation of probes for *in situ* hybridisation combined with flow cytometry [46]. New probes against members of the *Clostridium leptum* group as well as certain recently developed probes were shown to be reliable in tests against culture collection strains and this resulted in the definition of eighteen phylogenetic probes for a more comprehensive representation of the composition of the microbiota in healthy adults (Rigottier-Gois, unpublished observation).

Conclusions and perspectives

Enormous progress has been and is being made in our understanding of the dominant gut microbiota in human beings. The application of molecular techniques—which do not depend on anaerobic culture—is providing important information about how microbial ecology in the gut is affected by nutrition and pathology. Today, the most significant progress is in the field of high-volume analysis, as afforded by *in situ* hybridisation coupled with flow cytometry. And now, validation of 16S rDNA sequences cloned from human faecal matter is allowing us to develop DNA-based tools (macro-arrays and biochips) which can be used for the simultaneous investigation of hundreds of bacterial species in a single faecal specimen.

However, although the methods referred to above are providing us with a more accurate description of the intestinal microbiota, they are nevertheless all based on a single molecule (the 16S ribosomal RNA) which could never, on its own, cover all aspects of this complex ecological system. The activities going on in any ecosystem must depend on all the messenger RNAs, the proteins and the metabolites produced therein, and it can only be expected that over the next decade, our understanding of the colonic microbiota will continue to expand in other respects as a result of the broadening of the molecular approach with the tools of integrative biology. The full genome (or "metagenome") of the gut intestinal ecosystem and the mechanisms whereby the various genes are regulated will be studied, including the genes of many species that cannot as yet be grown *in vitro*.

Colonic microorganisms interact with host cells, notably through the immune response and *via* the metabolic products of fermentation processes. These interactions may be beneficial or detrimental for the host's state of health and nutritional status but very few precise mechanisms are as yet understood. It will only be possible to begin to describe the vast network of metabolic interactions (including those between host and microbiota) if we learn how to refer back to the ecosystem as a whole and use reductionist models based on the characteristics of newly isolated bacterial strains. Work already underway is looking at the interface between the genomes of gut bacteria and those of the gnotobiotic animals inside which they reside [47-52], and this approach will soon be extended to humans.

It is ultimately most important that all these technical and methodological advances lead to refinement and revision of our perceptions of how the digestive tract is colonized and how the microbiota adapts to the ecosystem that is the intestine, notably:

- the relative importance of genetic and ecological considerations in determining the diversity of dominant bacterial species—specific and stable for each subject;

- despite the fact the specific composition of the microbiota appears to vary enormously from individual to individual, it nevertheless fulfils very similar functions in everyone, a paradox which, in normal conditions, is greatly to the host's benefit.

Acknowledgements

The INRA work described here was partly funded by the Office of Genetic Resources and the European Union (Projects n° CT-97-3035 and CT-97-3181, QLK1-2000-00067 and QLK1-2000-00108).

Key points

- More than 50% of the dominant gut microbiota of the healthy adult (corresponding to 10^8-10^{11} bacteria per gram of faeces) cannot be cultured using traditional anaerobic culture techniques.

- Molecular approaches, especially those based on the use of 16S ribosomal DNA molecules as a phylogenetic marker are making exhaustive analysis of the dominant microbiota possible.

- Eighty percent of all the bacterial species which compose the dominant gut microbiota in the healthy adult are not represented in existing culture collections.

- Molecular approaches—denaturing gradient gel electrophoresis of 16S RNA molecules, *in situ* hybridisation coupled with flow cytometry and quantitative PCR—are making high-rate analysis of the composition of the gut microbiota possible thereby yielding information about the local microbial ecology.

- Technological progress in the field of integrative biology coupled with fuller molecular characterization will provide information about the functions fulfilled by the newly discovered, hitherto unculturable components of the gut microbiota.

References

1. Mai V, Morris JG Jr. Colonic bacterial flora: changing understandings in the molecular age. *J Nutr* 2004 ; 134 : 459-64.

2. Zoetendal EG, Collier CT, Koike S, Mackie RI, Gaskins HR. Molecular ecological analysis of the gastrointestinal microbiota: a review. *J Nutr* 2004 ; 134 : 465-72.

3. Hungate RE. A roll tube method for cultivation of strict anaerobes In : Norris JR, Ribbons DW, eds. *Methods in microbiology*, Vol. 3B. New York : Academic Press, 1969 : 117.

4. Freter R. Interactions between mechanisms controlling the intestinal microflora. *Am J Clin Nutr* 1974 ; 27 : 1409-16.

5. McCartney AL, Wenzhi W, Tannock GW. Molecular analysis of the composition of the bifidobacterial and lactobacillus microflora of humans. *Appl Environ Microbiol* 1996 ; 62 : 4608-13.

6. Mitsuoka T, Ohno K, Benno Y, Suzuki K, Namba K. The fecal flora of man. IV. Communication: comparison of the newly developed method with the old conventional method for the analysis of intestinal flora. *Zentralbl Bakteriol [Orig A]* 1976 ; 234 : 219-33.

7. Moore WE, Holdeman LV. Human fecal flora: the normal flora of 20 Japanese-Hawaiians. *Appl Microbiol* 1974 ; 27 : 961-79.

8. Finegold SM, Sutter VL, Mathisen GE. Normal indigenous intestinal flora. In : Hentges DJ, ed. *Human intestinal microflora in health and disease*. New York : Academic Press, 1983 : 3-31.

9. Moore WE, Cato EP, Holdeman LV. Some current concepts in intestinal bacteriology. *Am J Clin Nutr* 1978 ; 31 : S33-42.

10. Good IJ. The population frequencies of species and the estimation of population parameters. *Biometrica* 1953 ; 40 : 237-64.

11. Benno Y, Endo K, Mizutani T, Namba Y, Komori T, Mitsuoka T. Comparison of fecal microflora of elderly persons in rural and urban areas of Japan. *Appl Environ Microbiol* 1989 ; 55 : 1100-5.

12. Savage DC. Microbial ecology of the gastrointestinal tract. *Ann Rev Microbiol* 1977 ; 31 : 107-33.

13. Balch WE, Fox GE, Magrum LJ, Woese CR, Wolfe RS. Methanogens: reevaluation of a unique biological group. *Microbiol Rev* 1979 ; 43 : 260-6.

14. Nottingham PM, Hungate RE. Isolation of methanogenic bacteria from feces of man. *J Bacteriol* 1968 ; 96 : 2178-9.

15. Miller TL, Wolin MJ, de Macario EC, Macario AJ. Isolation of *Methanobrevibacter smithii* from human feces. *Appl Environ Microbiol* 1982 ; 43 : 227-32.

16. Pochart P, Doré J, Lemann F, Goderel I, Rambaud JC. Interrelations between populations of methanogenic archaea and sulfate-reducing bacteria in the human colon. *FEMS Microbiol Lett* 1992 ; 77 : 225-8.

17. Doré J, Morvan B, Rieu-Lesme F, Goderel I, Gouet P, Pochart P. Most probable number enumeration of H_2-utilizing acetogenic bacteria from the digestive tract of animals and man. *FEMS Microbiol Lett* 1995 ; 130 : 7-12.

18. Bernalier A, Rochet V, Leclerc M, Doré J, Pochart P. Diversity of H_2/CO_2-utilizing acetogenic bacteria from feces of non-methane-producing humans. *Curr Microbiol* 1996 ; 33 : 94-9.

19. Simmering R, Kleessen B, Blaut M. Quantification of the flavonoid-degrading bacterium *Eubacterium ramulus* in human fecal samples with a species-specific oligonucleotide hybridization probe. *Appl Environ Microbiol* 1999 ; 65 : 3705-9.

20. Hur HG, Beger RD, Heinze TM, *et al*. Isolation of an anaerobic intestinal bacterium capable of cleaving the C-ring of the isoflavonoid daidzein. *Arch Microbiol* 2002 ; 178 : 8-12.

21. Holdeman LV, Good IJ, Moore WEC. Human fecal flora: variation in bacterial composition within individuals and a possible effect of emotional stress. *Appl Environ Microbiol* 1976 ; 31 : 359-75.

22. Mitsuoka T, Ono K. Fecal flora of man. The fluctuation of the fecal flora of the healthy adult. *Zentralbl Bakteriol [Orig A]* 1977 ; 238 : 228-36.

23. Wilson KH, Blitchington RB. Human colonic biota studied by ribosomal DNA sequence analysis. *Appl Environ Microbiol* 1996 ; 62 : 2273-8.

24. Suau A, Bonnet R, Sutren M, *et al*. Direct analysis of genes encoding 16S rRNA from complex communities reveals many novel molecular species within the human gut. *Appl Environ Microbiol* 1999 ; 65 : 4799-807.

25. Langendijk PS, Schut F, Jansen GJ, *et al*. Quantitative fluorescence *in situ* hybridization of *Bifidobacterium* spp. with genus-specific 16S rRNA-targeted probes and its application in fecal samples. *Appl Environ Microbiol* 1995 ; 61 : 3069-75.

26. Olsen GJ, Woese CR. Ribosomal RNA: a key to phylogeny. *FASEB J* 1993 ; 7 : 113-23.

27. Olsen GJ, Lane DJ, Giovannoni SJ, Pace NR, Stahl DA. Microbial ecology and evolution: a ribosomal RNA approach. *Annu Rev Microbiol* 1986 ; 40 : 337-65.

28. Pace NR. New perspective on the natural microbial world: molecular microbial ecology. *ASM News* 1996 ; 62 : 463-70.

29. Stahl DA, Flesher B, Mansfield HR, Montgomery L. Use of phylogenetically based hybridization probes for studies of ruminal microbial ecology. *Appl Environ Microbiol* 1988 ; 54 : 1079-84.

30. Bonnet R, Suau A, Doré J, Gibson GR, Collins MD. Differences in rDNA libraries of faecal bacteria derived from 10- and 25-cycle PCRs. *Int J Syst Evol Microbiol* 2002 ; 52 : 757-63.

31. Ohkuma M, Kudo T. Phylogenetic diversity of the intestinal bacterial community in the termite *Reticulitermes speratus*. *Appl Environ Microbiol* 1996 ; 62 : 461-8.

32. Whitford MF, Forster RF, Beard CE, Gong J, Teather RM. Phylogenetic analysis of rumen bacteria by comparative sequence analysis of cloned 16S rRNA genes. *Anaerobe* 1998 ; 4 : 153-63.

33. Leser TD, Amenuvor JZ, Jensen TK, Lindecrona RH, Boye M, Moller K. Culture-independent analysis of gut bacteria: the pig gastrointestinal tract microbiota revisited. *Appl Environ Microbiol* 2002 ; 68 : 673-90.

34. Zoetendal EG, Akkermans AD, De Vos WM. Temperature gradient gel electrophoresis analysis of 16S rRNA from human fecal samples reveals stable and host-specific communities of active bacteria. *Appl Environ Microbiol* 1998 ; 64 : 3854-9.

35. Seksik P, Rigottier-Gois L, Gramet G, *et al*. Alterations of the dominant faecal bacterial groups in patients with Crohn's disease of the colon. *Gut* 2003 ; 52 : 237-42.

36. Marchesi JR, Sato T, Weightman AJ, *et al*. Design and evaluation of useful bacterium-specific PCR primers that amplify genes coding for bacterial 16S rRNA. *Appl Environ Microbiol* 1998 ; 64 : 795-9.

37. Woese CR, Kandler O, Wheelis ML. Towards a natural system of organisms: proposal for the domains Archaea, Bacteria, and Eucarya. *Proc Natl Acad Sci USA* 1990 ; 87 : 4576-9.

38. Amann R. Who is out there? Microbial aspects of biodiversity. *Syst Appl Microbiol* 2000 ; 23 : 1-8.

39. Sghir A, Gramet G, Suau A, Rochet V, Pochart P, Doré J. Quantification of bacterial groups within human fecal flora by oligonucleotide probe hybridization. *Appl Environ Microbiol* 2000 ; 66 : 2263-6.

40. Doré J, Gramet G, Goderel I, Pochart P. Culture-independent characterization of human fecal flora using rRNA-targeted hybridization probes. *Genet Sel Evol* 1998 ; 30S : S287-96.

41. Franks AH, Harmsen HJ, Raangs GC, Jansen GJ, Schut F, Welling GW. Variations of bacterial populations in human feces measured by fluorescent *in situ* hybridization with group-specific 16S rRNA-targeted oligonucleotide probes. *Appl Environ Microbiol* 1998 ; 64 : 3336-45.

42. Harmsen HJ, Wildeboer-Veloo AC, Raangs GC, *et al*. Analysis of intestinal flora development in breast-fed and formula-fed infants by using molecular identification and detection methods. *J Pediatr Gastroenterol Nutr* 2000 ; 30 : 61-7.

43. Harmsen HJM, Wildeboer-Veloo ACM, Grijpstra J, Knol J, Degener JE, Welling GW. Development of 16S rRNA-based probes for the *Coriobacterium* group and the *Atopobium* cluster and their application for enumeration of coriobacteriaceae in human feces from volunteers of different age groups. *Appl Environ Microbiol* 2000 ; 66 : 4523-7.

44. Thomas V, Rochet V, Boureau H, *et al*. Molecular characterization and spatial analysis of a simplified gut microbiota displaying colonization resistance against *Clostridium difficile*. *Microb Ecol Health Dis* 2002 ; 14 : 203-10.

45. Rigottier-Gois L, Le Bourhis AG, Gramet G, Rochet V, Doré J. Fluorescent hybridisation combined with flow cytometry and hybridisation of total RNA to analyse the composition of microbial communities in human faeces using 16S rRNA probes. *FEMS Microbiol Ecol* 2003 ; 43 : 237-45.

46. Rigottier-Gois L, Rochet V, Garrec N, Suau A, Doré J. Enumeration of *Bacteroides species* in human faeces by fluorescent *in situ* hybridisation combined with flow cytometry using 16S rRNA probes. *Syst Appl Microbiol* 2003 ; 26 : 110-8.

47. Hooper LV, Midtvedt T, Gordon JI. How host-microbial interactions shape the nutrient environment of the mammalian intestine. *Annu Rev Nutr* 2002 ; 22 : 283-307.

48. Hooper LV, Stappenbeck TS, Hong CV, Gordon JI. Angiogenins: a new class of microbicidal proteins involved in innate immunity. *Nat Immunol* 2003 ; 4 : 269-73.

49. Xu J, Bjursell MK, Himrod J, *et al*. A genomic view of the human-*Bacteroides thetaiotaomicron* symbiosis. *Science* 2003 ; 299 : 2074-6.

50. Hooper LV, Gordon JI. Commensal host-bacterial relationships in the gut. *Science* 2001 ; 292 : 1115-8.

51. Hooper LV, Gordon JI. Glycans as legislators of host-microbial interactions: spanning the spectrum from symbiosis to pathogenicity. *Glycobiology* 2001 ; 11 : 1R-10R.

52. Hooper LV, Wong MH, Thelin A, Hansson L, Falk PG, Gordon JI. Molecular analysis of commensal host-microbial relationships in the intestine. *Science* 2001 ; 291 : 881-4.

53. Zheng D, Alm EW, Stahl DA, Raskin L. Characterization of universal small-subunit rRNA hybridization probes for quantitative molecular microbial ecology studies. *Appl Environ Microbiol* 1996 ; 62 : 4504-13.

54. Amann RI, Krumholz L, Stahl DA. Fluorescent-oligonucleotide probing of whole cells for determinative, phylogenetic, and environmental studies in microbiology. *J Bacteriol* 1990 ; 172 : 762-70.

55. Doré J, Sghir A, Hannequart-Gramet G, Corthier G, Pochart P. Design and evaluation of a 16S rRNA-targeted oligonucleotide probe for specific detection and quantitation of human faecal *Bacteroides* populations. *Syst Appl Microbiol* 1998 ; 21 : 65-71.

56. Sghir A, Chow JM, Mackie RI. Continuous culture selection of bifidobacteria and lactobacilli from human faecal samples using fructooligosaccharide as selective substrate. *J Appl Microbiol* 1998 ; 85 : 769-77.

Establishment and Composition of the Gut Microflora

Anne Collignon[1], Marie-José Butel[2]

1. Service de Microbiologie, Hôpital Jean-Verdier, Assistance Publique-Hôpitaux de Paris et Département de Microbiologie, Faculté de Pharmacie, Université Paris-XI, France.
2. Département de Microbiologie, Faculté de Pharmacie, Université Paris-V, France.

The intestinal microbiota is both complex and diverse. Any individual's microbiota varies from one segment of the gut to another and also over time—the microbiota of a newborn is quite different from that of an adult which is in turn quite different from that of an elderly person. Similarly, composition varies along the digestive tract with the overall density rising from the mouth towards the anus. However, once established in a healthy person, the intestinal microbiota varies relatively little in normal conditions, although it is affected by environmental factors such as diet and the taking of antibiotics [1, 2].

In humans, the intestinal microbiota consists of about 10^{14} bacteria, corresponding to more than ten times the number of the body's own cells. Over four hundred different species have been identified [1-4]. Apart from representing a significant biomass, this microbiota mediates many key functions. Comprehensive bacteriological analysis of total intestinal microbiota—99% of which are obligate anaerobes and varied species— represents an enormous amount of exacting work if traditional culture-based methods are used; in addition, about 50% of the species present cannot be cultivated, as revealed in recent years by the application of molecular approaches based on analysis of ribosomal RNA molecules (rRNA) and their genes (rDNA) [5, 6].

The intestinal microbiota cannot be studied independently of its environmental context, i.e., the host and its diet. Taken altogether, these components constitute the digestive microbial ecosystem, the homeostasis of which is a key determinant in human health. Any change in any of the relevant parameters might disrupt the whole system leading to impaired function.

Digestive tract colonization: microbiota-host interactions, and bacteria-bacteria interactions

To simplify, the normal microbiota could be defined as all the species in the ecosystem which are involved in symbiotic relationships with the host [7-9].

In the colon microbiota, a distinction is made between the resident (also called autochtonous) microbiota and the transient (also called allochtonous) microbiota. The former includes all the species that are permanently present in the ecosystem of the digestive tract, species that have colonized some specific spot and are capable of multiplying there. These species have a cellular and tissue-specific tropism and can be isolated regularly from a person's microbiota over a long period of time: they are characteristic of their specific host. In contrast, transient species which can only establish on a temporary basis are found in the local microbiota for a limited amount of time; they constitue the allochtonous microbiota. These bacteria derive from ingested food and may belong to different bacterial groups. In adults, certain strains of *Escherichia coli* may persist in the intestinal microbiota for some time (months or even years) whereas other strains of the same species may appear or disappear in consecutive samples. Similarly, certain bifidobacterial ribotypes are always found in the digestive tract whereas others are transient [9]. Among these transient species are the so-called probiotics, most of which actually do not colonize the digestive tract although they survive during their transit [7, 8].

The ability of a species to colonize and persists in the digestive tract depends on a complex series of interactions between bacterium and host as well as between different bacteria. Colonizing potential and survival in this ecosystem may depend on binding capacities to the intestinal mucus or enterocytic membranes and on ability to metabolize some substrates [9-11]. Van de Merwe *et al.* compared digestive microbiotas in ten pairs of twins of between two and eighteen years of age, using a classification system based on seven different morphotypes together with Gram staining patterns [12]: they hypothesise that there is a host genetic component—encoding receptors and/or endogenous substrates—determining the bacterial profile in the gut since the faecal microbiotas of homozygous twins resembled one another more closely than those of dizigote twins which were in turn more similar than those of unrelated subjects. A genetic component has been reported to influence the nasal microbiota [13] and a link with blood group has been suggested by Hoskins & Boulding [14].

Since the first strain to become established does not need to compete for its niche, nutrients or growth factors, it has an ecological advantage. Then a microbiota barrier establishes inhibiting colonization by next species. Recent research has shown that colonizing bacteria can interact (cross-talk) with the host, resulting in the expression of host genes that tend to create a favourable environment for their establishment [15], e.g. in gnotoxenic animals, *Bacteroides thetaiotaomicron* modifies glycosylation of the digestive mucosa by regulating host glycosyltransferase expression—the intestinal surface is fucosylated which generates a specific ecological niche for this species. Other bacteria or their culture supernatants have also been shown to be able to change glycosylation of the intestinal mucosa [16]. Therefore, bacterium-host and bacterium-bacterium communication and interactions underlie waves of colonization in which particular ecological niches are created and suitable nutrients are imported for the various bacterial species which can colonize the digestive tract.

Composition and topographical of intestinal microbiota distribution in adults

The microbiota not only varies along the length of the digestive tract but also radially, between lumen and mucosa. Depending on the intestinal levels, the microbiota found is quite different, corresponding to different habitats or specific ecological niches.

Data from culture-based bacteriological methods

Using traditional culture-based methods, it has been shown that bacterial density steadily rises from the highly motile small intestine through the less motile colon.

Small intestine

After passing out of the acidic stomach, the pH of the gut contents is brought back up to neutral, the oxygen tension falls and surviving bacteria begin to multiply so their numbers steadily rise through the duodenum to the ileum. There are no more than 10^4-10^6 CFU per gram of contents in the duodenum and jejunum, essentially aerobes and facultative anaerobes (*Streptococcus, Lactobacillus, Enterobacteriaceae*) corresponding to the transient microbiota. In the ileum, numbers rise, reaching 10^5-10^7 CFU per gram of contents in which strict anaerobes belonging to the genus *Bacteroides* predominate although some facultative anaerobes are still present. This relatively sparse microbiota does not mediate any important functions apart from in certain pathological situations [1-4].

Colon

Bacterial densities are highest in the colon with numbers of 10^9-10^{11} CFU per gram of contents. These high densities of anaerobic bacteria are possible because of the slow transit and low redox potential in this segment of the gut. The colon, in which competition for space and nutrients underlies the stability of the microbiota, is the only segment of the digestive tract which is colonized on a permanent basis by a resident microbiota [1-4].

The predominantly anaerobic intestinal microbiota could be seen as a distinct organ—albeit microbial—which performs a whole set of functions which are beneficial to the host:
- metabolic functions such as the fermentation of residual, undigestible food and host-derived materials, yielding energising short-chain fatty acids and vitamins;
- trophic activity at the intestinal mucosa, stimulation of intestinal angiogenesis *via* Paneth cells, and local development of the immune system;
- colonization resistance: a barrier function combating the establishment of pathogenic bacteria [7, 8].

Investigation of the microbiota in the right human colon is complicated by the fact that sample-taking is difficult in this segment and sophisticated methods are required to gain access to the contents, such as pyxigraphy or intubation. One study using pyxigraphic sampling showed that there are one hundred times fewer strict anaerobes in the caecum than there are in the faeces [17], although the density of facultative aero-anaerobes is higher. The density of methanogenic bacteria was also found to be low in the caecum compared with that in the faeces.

Faeces

It is the faecal microbiota that has been studied most extensively. The faeces contain 10^9-10^{11} CFU per gram, and microorganisms account for about 40% of their weight [1-4].

In addition to the resident microbiota (including the dominant and the subdominant microbiota), the faeces also contain the transient microbiota (Figure 1).

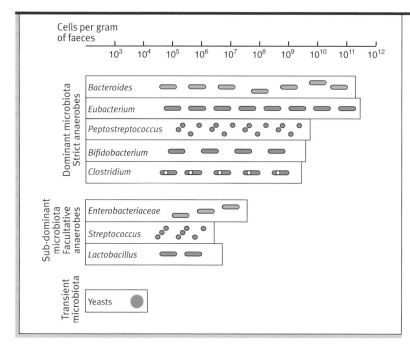

Figure 1.
Faecal microbiota: composition according to culture-based methods (taken from [3])

The dominant microbiota (10^9-10^{11} CFU per gram) is almost entirely composed of strict anaerobes, including large numbers of Gram-negative bacilli belonging to the genus *Bacteroides*, Gram-positive bacilli belonging to the genera *Eubacterium*, *Bifidobacterium* and *Clostridium*, and Gram-positive cocci such as *Peptostreptococcus* and *Ruminococcus*.

The subdominant microbiota (10^6-10^8 CFU per gram) is composed of facultative anaerobes belonging to various species of the *Enterobacteriaceae* family (notably *Escherichia coli*) and the genera *Streptococcus*, *Enterococcus* and *Lactobacillus*, etc. Uncontrolled, exuberant proliferation of this part of the microbiota can lead to pathology [8].

The transient microbiota varies and does not become established in the digestive tract in non-pathological conditions. This microbiota which accounts for less than 10^6 CFU per gram is extremely variable and may include *Enterobacteriaceae* of the genera *Citrobacter, Klebsiella, Proteus* and *Enterobacter* as well as *Pseudomonas*, staphylococci and yeasts (mainly belonging to the genus *Candida*).

Data from molecular methods

In fact, the biodiversity of the faecal microbiota is actually far richer than traditional culture-dependent methods can reveal since 15-85% (depending on the authors) of all the anaerobic organisms present can be cultured out [5, 6]. These days, molecular methods based on the cloning and sequencing of 16S rDNA molecules are showing that less than half of all the dominant species are identifiable by methods which are dependent on an anaerobic culture step [5, 6].

Suau *et al.* characterized the faecal microbiota of a healthy adult by cloning and sequencing the genes encoding 16S rRNA molecules from extracted faecal DNA of a healthy adult [6]. Three major phylogenetic lineages accounted for 95% of the clones generated, namely the *Bacteroides-Porphyromonas-Prevotella* group [18], the *Clostridium coccoides* sub-group (*Clostridium* cluster XIV in Collins' terminology) and the *Clostridium leptum* group (or *Clostridium* cluster IV) [19]. Many other clones were isolated representing unique molecular species, bearing witness to the huge diversity of the intestinal microbiota. About 75% of the sequences correspond to no known, culturable species.

On the basis of knowledge of sequences corresponding to bacterial groups or molecular species, probes have been constructed which match 16S rRNA molecules. These probes target an entire domain (e.g. the *Bacteria*), a major bacterial group or sub-group (e.g. the *Bacteroides-Porphyromonas-Prevotella* group, the *Clostridium coccoides* group, the *Clostridium leptum* sub-group, *Bifidobacterium, Lactobacillus* or the *Enterobacteriaceae*) or a single species [20]. These probes can be radiolabelled for use in a quantitative dot-blot assay after extraction of faecal RNA, or fluorochrome-labelled for fluorescence *in situ* hybridization (FISH) directly on faecal material containing whole, permeabilised bacterial cells (Figure 2).

Sghir *et al.* [21] used a universal probe targeting the domain *Bacteria* together with six group-specific probes—targeting respectively *Bacteroides, Clostridium leptum, Clostridium coccoides, Enterobacteriaceae, Lactobacillus-Streptococcus-Enterococcus* and *Bifidobacterium*—in dot blots experiments to study the faecal microbiota from twenty-seven healthy adults. The six group probes recognized more than 70% of all the organisms hybridised by the *Bacteria* probe. The *Bacteroides* group accounted for 37 ± 16% of total rRNA; the groups *Clostridium leptum* and *Clostridium coccoides* accounted for respectively 16 ± 7% and 14 ± 6%; *Bifidobacterium, Lactobacillus* and the *Enterobacteriaceae* accounted for less than 2%.

In situ hybridisation combined with microscopic detection (epi-fluorescence) gives similar results, e.g. Rochet *et al.* [22] found that a probe targeting the domain *Bacteria* recognized 80 ± 11% of all the DAPI-labelled cells; the *Clostridium coccoides-Eubacterium rectale* group was the most abundant (36 ± 7%) followed by the *Bacteroides* group (17 ± 5%),

Bifidobacterium (15 ± 9%) and *Fusobacterium prausnitzii* (23 ± 5%). The last belongs to the *Clostridium leptum* sub-group and represents one-third of the rRNA of this group [23].

The percentage detection rate rises if more specific probes—against sub-groups or individual species—are used. Using six species- and group-specific probes for *in situ* hybridisation combined with image analysis, Franks *et al.* [24] could detect two-thirds of organisms found in the faecal microbiota. Together, the *Bacteroides fragilis* and *Bacteroides distasonis* probes recognized 20%, and the *Clostridium coccoides-Eubacterium rectale* group probe 29%: these two groups therefore account for nearly half of the microbiota and are the most common constituents. The *Bifidobacterium* probe detected only 3% of the organisms present. Probes for the lactococci-streptococci group, *Clostridium lituseburense* and *Clostridium histolyticum* recognized under 1% of the organisms present but serve as a measure of the diversity of the microbiota.

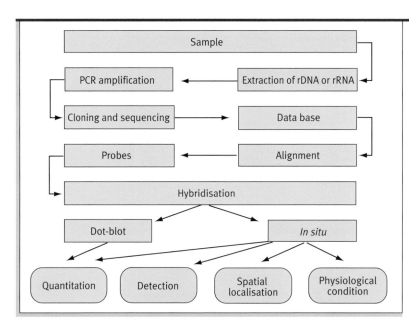

Figure 2.
Molecular methods
for studying
the gut microbiota

In situ hybridisation combined with microscope detection is a demanding technique even though the counting step can be automated [21]: combination with a flow cytometry detection makes reading results easier and speeds up the counting process so the technique can be used to study multiple samples (Figure 3) [11, 25]. Similarly, methods based on the analysis of denaturing gradient gel electrophoretic profiles after rRNA amplification are suitable for large-scale studies [26].

Molecular approaches are confirming the results from culture-based methods concerning the longitudinal and transversal variability in microbiotal composition. Using 16S rRNA probes, Marteau *et al.* have shown that the groups *Bacteroides* (*Bacteroides-Porphyromonas-Prevotella*) and *Clostridium*

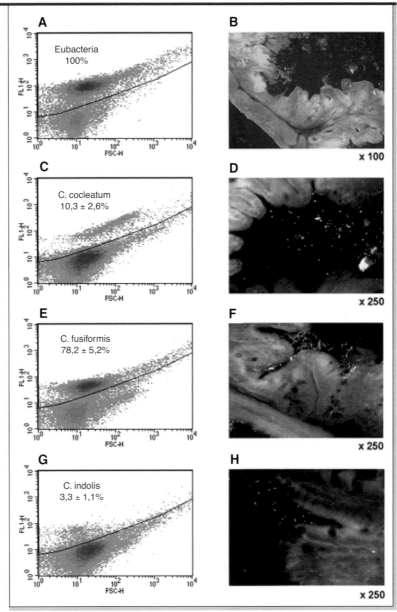

Figure 3.
In situ hybridisation of trixenic microbiota in the mouse. Analysis by flow cytometry (A, C, E, G) and image analysis (B, D, F, H).
A, B : Eubacteria probe
C, D : Clostridium cocleatum probe
E, F : Clostridium fusiformis probe
G, H : Clostridium indolis probe
(taken from [11])

(the *Clostridium coccoides* group and the *Clostridium leptum* sub-group) account for 44% of bacterial rRNA in faeces but only 13% in the contents of the caecum [27]. Facultative anaerobes (*Lactobacillus-Enterococcus* and *Escherichia coli*) represent 50% of the caecal microbiota (as against only 7% of the faecal microbiota) and probably play an important role in fermentation processes in the caecum. Transversal distribution was studied at the molecular level by Zoetendal *et al.* [28] on faeces and biopsies taken from ten volunteers, some healthy and some with pathology at various points along the colon (localized in the ascending, descending or transverse segments). Biopsies taken after evacuation of the contents of the colon seem to give a good idea of the microbiota associated with the mucus layer and the mucosa where bacterial cells are intimately associated with the host's cells. Flow cytometry analysis after propidium iodide staining showed a total of 10^5-10^6 bacteria in biopsy material (which are therefore probably associated with the host's mucosal tissue). Denaturing gradient gel electrophoresis (DGGE) has shown that every individual has his or her own distinct microbiota (in a single individual, the profiles at different levels of the colon are similar). On the other hand, the faecal profiles are quite different from that of biopsy materials. The specificity of the mucosal microbiota is strong evidence that host-dependent factors may be important in determining its composition of the intestinal microbiota [28].

In situ hybridisation on tissue sections combined with image analysis is another way of studying the horizontal distribution of species going from the intestinal lumen to the colonocytes through the mucus layer. Figure 4 shows this distribution on a section of caecal tissue colonized of a human microflora-associated mouse, including the signals generated with probes against the domain *Bacteria*, and the *Bacteroides-Prevotella-Porphyromonas* and *Clostridium coccoides-Eubacterium rectale* groups (personal data).

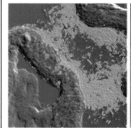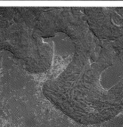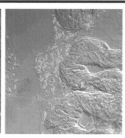

A. Bacteria   B. Bacteroides   C. Eubacterium rectale

Figure 4.
Fluorescence in situ hybridisation combined with image analysis on caeca sections of human microflora-associated mice.
A : Bacteria probe
B : Bacteroides-Porphyromonas-Prevotella group probe
C : Clostridium coccoides-Eubacterium rectale probe

Variability of the intestinal microbiota over time

The composition of the microbiota varies from individual to individual and may also vary with changing physiological and pathological conditions.

Zoetendal *et al.* [26] estimate that a DGGE profile reveals between 90% and 99% of the bacteria present. In sixteen adults, they described highly variable profiles with differences in both the number and positions of bands.

In contrast, the profile for any given individual remained very stable over time, suggesting that every healthy person has a distinct but fairly constant microbiota. A few bands were common to all subjects, and sequence analysis of these bands revealed strong homologies to *Ruminococcus obeum*, *Eubacterium hallii* and *Fusobacterium prausnitzii*; these species are therefore often found in the human microbiota and probably play important functional roles [6, 25].

Franks *et al.* used *in situ* hybridisation combined with image analysis to study microfloral variability in 78 samples prepared at different times from a total of nine subjects. There was more variability in the *Bacteroides* group than in the *Clostridium coccoides* group and in every single subject, it was the *Bifidobacterium* group which varied the most [24]. Another study focused on temporal variations in *Bifidobacterium* in five adults: profiles proved to be host-specific and remained stable over the four weeks of the experiment [29]. DGGE has shown that *Lactobacillus* populations remain more constant in adults than they do in babies [30].

Finally, a few studies have focused on the intestinal microbiota in the elderly. Mitsuoka [31] showed rises in clostridia, enteric bacteria and enterococci. In the same vein, a more recent study combining a molecular dot-blot approach with fatty acid analysis showed that the number of anaerobes falls and the number of *Enterobacteriaceae* rises with age [32]. It has also been shown that microbiota diversity tends to increase with age, with routine probes only detecting about 50% of the microbiota of an elderly subject (compared with 80% in a normal adult) suggesting that many species remain to be identified [33].

Establishment of the intestinal microbiota in the newborn

At birth, the digestive tract is sterile and the adult microbial ecosystem will not become definitively established for years.

The dynamics of colonization

The kinetics of microbiotal establishment following birth are relatively well characterized, although the process is so complex that it is far from being fully understood. *In utero*, the digestive tract is normally sterile and colonization only begins once the foetal membranes have been broached, when suddenly the baby finds itself plunged into a universe full of bacteria of a multitude of different sorts. Colonization begins with a simple range of microorganisms derived from the mother's vaginal, intestinal and skin microbiotas together with some environmental species. Continually exposed to novel bacteria, the baby's microbiota subsequently diversifies until a profile considered as more or less identical to that of an adult is established by the age of about two [34].

Although a baby is exposed to a myriad of different bacterial species, few are capable of establishing in the digestive tract. Interactions with the host and other bacteria may be required for a species to become established. In normal conditions, the colonic redox potential is high at this stage of life, so strict anaerobes cannot grow and the first colonizing bacteria are aerobic species or facultative anaerobes (staphylococci, enterococci and enteric bacteria). These proliferate rapidly in the colon to reach a level of 10^{10}-10^{11} CFU per gram of contents. They consume oxygen thereby leading to a drop in the local redox potential: after about one week of life, strictly anaerobic species such as *Bifidobacterium, Bacteroides* and *Clostridium* colonize the colon. Conversely, oxygen level falls and density of aerobes dicreases [34, 35].

Although colonization is rapid in the newborn gut, all bacteria are not capable of surviving or establishing there. That bacteria are transmitted from the mother's vaginal and faecal microbiota has been definitively demonstrated, with the latter appearing to predominate—it is enteric bacteria and bifidobacteria from the faeces rather than lactobacilli from the vagina which establish most efficiently [36]. In addition to the mother, the baby may be exposed to bacteria *via* the hands of health care providers, and general hygiene conditions may have a major influence on digestive colonization in babies.

The factors which determine whether or not a given bacterial strain can become established are poorly understood. A study of *Escherichia coli* implantation showed that certain strains persist in the newborn gut for months or even more than a year (resident strains) whereas others disappear within weeks (transient strains) [37]. Resident strains share certain characteristics such as genes encoding *fimbriae* (or pili) and haemolysins, factors which may be key in their ability to establish.

The effects on children's health of different colonization patterns are also poorly understood. Some genera (notably *Bifidobacterium*) which are typically dominant in babies born at term and breast-fed are considered as beneficial. It has long been recognized that the digestive microbiota is a key contributor to the ability to resist infection by pathogenic species (the so-called colonization resistance or barrier effect) [38] as well as to the development of mucosal immunity [39].

Exogenous factors involved in colonization

Many exogenous factors are known to affect the dynamics and outcome of colonization, including route of delivery, gestational age at birth, diet, general environmental factors and, in particular, any antibiotics taken by the mother prior to delivery and/or administered to the baby after birth.

Route of delivery

The majority of bacteria first encountered by babies born by Caesarean section are those in the environment—from the air or transmitted by health care providers. This markedly affects the dynamics of colonization. The first bacteria to establish are always facultative anaerobes (enteric bacteria, enterococci and staphylococci) with strict anaerobes (notably *Bifidobacterium* and *Bacteroides*, enteric in origin) not becoming established until much later (however, anaerobic species which are capable of sporulating and are therefore present in the environment such as *Clostridium* can establish themselves rapidly) [40]. This lag *vis-à-vis* the establishment of a normal microbiota may last for months [41].

Term

There is relatively little evidence about intestinal microbiota establishment in premature babies who are known to be at particularly high risk of gastrointestinal infection. The key features are significantly delayed colonization (compared with babies born at term) and a reduced variety of species. Although the premature baby's gut is colonized fairly rapidly by aerobic bacteria, anaerobic species (notably *Bifidobacterium* and *Bacteroides* species) take longer to establish and the more premature the baby, the longer the lag. Bifidobacteria begin to appear after an average of ten days and do not become dominant until two to three weeks after delivery [42]. This sequence may be due to the fact that children are born by Caesarean section, are more often separated from their mother and kept in an aseptic, intensive care setting; they are also more commonly treated with broad-spectrum antibiotics. As a result, they are more likely to become colonized by environmental bacteria than directly from their mother's enteric microbiota.

Diet

Diet has been the most extensively studied parameter. The microbiota of the breast-fed newborn is less diverse than that of the bottle-fed baby because breast-feeding promotes the establishment of a dominant microbiota based on members of the *Bifidobacterium* genus. This is associated with delayed or lower-level colonization by *Enterobacteriaceae*, *Clostridium* and *Bacteroides* [35, 43-45]. However, as soon as the diet is diversified, the microbiota quickly changes to one resembling that of the bottle-fed baby. This differential colonization pattern would be due to the absence of the buffering activity of breast milk which lowers the pH in the colon (to 5 or 6) which favours the growth of bifidobacteria and lactobacilli at the expense of other genera. Some studies have reported high-level colonization by bifidobacteria in children fed on high-quality formula but the dominant species seem to be different in these children. Today, the differences between bottle-fed and breast-fed babies seem to be diminishing, partly because of improvements in formula (notably the inclusion of bifidogenic factors such as oligosaccharides) but also because of changes in other conditions [34].

When the diet is diversified, the differences disappear between the two groups, both of which are carrying a more or less adult-like microbiota by the age of two [34].

Antibiotics

Antibiotics select for resistant microbes and affect the barrier microbiota in such a way as to undermine the mechanisms that underlie resistance to colonization by pathogenic species. Since few studies have analysed the microbiota as a whole (or even the global anaerobic microbiota), exactly what antibiotics do is difficult to evaluate. Most of the relevant studies have been conducted in intensive care units and some of these have shown that a long course of a broad-spectrum antibiotic is a risk factor for colonization by resistant *Enterobacteriaceae* [46] although other studies have revealed no such link: nevertheless, a policy of cutting down antibiotic prescription has successfully curtailed several epidemics due to multi-drug-resistant bacteria. Colonization by drug-resistant bacteria is associated with longer hospital stays, low birth age and low birth weight [47, 48].

The effects of antibiotics on the overall microbiota implantation has not been extensively investigated. Goldman *et al.* [49] observed no changes in the microbiota of newborns even after courses of treatment lasting more than three days, although this study only looked at aerobic species. In a study conducted by Bennet [50], there were no more than 10^6 anaerobic bacteria per gram in the faeces of 60-80% of a group of children who had taken an antibiotic whereas the density in 100% of a parallel group of untreated children was at least 10^7 per gram.

Environmental factors and hygiene

The environment may affect intestinal colonization. The intestinal microbiota of children born in developing countries differs from that of those from the first world and differences have been detected between children born in the country and town, and between those delivered at home and in a hospital [51, 52].

Over the last ten years, changes have been observed in the pattern of establishment of the intestinal microbiota with the normal microbiota tending to appear later: enteric bacteria (*Enterobacteriaceae*, *Bacteroides*, *Bifidobacterium*) are no longer necessarily established in the gut by one week of age [42, 53]. In a study comparing Swedish and Estonian newborns all delivered *via* the vaginal route at term and breast-fed [53], only 50% of the Swedish babies were carrying *Bifidobacterium* (at a median density of 10^3 per gram of faeces) by the age of one month. This delay is probably due to the strict hygiene of the delivery process in Sweden, resulting in reduced exposure to the maternal microbiota which paves the way for colonization by bacteria from the environment. A similar trend has been observed in premature newborns in whom the delay is far longer these days than it used to be. Two recent studies showed that beyond one month, the digestive tract of this population of babies were colonized by only two to four different bacterial species with seriously delayed establishment of enteric bacteria [54, 55], notably members of the genus *Bifidobacterium* [54].

These differences boil down to delayed establishment of maternally derived enteric bacteria (including those belonging to the genus *Bifidobacterium*) to the benefit of environmental bacteria. The most likely explanation for this is related to the ever-increasingly stringent hygiene of delivery protocols, including antiseptic treatment of the vaginal cavity coupled with more widespread prescription of prophylactic antibiotics. By way of example, one study showed that prophylactic antibiotics affected the establishment of the intestinal microbiota by cutting down colonization by *Bifidobacterium* and *Clostridium* which are susceptible to the drugs routinely used [56]. Such changes could compromise the barrier effect and promote colonization by resistant strains; supporting this hypothesis, a rise has been documented in neonatal infections with bacteria resistant to the antibiotic administered during delivery [57]. A worrying fact is that the long-term consequences of this type of change are unknown, e.g. the rising prevalence of allergic disease in Europe could be related to new patterns in the establishment of the intestinal microbiota causing a harmful shift in the intestinal immune response [58].

Data from molecular approaches

The new methods have confirmed much of the data obtained using culture-based techniques about how the microbiota becomes established. In experiments exploiting the FISH technique with probes targeting different bacterial groups, it has been confirmed that members of the genus *Bifidobacterium* dominate in breast-fed babies but not in adapted formula-fed infants [59].

Such approaches have extended our knowledge about bacteria which have hitherto been difficult or impossible to culture *in vitro*, as well as about the dynamics of establishment of the microbiota. Using probes targeting the *Coriobacterium* group and the *Atopobium* cluster, Harmsen *et al.* [60] studied the faecal microbiotas of children of different ages: *Coriobacterium* species were more common in bottle-fed babies than in breast-fed babies and diversity within the *Atopobium* cluster increased with age.

The DGGE method has also been applied to the study of the intestinal microbiota of two children from birth to ten months of age. In parallel, with a view to identifying the dominant species, a 16S rDNA bank was generated from faecal samples [61]. The results of this approach confirmed some of the results previously obtained using culture-based methods: during the days following birth, the DGGE profile was simple, subsequently becoming more complex as the established microbiota diversifies. Another change in faecal profiles was observed at the moment of weaning. The bacteria identified by cloning and sequencing included members of the genera *Bifidobacterium*, *Ruminococcus*, *Enterococcus*, *Clostridium* and *Enterobacteriaceae*. Species belonging to the genera *Bifidobacterium* and *Ruminococcus* were dominant in terms of numbers over time in both children although no *Bacteroides* species were among the dominant bacteria in these children. The same method used on samples from hospitalized, premature newborns showed that the diversity of the microbiota drops with the length of the hospital stay pointing to the importance of the environment (compared with other variables) in establishment of the intestinal microbiota—a fact that does not apply to newborn babies born at term [62].

Key points

- In humans, the intestinal microbiota consists of about 10^{14} bacterial cells, i.e., ten to twenty times as many cells as there are of the body itself. It varies from segment to segment of the digestive tract with numbers really escalating between the small intestine and the colon where densities of the order of 10^9-10^{11} CFU per gram of contents are found.

- Faecal analysis gives a misleading picture of the composition of the colonic microbiota which comprises: the dominant resident microbiota composed of strictly anaerobic bacteria; the sub-dominant resident microflora composed of facultative anaerobes; and the transiting allochtonous microbiota. Over 50% of the dominant microbiota cannot be cultured.

- Every host has his or her own distinctive faecal microbiota, the composition of which remains relatively constant over time. In contrast, the microbiota varies enormously from one person to another. In reality, the gut microbiota is far more diverse than can be revealed by culture-based methods. Microbiotal diversity increases with age.

- Colonization of the digestive tract begins when the foetal membranes are broached. The main source is the mother (from the vaginal and faecal material). The initial microbiota is simple, reaching a density of 10^{10}-10^{11} CFU per gram of contents within about ten days.

- Various factors—including the route of delivery, diet (formula or breast-feeding), and gestational age at birth—can affect the dynamics of the establishment of the intestinal microbiota. The ever-increasingly strict hygiene of delivery in industrialized countries is associated with delayed colonization by bacteria from the mother, leading to the establishment of bacteria from the environment.

References

1. Simon GL, Gorbach SL. Intestinal flora in health and disease. *Gastroenterology* 1984 ; 86 : 174-93.

2. Moore WE, Holdeman LV. Human fecal flora: the normal flora of 20 Japanese-Hawaiians. *Appl Environ Microbiol* 1974 ; 27 : 961-79.

3. Ducluzeau R, Raibaud P. Écologie microbienne du tube digestif. In : *Actualités scientifiques de l'INRA*. Paris : Masson, 1979.

4. Finegold SM, Sutter VL, Mathisen GE. Normal indigenous intestinal microflora. In : Hentges DJ, ed. *Human intestinal microflora in health and disease*. New-York : Academic Press, 1983 : 3-31.

5. Wilson KH, Blitchington RB. Human colonic biota studied by ribosomal DNA sequence analysis. *Appl Environ Microbiol* 1996 ; 62 : 2273-8.

6. Suau A, Bonnet R, Sutren M, *et al.* Direct analysis of genes encoding 16S rRNA from complex communities reveals many novel molecular species within the human gut. *Appl Environ Microbiol* 1999 ; 65: 4799-807.

7. Bourlioux P, Koletzko B, Guarner F, Braesco V. The intestine and its microflora are partners for the protection of the host: report on the Danone symposium « The intelligent intestine ». *Am J Clin Nutr* 2003 ; 78 : 675-83.

8. Guarner F, Malagelada JR. Gut flora in health and disease. *Lancet* 2003 ; 360 : 512-9.

9. Adlerberth I, Cerqueti M, Poilane I, Wold A, Collignon A. Mechanisms of colonisation and colonisation resistance of the digestive tract. Part 1. Bacteria/Host interactions. *Microbial Ecol Health Dis* 2000 ; suppl 2 : 223-39.

10. Fons M, Gomez A, Karjalainen T. Mechanisms of colonisation and colonisation resistance of the digestive tract. Part 2. Bacteria/Bacteria interactions. *Microbial Ecol Health Dis* 2000 ; suppl 2 : 240-6.

11. Thomas V, Rochet V, Boureau H, *et al.* Molecular characterization and spatial analysis of a simplified microbiota displaying colonization resistance against *Clostridium difficile*. *Microbial Ecol Health Dis* 2002 ; 14 : 203-10.

12. Van de Merwe JP, Stegeman JH, Hazenberg MP. The resident faecal flora is determined by genetic characteristics of the host. Implications for Crohn's disease? *Antonie Van Leeuwenhoek* 1983 ; 49 : 119-24.

13. Hoeksma A, Winkler KC. The normal flora of the nose in twins. *Acta Leiden* 1963 ; 32 : 123-33.

14. Hoskins LC, Boulding ET. Degradation of blood group antigens in human colon ecosystems. II. A gene interaction in man that affects the fecal population density of certain enteric bacteria. *J Clin Invest* 1976 ; 57 : 74-82.

15. Hooper LV, Gordon JI. Commensal host-bacterial relationships in the gut. *Science* 2001 ; 292 : 1115-8.

16. Freitas M, Axelsson LG, Cayuela C, Midtvedt T, Trugnan G. Microbial-host interactions specifically control the glycosylation pattern in intestinal mouse mucosa. *Histochem Cell Biol* 2002 ; 118 : 149-61.

17. Pochard P, Léman F, Flourié B, Pellier P, Goderel I, Rambaud JC. Pyxigraphic sampling to enumerate methanogens and anaerobes in the right colon of healthy humans. *Gastroenterology* 1993 ; 108 : 1281-5.

18. Paster BJ, Dewhirst FE, Olsen I, Fraser GJ. Phylogeny of *Bacteroides, Prevotella*, and *Porphyromonas spp.* and related bacteria. *J Bacteriol* 1994 ; 176 : 725-32.

19. Collins MD, Lawson PA, Willems A, *et al.* The phylogeny of the genus *Clostridium*: proposal of five new genera and eleven new species combinations. *Int J Syst Bacteriol* 1994 ; 44 : 812-26.

20. Vaughan EE, Schut F, Heilig H GHJ, Zoetendal EG, De Vos WM, Akkermans ADL. A molecular view of the intestinal ecosystem. *Curr Issues Intest Microbiol* 2000 ; 1 : 1-12.

21. Sghir A, Gramet G, Suau A, Rochet V, Pochart P, Doré J. Quantification of bacterial groups within human fecal flora by oligonucleotide probe hybridization. *Appl Environ Microbiol* 2000 ; 66: 2263-6.

22. Rochet V, Rigottier-Gois L, Béguet F, Doré J. Composition of human intestinal flora analysed by fluorescent *in situ* hybridisation using group-specific 16S rRNA-targeted oligonucleotide probes. *Genet Sel Evol* 2001 ; 33 : S339-52.

23. Suau A, Rochet V, Sghir A, *et al. Fusobacterium prausnitzii* and related species. *Syst Appl Microbiol* 2001 ; 24 : 139-45.

24. Franks AH, Harmsen HJM, Raangs GC, Jansen GJ, Schut F, Welling GW. Variations of bacterial populations in human feces measured by fluorescent *in situ* hybridization with group-specific 16S rRNA-targeted oligonucleotide probes. *Appl Environ Microbiol* 1998 ; 64 : 3336-45.

25. Zoetendal EG, Ben-Amor K, Harmsen HJM, Schut F, Akkermans ADL, De Vos WM. Quantification of uncultured *Ruminococcus obeum*-like bacteria in human fecal samples by fluorescent *in situ* hybridization and flow cytometry using 16S rRNA-targeted probes. *Appl Environ Microbiol* 2002 ; 68 : 4225-32.

26. Zoetendal EG, Akkermans ADL, De Vos WM. Temperature gradient gel electrophoresis analysis of 16S rRNA from human fecal samples reveals stable and host-specific communities of active bacteria. *Appl Environ Microbiol* 1998 ; 64 : 3854-9.

27. Marteau P, Pochard P, Doré J, Béra-Maillet C, Bernalier A, Corthier G. Comparative study of bacterial groups within the human cecal and fecal microbiota. *Appl Environ Microbiol* 2001 ; 67 : 4939-42.

28. Zoetendal EG, Von Wright A, Vilpponen-Salmela T, Ben-Amor K, Akkermans ADL, De Vos WM. Mucosa-associated bacteria in the human gastrointestinal tract are uniformly distributed along the colon and differ from the community recovered from feces. *Appl Environ Microbiol* 2002 ; 68 : 3401-7.

29. Satokari RM, Vaughan EE, Akkermans ADL, Saarela M, De Vos WM. Bifidobacterial diversity in human feces detected by genus-specific PCR and denaturing gradient gel electrophoresis. *Appl Environ Microbiol* 2001 ; 67 : 504-13.

30. Heilig HG, Zoetendal EG, Vaughan EE, Marteau P, Akkermans ADL, De Vos WM. Molecular diversity of *Lactobacillus spp.* and other lactic acid bacteria in the human intestine as determined by specific amplification of 16S ribosomal DNA. *Appl Environ Microbiol* 2002 ; 68 : 114-23.

31. Mitsuoka T. Intestinal flora and aging. *Nutr Rev* 1992 ; 50 : 438-46.

32. Hopkins MJ, Sharp R, Macfarlane GT. Age and disease related changes in intestinal bacterial populations assessed by cell culture, 16S rRNA abundance and community cellular fatty acid profiles. *Gut* 2001 ; 48 : 198-205.

33. Saunier K, Doré J. Gastrointestinal tract and the elderly: functional foods, gut microflora and healthy ageing. *Dig Liver Dis* 2002 ; 34 Suppl 2 : S19-24.

34. Mackie R, Sghir A, Gaskins HR. Developmental microbial ecology of the neonatal gastrointestinal tract. *Am J Clin Nutrit* 1999 ; 69 : 1035S-45S.

35. Heavey PM, Rowland IR. The gut microflora of the developpong infant: microbiology and metabolism. *Microbial Ecol Health Dis* 1999 ; 11 : 75-83.

36. Tannock GW, Fuller R, Smith SL, Hall MA. Plasmid profiling of members of the family Enterobacteriaceae, lactobacilli, and bifidobacteria to study the transmission of bacteria from mother to infant. *J Clin Microbiol* 1990 ; 28 : 1225-8.

37. Nowrouzian F, Hesselmar B, Saalman R, *et al.* Escherichia coli in infants' intestinal microflora: colonization rate, strain turnover, and virulence gene carriage. *Pediatr Res* 2003 ; 54 : 8-14.

38. Ducluzeau R. L'etablissement de la flore du tractus gastro-intestinal chez le nouveau-né humain. *Rech Gynecol* 1990 ; 2 : 71-5.

39. Moreau MC, Gaboriau-Routhiau V. Influence of resident intestinal microflora on the development and functions of the Gut-Associated Lymphoid Tissue. *Microbiol Ecol Health Dis* 2001 ; 13 : 65-86.

40. Bezirtzoglou E, Romond C. Occurence of *Bifidobacterium* in the feces of newborns delivered by cesarean section. *Biol Neonate* 1990 ; 58 : 247-51.

41. Grönlund MM, Lehtonen OP, Eerola E, Kero P. Fecal microflora in healthy infants born by different methods of delivery: permanent changes in intestinal flora after cesarean delivery. *J Pediat Gastroenterol Nutr* 1999 ; 28 : 19-25.

42. Sakata H, Yoshioka H, Fujita K. Development of the intestinal flora in very low birth weight infants compared to normal full-term newborns. *Eur J Pediatr* 1985 ; 144 : 186-90.

43. Ducluzeau R. Installation, équilibre et rôle de la flore microbienne chez le nouveau-né. *Ann Pédiatr* 1993 ; 40 : 13-22.

44. Hudault S. Microbial colonization of the intestine of the newborn. In : Bindels JG, Goedhart AC, Visser HKA, eds. *Recents developments in infant nutrition*. Dordrecht : Kluwer Academic Publishers, 1996 : 307-17.

45. Gothefors L. Effects of diet on intestinal flora. *Acta Poediatr Scand 1989* ; Suppl 351 : 118-21.

46. de Man P, Verhoeven BA, Verbrugh HA, Vos MC, van den Anker JN. An antibiotic policy to prevent emergence of resistant bacilli. *Lancet* 2000 ; 355 : 973-8.

47. Toltzis P, Dul MJ, Hoyen C, *et al*. Molecular epidemiology of antibiotic-resistant gram-negative bacilli in a neonatal intensive care unit during a nonoutbreak period. *Pediatrics* 2001 ; 108 : 1143-8.

48. Almuneef MA, Baltimore RS, Farrel PA, Reagan-Cirincione P, Dembry LM. Molecular typing demonstrating transmission of gram-negative rods in a neonatal intensive care unit in the absence of a recognized epidemic. *Clin Infect Dis* 2001 ; 32 : 220-7.

49. Goldmann DA, Leclair J, Macone A. Bacterial colonization of neonates admitted to an intensive care environment. *J Pediatr* 1978 ; 93 : 288-93.

50. Bennet R, Eriksson M, Nord CE, Zetterstrom R. Fecal bacterial microflora of newborn infants during intensive care management and treatment with five antibiotic regimens. *Pediatr Infect Dis* 1986 ; 5 : 533-9.

51. Adlerberth I, Carlsson B, de Man P, *et al*. Intestinal colonization with *enterobacteriaceae* in Pakistani and swedish hospital-delivered infants. *Acta Paediat Scand* 1991 ; 80 : 602-10.

52. Simhon A, Douglas JR, Drasar BS, Soothill JF. Effect of feeding on infants' faecal flora. *Arch Dis Child* 1982 ; 57 : 54-8.

53. Sepp E, Naaber P, Voor T, Mikelsaar M, Björkstén B. Development of intestinal microflora during the first month of life in Estonian and Swedish infants. *Microbiol Ecol Health Dis* 2000 ; 12 : 22-6.

54. Butel MJ. La flore du prématuré. In : Dupont C, Gauthier F, Goulet O, Moktari M, Vodovar M, eds. 16e séminaire Guigoz, Deauville 14-16 octobre 2001. Noisiel : Guigoz Editions, Groupe d'Études en Néonatologie - Ile de France, 2001 : 111-42.

55. Gewolb IH, Schwalbe RS, Taciak VL, Harrison TS, Panigrahi P. Stool microflora in extremely low birthweight infants. *Arch Dis Child Fetal Neonatal* 1999 ; 80 : F167-73.

56. Jaureguy F, Doucet-Populaire F, Panel P, Butel MJ, Ghnassia JC. *Conséquences de l'antibioprophylaxie per partum à l'amoxicilline sur la flore intestinale du nouveau-né*. 20e Réunion Interdisciplinaire de Chimiothérapie Anti-Infectieuse. Paris, 7-8 décembre 2000.

57. Stoll BJ, Hansen N, Fanaroff AA, *et al*. Changes in pathogens causing early-onset sepsis in very-low-birth-weight infants. *N Engl J Med* 2002 ; 347 : 240-7.

58. Bjorksten B. Allergy priming early in life. *Lancet* 1999 ; 353 : 167-8.

59. Harmsen HJ, Wildeboer-Veloo AC, Raangs GC, *et al*. Analysis of intestinal flora development in breast-fed and formula-fed infants by using molecular identification and detection methods. *J Pediatr Gastroenterol Nutr* 2000 ; 30 : 61-7.

60. Harmsen HJ, Wildeboer-Veloo AC, Grijpstra J, Knol J, Degener JE, Welling GW. Development of 16s rRNA-based probes for the *Coriobacterium* group and the *Atopobium* cluster and their application for enumeration of *Coriobacteriaceae* in human feces from volunteers of different age groups. *Appl Environ Microbiol* 2000 ; 66 : 4523-7.

61. Favier CF, Vaughan EE, De Vos WM, Akkermans ADL. Molecular monitoring of succession of bacterial communities in human neonates. *Appl Environ Microbiol* 2002 ; 68 : 219-26.

62. Schwiertz A, Gruhl B, Lobnitz M, Michel P, Radke M, Blaut M. Development of the intestinal bacterial composition in hospitalized preterm infants in comparison with breast-fed, full-term infants. *Pediatr Res* 2003 ; 54 : 393-9.

Factors Controlling the Bacterial Microflora. Definitions and Mechanism of Action of Probiotics and Prebiotics

Philippe Marteau

Service de Gastro-entérologie, Hôpital Européen Georges Pompidou, et Université Paris-V, Paris, France.

The intestinal bacterial microflora exerts many physiological functions, in particular fermentation and the "barrier effect" (term referring to the physiological capacity of the endogenous bacterial microflora to inhibit colonization of the intestine by pathogenic microorganisms). These functions are often beneficial for the host but are sometimes harmful: thus a deleterious role of the microflora (called imbalanced intestinal microflora) is suspected in the pathogenesis of acute or chronic intestinal disorders such as diarrhoea, irritable bowel syndrome, Crohn's disease and cancers of the colon. Thus controlling the microflora becomes an objective.

Over the last fifteen years, specialists interested in the ecology of the human gastrointestinal tract have acquired a very significant body of knowledge based on observations of other ecosystems including the seabed, silage, the soil or the digestive tract of other animals (in particular ruminants). To understand and attempt to influence the balance of an ecosystem, the ecologists' vision should not be limited only to that of living organisms (biotic elements) but also should encompass that of their medium (abiotic elements). In the intestine, the primary abiotic ecological factors are pH, degree of anaerobiosis, bile acids, pancreatic enzymes, availability of endogenous or exogenous (food-derived) substrates, the potential sites of adherence of microorganisms to the epithelium or the mucus and the "intestinal flow" (intestinal motility). Since such factors are stable neither throughout the digestive tract nor over time, each section of the gastrointestinal tract must be studied as an original ecosystem. For example, the ascending colon, which receives more food-derived substrate and bacteria than the descending colon, is more acidic and contains a higher quantity of short-chain fatty acids, etc. and so it is therefore not surprising that its bacterial microflora differs from that of the descending colon [1].

Modifying the colonic ecosystem for therapeutic purposes, especially preventive ones, has long been a conceptual aim. The balance of the intestinal ecosystem can be affected primarily by acting either on its biotic elements or on its abiotic factors (Figure 1). Modulation of biotic factors can be done by adding new microorganisms (probiotics, *see below*) or by removing them (by use of antibiotics); it can also be done by providing different nutritional factors to endogenous microorganisms (dietary fiber, resistant starches or prebiotics, *see below*). Although the extensive systematic practice of administering enemas and purgatives is no longer widespread in Europe or

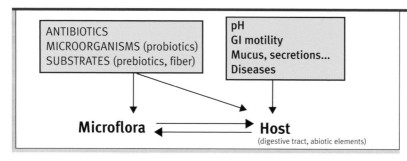

ANTIBIOTICS MICROORGANISMS (probiotics) SUBSTRATES (prebiotics, fiber)	pH GI motility Mucus, secretions... Diseases

Microflora ⇄ **Host**
(digestive tract, abiotic elements)

Figure 1.
Modulation of the
intestinal ecology

North America, it continues to be practiced in many developing countries. As soon as they were discovered, antibiotics were widely used to treat intestinal infectious diseases and also to have an impact on the resident bacterial microflora and to decrease the risk of disease [2]. In livestock, the systematic use of antibiotic therapy has decreased the mortality in animals at time of weaning and has promoted their growth. Nevertheless, there is the other side of the coin to consider: the dissemination of antibiotic resistance, a practice which today has been abandoned due to the ecological risk involved. Except for curative therapies for intestinal infections, today the indications for antibiotics to modulate the intestinal microflora in humans are relatively limited (Table I).

- Prevention of traveller's diarrhoea in high risk subjects
- Prophylaxis of ascitic fluid infection in case of cirrhosis with risk factors
- Intestinal decontamination in aplastic anemia patients or immuno-compromised subjects in the initial period after bone marrow grafting
- Decontamination before certain surgical procedures on the GI tract
- Antibiotic prophylaxis of endoscopic procedures in the GI tract in high risk subjects
- Crohn's disease

Table I.
Uses of antibiotic
therapies to modulate
the intestinal microflora
in humans except for
treatment of reported
intestinal infections or
the stagnant loop
syndrome

Administering special microorganisms to modulate the endogenous microflora is also an idea of long standing. Elie Metchnikoff (Figure 2) obtained the Noble Prize in 1908 for his work on phagocytosis, and published a thesis on the assumed influence of lactic bacteria present in the early form of modern yogurt on the intestinal microflora and the longevity of Bulgarian subjects [3].

The concept of probiotics was born and several medications were developed in the 1950's and 1960's. However, a few years later, since data on the clinical efficacy of many probiotics were not obtained based on rigorous assays, their use gradually waned, except for a few probiotics, whose properties had been confirmed. Scientists also criticized the poor

Figure 2.
Elie Metchnikoff

microbiological quality or stability of certain food products which was sometimes major; some scientists even doubted their efficacy because of the probability (not studied up until then) that such microorganisms and their active substances would be destroyed as soon as they entered the stomach. At the same time, study results were coming in, attesting to the stability of the faecal microflora in a given subject and the apparent impossibility of changing this balance by diet or the administration of microorganisms. These results led to the development of the concept known as the "barrier effect", proposed in France by Raibaud and Ducluzeau, and of "colonization resistance" proposed simultaneously in the Netherlands by van der Waaij. The search for alternatives to antibiotic therapy in livestock animals, and the improvement in knowledge on the mutual relations between the intestinal microflora and the host organism that harbors them, brought about a renewed interest in probiotics. The more recent concept of prebiotics is based on the modulation of the microflora by providing it with new nutritional substrates which can selectively stimulate beneficial endogenous bacteria.

The aim of this chapter is to describe the factors controlling the intestinal microflora, the present state of knowledge concerning their mechanisms of action and their possible adverse effects. Their therapeutic applications, demonstrated for some of them in randomised, controlled, double-blind trials (and thus with a high level of evidence) are discussed in the chapter entitled "Probiotics and Digestive Problems". The pharmacological and clinical data on *Saccharomyces boulardii* are described in detail in the chapter entitled "Example of an Efficient Medicinal Probiotic: Lyophilised *Saccharomyces boulardii*".

Abiotic factors controlling the microflora

Acidity, bile, pancreatic, and intestinal secretions, mucus, defensins

Gastric acid secretion is a major defense factor against downstream colonization of the GI tract by pathogens [4]. The risk of intestinal infections is moderately but significantly increased in cases of achlorohydria or administration of antisecretory therapies, because the number of bacteria needed to trigger an infection is thus also reduced [5]. Since the risk remains low in normal clinical situations, this indicates the presence of other antimicrobial factors in the digestive tract and the role of GI motility. Resistance to acid differs greatly among microorganisms, and some (among which probiotics are selected) completely or partially survive passage through the stomach [4]. Biliary acids also have significant antimicrobial properties on bacterial membranes [6]. Fairly minor fluctuations in these acid levels in the intestine significantly influence, for example, the survival of lactobacilli or bifidobacteria ingested [6]. Experimental results suggest that the pancreatic juice can also have an antimicrobial effect [7]. Nevertheless, the clinical consequences of this observation remain uncertain. The influence of other digestive secretions, such as mucus or defensins, is only partially understood. Mucus forms a physical barrier between the lumen and epithelial cells of the stomach, small intestine, and the colon. This 50-450 μM thick clear gel adheres to the mucosa; it is viscous, composed of mucoglycoprotein polymers secreted by the goblet cells of the epithelium [8]. Its composition and properties vary among different sites in the GI tract and are under the control of at least nine genes ($MUC_{1,2,3,4,5AC,5B,6,7,8}$). MUC_2 is the predominant mucin in the colon and MUC_5 and MUC_6 are the predominant mucins of the stomach. Mucus secretion is decreased by fasting and total parenteral feeding [7, 8]. The bacterial microflora can change its composition and properties not only by partial degradation (which has long been established) but also, as demonstrated in a recent and exciting discovery, by influencing its synthesis. This finding was the first example of the existence of cross-talk, i.e., the exchange of information between the microflora and the mucosa [9]. The mucus not only forms a physical barrier on the surface of the epithelium, but it also concentrates many antimicrobial substances such as secretory immumoglobulin A (IgA), lactoferrin, lactoperoxidase and lysozyme in its web. It also has the ability to bind various microorganisms due to some of its sugars which mimic bacterial receptors. Defensins are antimicrobial peptides that are secreted in the intestinal crypts by Paneth cells which colonize their basal part. They act by destroying the bacterial cell membrane and in particular are active against *Escherichia coli, Listeria monocytogenes, Salmonella* and *Candida albicans* [10]. Their possible action on the saprophytic microflora is not known.

Immune system

The function of the intestinal immune system in controlling the pathogenic intestinal microflora is supported by the observation of disturbances in this pathogenic microflora in immune-deficient hosts. Thus, in the course of IgA selective deficiency or common variable immunodeficiency (hypogammaglobulinemias), an increased risk of recurrent intestinal infection is observed, especially giardiasis (a parasitic disease, also known as lambliasis). Depending on the severity of the immune deficiency in untreated acquired immunodeficiency syndrome (AIDS), an increased risk of bacterial colitis (*Campylobacter jejuni* and *coli*, Salmonella, *Clostridium difficile*), and then (more serious deficiency), cytomegalovirus infections, infections with different protozoa, mycobacteria, or fungi is observed. The complex interactions between the resident microflora and the intestinal and systemic immunity are described in the chapter entitled "Influence of the Intestinal Microflora on Host Immunity".

Intestinal motility and redox potential

Differences in the motility of the small intestine and the colon account for the primary localization of intestinal microflora in the colon (*see chapter entitled* "Microflora and Colonic Motility. Physiological Data and Irritable Bowel Syndrome"). In particular, interdigestive migratory motor complexes play the role of "housekeeper" in the small intestine [11] and account for the lack of microflora in this organ, except for the terminal ileum [12]. All stasis factors in the small intestine produce abundant bacterial colonization by a microflora intermediate between that of the oropharynx and the colon [12].

Lastly, a very low redox potential present in the colon explains the colonic predominance of the anaerobic bacterial microflora.

Dietary factors

The ecosystem in the human distal colon and the faecal bacterial microflora have long known to be relatively stable under physiological conditions and apparently independent of changes in eating habits (*see chapter entitled* "Establishment and Composition of the Gut Microflora"). The factors for stability include stable temperature and strict anaerobiosis and wide biodiversity in the endogenous microflora and high concentrations of microorganisms which comprise it, and also the low levels of available exogenous substrates (unfermented food residue in the proximal colon) compared with endogenous substrates which are found at much more constant levels over time. Reaching the distal colon is difficult for fermentable food substrates because many nondigestible carbohydrates are fermented in the ascending colon if at low doses or are responsible in the distal colon for an osmotic effect (i.e., a risk of diarrhoea) when at high doses [13].

In the 1980's, many studies showed that although the balance in the faecal bacterial microflora seemed to be unchanged by food, certain enzymatic activities in the faecal microflora such as that of β-glucuronidase or 7α-dehydroxylase could be significantly affected, which possibly reflects the activity of the bacterial microflora in the ascending colon [1].

The ecosystem in the proximal colon (ascending colon) has been markedly less studied in humans because it is difficult to access; it differs from the distal ecosystem because it still receives oxygen and especially much higher quantities of varied exogenous substrates. Studies have shown its original features and its instability from one day to another [1].

Purgatives, clysters and antibiotics

The idea of "detoxifying" the body by the rectal administration of various substances ranging from water ("hydrotherapy", "rectal irrigation", "intestinal gardening", etc.) to other liquid agents, solids, or even gaseous products, goes back to the beginning of times and has been depicted by artists on Mayan pottery [14] and Egyptian frescos. Naturally, advocates of such practices accounted for the existence of intestinal microflora in their theories after its discovery. But the ability of such practices to modify the microflora did not go beyond that of hypotheses (in light of the information which we have been able to obtain, in particular on the internet). Similarly, reduction of the faecal microflora during preparation of the colon with polyethylene glycol is transient in nature, as evidenced by the hydrogen breath test using lactulose as the substrate.

Many antibiotics reach the colon directly and/or after entering an enterohepatic cycle, where they have an impact on the microflora. This influence depends on the antimicrobial spectrum and the pharmacokinetics of the antibiotic (which determine the concentrations obtained in the colon). As a result, adverse effects may occur: in particular decreased capacity for fermentation (responsible for an increased risk of diarrhoea), a decrease in the barrier effect (responsible for an increased risk of the emergence of pathogens, chief among which is *Clostridium difficile*), and also the occurrence and dissemination of antibiotic resistance (*see chapter entitled* "Microflora and Diarrhoea: Antibiotic-Associated Diarrhoea"). Several antibiotics and in particular those used at relatively low doses have demonstrated an ability to decrease the mortality of different livestock animals and to improve their growth (i.e., "zootechnological yield") but at the expense of ecological risks which has led the condemnation of these practices [2]. In humans, the use of antibiotics with the aim of modulating the endogenous microflora is intended mainly to reduce the risk of infections starting in the intestine in high-risk subjects (Table I). The quinolones are the most widely used agents in the prevention of traveler's diarrhoea and the prophylaxis of infection of ascitic fluid in case of cirrhosis associated with risk factors. Antibiotic prophylaxis of endoscopic procedures on the digestive tract in high-risk subjects and that performed in certain procedures on the GI tract generally use cefazolin [15]. Metronidazole is recommended during proctological medical procedures.

Probiotics

Definitions

The definition of the term probiotic has changed over time and as a result of the discussion by researchers, industrialists, and specialists in communication with the general public. Lilly and Stillwell were apparently the first, in 1965, to use this term to designate "factors which promote growth produced by microorganisms" [16]. Parker, in 1974 [17], proposed expanding the definition to "organisms and substances which contribute to the balance of the microflora". However, in 1991, Fuller criticized Parker's definition for being too broad and potentially including antibiotics and proposed "microorganisms added to food and having a beneficial effect on the host by improving the balance of his intestinal microflora" [18]. Since then, three items have contributed to further modify this definition. The first was that some microorganisms can have effects on the host without necessarily modifying his microflora (enzymatic direct effects or by immunomodulation). The terms "transiting microorganisms" [19] and "biotherapeutic agents" [20] were then proposed and appear more strongly "evidence-based" since they do not predetermine the mechanism of action. The second item was the interest of certain industrialists to not denominate "generic" microorganisms as "probiotics", in particular those found in standard yogurt, and to reserve this denomination for products with similar appearance and taste, but containing microorganisms whose added value justified a higher cost. The third item was the desire of certain researchers and many food industrialists to exclude dead microorganisms from the definition. Certain dead microorganisms (particularly those killed by heat) can exert certain beneficial effects for the host, although studies have demonstrated that these effects were often less pronounced than those of ingested living microorganisms. The Food and Agriculture Organization (FAO) of the United Nations and the World Health Organization (WHO) established guidelines in 2001 for the proper use of the term "probiotic" in foods [21] and formulated the following definition: "probiotics are live microorganisms which when administered in adequate amounts confer a health benefit on the host."

Composition

Probiotics are living bacteria or yeast, though a few parasites have been studied in animals. They are present in certain foods, particularly fermented dairy products, whether they participate in their production or have been added to them in food supplements or in medicinal products and preferably in lyophilised form (Table II).

Table II. *Examples of available probiotic strains in the form of dietary supplements or medicinal products*	**Lactic bacteria and bifidobacteria**	
	Bifidobacteria	*Bifidobacterium lactis* Bb12 *Bifidobacterium animalis* DN 173 010
	Lactobacillus	*Lactobacillus rhamnosus* strain GG *Lactobacillus johnsonii* La1 *Lactobacillus casei* DN 114 001 *Lactobacillus casei shirota* *Lactobacillus salivarius* UCC118 *Lactobacillus reuteri*
	Enterococcus	*Enterococcus faecium* SF 568
	Escherichia coli	*Escherichia coli* Nissle 1917
	Yeasts	
	Saccharomyces	*Saccharomyces boulardii*

Regulations applicable to the presentation of each of these products are very different, particularly regarding labeling and level of evidence to be provided to authorize certain claims. The number of living microorganisms present in each product is often greater than 10^7/g. The microbial quality of each product is an essential characteristic. Several recent studies (after year 2000) have also criticized the inadequate microbial quality and the improper labeling of several products marketed, but fortunately these criticisms do not apply to many products, whose quality is regularly verified [22], nor do they apply, naturally, to medicinal products.

Pharmacokinetics

Probiotics can be considered as a vehicle for transporting active substances (enzymes, components of the cell wall, peptides or nucleotides, immunomodulators, antimicrobial proteins, etc.) to their targets of action in the GI tract. The majority of pharmacological studies have described the fate of probiotics, i.e., their survival in the intestinal tract. Indeed, the active substances are still infrequently known (*see below*) except for lactase enzyme which is contained in the yogurt bacteria [23, 24].

Methods of study

The majority of *in vivo* studies have investigated the survival of probiotics in stools [24]. Researchers interested in the effects of probiotics in the small intestine have used intubation to study the pharmacokinetics of probiotics in the duodenum and the terminal ileum. The survival of probiotics is compared to that of an inert marker ingested simultaneously. Spores of *Bacillus stearothermophillus* are also used as markers of intestinal motility because they do not multiply and are not destroyed in the GI tract [24].

After ingestion, their elimination in the stool is described by an exponential curve and they become undetectable in five to nine days. The sensitivity of the bacteriological methods to detect and identify a probiotic in an endogenous ecosystem is also a critical point in survival studies. The use of specific characteristics is often necessary. The method of expressing the results is also an important point. The usual criterion is the concentration of the probiotic or its active substances in the anticipated target site of action. It is often considered, but rarely observed, that concentrations of probiotics should be higher than 10^5 colony-forming units (CFU)/ml in the small intestine and 10^7 CFU/g in the stool. Such concentrations in the small intestine have been proposed because they are observed in patients with chronic pathological colonization of the small intestine with clinical manifestations [12, 19]. Concentrations in the stool which have been proposed are those of bacteria in the dominant microflora. The expression of results on survival as a percentage of ingesta is often used because it allows comparison of different probiotics.

The adherence to the wall of the colon (mucus, epithelium) of probiotics has been studied by biopsy cultures and ultrastructural methods. Some bacteria can survive much longer than after their disappearance from the stool.

Survival of ingested probiotics in the gastrointestinal tract and colonization

The survival of ingested microorganisms differs among microbial genera, species and even strains (*in* [24]). Some microorganisms are destroyed as soon as they pass into the stomach while other microorganisms have a high survival capacity as measured by recovery in the stools. Yogurt bacteria, *Lactobacillus delbrueckii subsp. bulgaricus* and *Streptococcus thermophilus*, are low acid resistant and are quickly destroyed within a few minutes at a pH near 1. Pochart *et al.* observed that duodenal concentrations of viable starter bacteria in yogurt in healthy subjects who had ingested 430 g of yogurt containing 10^7 CFU/mL were approximately 10^5 CFU/mL at time of peak level of passage through the duodenum [25]. Some authors have observed the survival of a few yogurt bacteria up to the end of the terminal ileum in some of the study volunteers. *Lactococcus lactis* also has a low rate of survival in the intestine, due to its sensitivity to acid and bile. This sensitivity was used to good advantage as a delivery vector for the small intestine [26].

Some bifidobacteria, ingested in fermented dairy products, as well as *Lactobacillus plantarum* NCIB 8826 have a significant rate of survival in stool, with faecal concentrations greater than 10^8/g being observed [24]. Significant survival rates, although lower, at concentrations of 10^6 CFU/g have been observed with *Lactobacillus acidophilus*, *reuteri* and *rhamnosus*, in particular the GG strain [24]. In humans, after administration of 1 g/day of lyophilised *Saccharomyces boulardii,* a steady state of faecal elimination is achieved at approximately 10^7 to 10^8 living cells per day or 10^5 to 10^6 cells per gram of stool [27].

Probiotics are usually excreted in the stool within a few days after their ingestion, in similar fashion, if not more quickly, than that of a transit marker, which confirms the usual absence of sustained colonization. However, in a few subjects, some authors have observed a prolonged persistence of probiotic strains in the stool or intestinal mucosa in particular [28]. Johanson *et al.* fed healthy volunteers a soup containing nineteen different lactobacilli and observed that, eleven days after ingesting this product, two strains of *Lactobacillus plantarum* (Lp299 and Lp299v)) were still present in biopsies collected from the jejunum or the rectum [29]. Alander *et al.* demonstrated in healthy subjects who ingested a fermented dairy product containing *Lactobacillus rhamnosus* GG, that this strain could be found in colonic biopsies collected twelve days later [30].

To date, few studies are available on the pharmacokinetics of the active substances transported by probiotics [24]. The pharmacokinetics of lactase enzyme contained in yogurt bacteria were studied in healthy, lactase-deficient subjects using the intestinal perfusion method [23]. As demonstrated in Figure 3, yogurt ingestion increased the lactase enzyme activity in the intestine for more than 2 hours. Approximately one fifth of the lactase enzyme present in the yogurt at the time of ingestion was recovered in the terminal ileum, and the quantity of undigested lactose that remained following the ingestion of the yogurt was significantly lower than after ingestion of pasteurized yogurt.

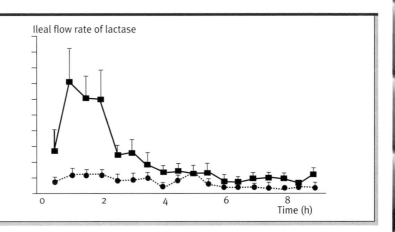

Figure 3.
Ileal flow rate of lactase at the end of the small intestine in eight subjects who ingested yogurt (squares) or pasteurized yogurt without lactase (circles)

Ileal flow rate of lactase

Time (h)

Demonstrated or postulated mechanisms of action of probiotics

Although they share the common point of being non-pathogenic microorganisms, probiotics differ considerably from one another. The diversity of clinical situations in which their efficacy has been demonstrated is also very significant. This suggests that a single mechanism of action is unlikely and that, on the contrary, multiple mechanisms of action are involved. Probiotics can produce direct effects on the chyme, microflora, or intestinal mucosa (enterocytes or immunocompetent cells). They can also have indirect effects related to changes in the microbial ecosystem (Figure 4).

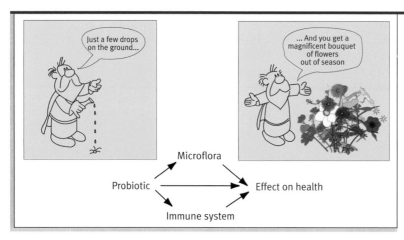

Figure 4.
The direct
and indirect effects
of probiotics

Direct effects

The direct effects of probiotics in the lumen or on the intestinal wall are easier to study and to predict. As mentioned earlier, the lactase enzyme contained in yogurt bacteria takes part in the digestion of lactose in the intestine and this accounts for the excellent digestion of yogurt lactose in lactase-deficient subjects [23]. In similar fashion, one study has demonstrated that the ingestion of *Saccharomyces cerevisiae* (which contains a saccharase) helped the digestion of saccharose in saccharase-deficient children [31]. Bile-sensitive bacteria were used in order to deliver their enzymatic contents in the duodenum [24]. Drouault *et al.* thus showed that lactococci, genetically modified to contain high quantities of intracellular lipase (by inserting the *Staphylococcus hiicus* gene) aided in the digestion of lipids in an animal model for pancreatic insufficiency obtained in the pig by ligation of the pancreatic canal [26]. Sidhu *et al.* [32] showed that force-feeding rats with *Oxalobacter formigenes* (a bacterium capable of breaking down oxalate) decreased the urinary excretion of oxalate; consequently, studies on prevention of renal oxalate lithiases were conducted in humans. Lactic bacteria, genetically modified to contain vaccinal epitopes in order to release them in the intestine, are the subject of studies. Steidler *et al.* [33] have designed a genetically modified lactococcus capable of secreting interleukin 10 (IL-10). This cytokine has anti-inflammatory properties in the intestine and is arousing therapeutic interest for some conditions such as Crohn's disease. The authors have demonstrated that oral administration of *Lactococcus lactis* genetically modified to secrete IL-10 improved experimentally-induced colitis in animals using dextran-sulphate or knocking out the IL-10 gene. A clinical study in humans is underway in the Netherlands (using a genetically modified strain constructed with confinement systems to prevent environmental dissemination, in particular the addition of suicide genes). Other probiotics with other therapeutic activities are currently being tested in inflammatory bowel diseases models, such as lactococci and *Lactobacillus plantarum* genetically modified to produce superoxide dismutase or trefoil peptides.

Several probiotics, and *Saccharomyces boulardii* in particular, have direct effects on the small intestine mucosa, its trophicity and its enzymatic stores [34, 35]. At this level, one (or more) of the active substances seem(s) to be polyamines contained in this yeast (*see chapter entitled* "Example of an Efficient Medicinal Probiotic: Lyophilised *Saccharomyces boulardii*").

Indirect effects

The effects of probiotics on the colonic microflora are paradoxically relatively poorly understood, except for the survival rate of the probiotic itself. It has been shown that the ingestion of certain strains of lactobacilli or bifidobacteria could modify, in a reproducible manner, certain faecal bacterial enzymatic activities, such as β-glucuronidase, azoreductase and nitroreductase [4]. Attempts to modulate the production of short-chain fatty acids or intracolonic pH by probiotics, have on the other hand been fruitless up until now; however studies were performed on stools and not on the contents of the ascending colon, accessible in humans through intubation or pixigraphy.

Many studies conducted in animals have found that the oral administration of various probiotics could modulate the mucosal immune barrier and/or the systemic immune barrier ([36], *see chapter entitled* "Influence of the Intestinal Microflora on Host Immunity: Normal Physiological Conditions"). Pioneering studies have demonstrated that the ingestion of very high quantities of yogurt bacteria increased the ability of circulating lymphocytes in the blood to secrete various cytokines, and interferon γ in particular. The clinical consequences of this biological effect are questionable and attempts to demonstrate a decrease in infections or an increase in the efficacy of oral vaccines under the effect of yogurt to date have failed. A study has shown that the strain *Lactobacillus rhamnosus* GG, administered to children with gastroenteritis due to rotavirus, increased the number of circulating cells able to secrete immunoglobulins [37]. During convalescence, 90% of the infants in the group receiving the probiotic *versus* 46% of those receiving a placebo had developed a specific IgA antibody response to the rotavirus. The same authors reported that the immunogenicity of an antirotavirus oral vaccine could be slightly enhanced by the simultaneous administration of *Lactobacillus rhamnosus* GG [38]. This effect was not observed with a strain of

Lactobacillus reuteri, but this did not prevent it from significantly shortening the rotavirus diarrhoea episode in children. The oral administration of *Lactobacillus johnsonni* strain LA1 increased the antibody response during oral vaccination with *Salmonella typhi* Ty 21a in humans [39]. This probiotic was also responsible for stimulating the phagocytic activity of circulating granulocytes and, in two independent studies, for slightly increasing plasma IgA levels [39]. Several teams are working on the use of genetically modified probiotics, allowing them to be used as vectors loaded with antigens having adjuvant properties and low intrinsic immunogenic properties.

The active substances in probiotics and the molecular details of host-microflora interactions are still poorly understood. Microbial signals identified to date include formylated peptides, lipopolysaccharides, peptidoglycans, components of the cell wall, and nucleotides [24]. The host differentiates signals transmitted by microorganisms *via* toll-like receptors (TLR) present in intestinal epithelial cells and on peripheral antigens presenting cells [40]. Cells use several TLRs to simultaneously detect different signals from the same microorganism. TLR 2 recognizes lipoproteins and peptidoglycans and triggers a response to Gram-positive bacteria and yeasts. TLR 4 mediates the response to the lipopolysaccharides of Gram-negative bacteria, but is little expressed in the colon. TLR1 and TLR 6 take part in the activation of macrophages by Gram-positive bacteria, while TLR 5 and TLR 6 recognize flagellin and bacterial DNA CpG (cytosine phosphoryl guanine) respectively [41]. Bacterial DNA and oligo-nucleotides containing non-methylated CpG stimulate lymphocytes, while eucaryote DNA and methylated oligo-nucleotides do not [41-43]. The stimulation of dendritic cells by DNA CpG is associated with the production of Th1-type cytokines. Rachmilevitz *et al.* recently demonstrated that the administration of bacterial DNA CpG has a therapeutic effect in models of experimentally-induced colitis [42, 43]. They demonstrated that the beneficial effects of a probiotic mixture VSL#3 in this model were due to non-methylated DNA, while the methylated DNA of the probiotic and the control DNA from the calf thymus were ineffective. *In vitro* studies have demonstrated that the response of immunocompetent cells to different pathogenic microorganisms or probiotics was not the same and that various probiotics were able to inhibit TNFα production in *ex vivo* biopsies collected from the mucosa of subjects presenting with Crohn's disease [44, 45]. Probiotics might also have an impact in the development of regulatory T cells, which would help us to explain their apparent clinical efficacy in immune disorders involving the TH2 and TH1 immune response and to expect a therapeutic benefit in the context of atopy.

Observed or theoretical side effects of probiotics

The safety of use of probiotics developed until now has been excellent [24]. However, four types of potential adverse effects deserve consideration: infections, harmful metabolic activity, excessive immunomodulation and gene transfer.

Infections

Probiotics are not selected among pathogens, so the risk of infections is particularly low. Rare cases of local or systemic infections, including septicemia or endocarditis, due to lactobacilli, bifidobacteria, or other lactic bacteria have been reported. *Enterococcus faecium* and *Enterococcus fecalis* are most often involved and arouse very special attention because of the emergence of vancomycin-resistant strains. In most cases, it was difficult to separate the role they played from that of endogenous infection. However, in some cases, the responsibility of the probiotic itself was implicated. Thus, about thirty cases of fungemia were reported in patients treated with *Saccharomyces boulardii* [46-48], and cases of infection were attributed to *Lactobacillus rhamnosus* [49, 50]. The number of cases of fungemia which occurred during treatment with *Saccharomyces boulardii* should be compared to its extensive use worldwide, in particular in the hospital setting, and to its status as a medicinal product which leads to its use in patients who are often in frail health and present with a broad spectrum of risk factors. All subjects who had *Saccharomyces boulardii*-related fungemia had a central venous catheter [46]. Bacterial colonization of catheters, which takes place following the opening of probiotic sachets through hand-borne transmission, has been demonstrated. Another mechanism may be translocation of yeast; however, this mechanism was not observed in patients presenting with intestinal ulcerations who received yeast in clinical trials.

The risk of probiotics in patients with immunocompromised function is poorly established. On the contrary, *Saccharomyces boulardii* has demonstrated protective effect against intestinal pathogens in immunosuppressed mice [51]. On the other hand, it is likely that *Lactobacillus rhamnosus* infections were due to translocation. Translocation is defined as the passage of microorganisms or their products, endotoxins or exotoxins, from the GI tract to non-intestinal sites such as mesenteric lymph nodes, the liver, spleen or blood. Endogenous bacteria continuously translocate in very small quantities, including in immunocompetent subjects; however, these bacteria are quickly destroyed in the lymphoid organs. Bacterial translocation may result from intestinal microbial overgrowth, enhanced mucosal permeability or an immune deficiency. A 74-year-old woman, presenting with non-insulin dependent diabetes mellitus, and who regularly ingested the probiotic *Lactobacillus rhamnosus* GG, suffered from liver abscess related to lactobacilli impossible to differentiate from the probiotic strain [49]. The other case of infection probably due to *Lactobacillus rhamnosus* ingested in the form of a probiotic was observed in a 67-year-old man presenting with minimal mitral regurgitation, and who had the habit of chewing a mixture of probiotics containing *Lactobacillus rhamnosus*, *Lactobacillus acidophilus* and *Streptococcus faecalis* [50]. A few days after a tooth extraction associated with amoxicillin antibiotic therapy, *Lactobacillus rhamnosus*-associated endocarditis occurred. The lactobacillus isolated from the blood was entirely identical to one of the microorganisms present in the probiotic preparation. However, infections with endogenous lactobacilli with no relation to the probiotic are also possible, and in particular one case of infection with *Lactobacillus rhamnosus* in a patient presenting with ulcerative colitis has been published [52]. Salminen *et al.* have studied the prevalence of bacteremia associated with lactobacilli in southern Finland, during two consecutive four- and six-year periods. They compared the characteristics of positive blood cultures (twenty over the ten years) to the strains of probiotics in commercial dairy products. In no cases were there any similarities between the infectious strains and the probiotic strains [53].

In summary, the risk of infection is very low and there is no evidence that probiotics pose a higher risk of infection than commensal strains. In practice, all the infections were observed in subjects with predisposing conditions, especially valvular abnormalities in cases of endocarditis, or the existence of central catheters in cases of septicemia. The data regarding the risks or benefits of probiotics in cases of immune deficiency are still insufficient.

Metabolic side effects

If it is recognized that probiotics can transport or promote beneficial activities in the GI tract, they can also have negative effects on health through the same mechanism [24]. The concentrations of microorganisms passing through the small intestine after the ingestion of probiotics are often of the same order of magnitude as those observed during chronic bacterial colonization of the small intestine. One study drew attention to a potential risk of excessive deconjugation or dehydroxilation of bile acids in the small intestine by probiotics [54]. Indeed, the study showed that in subjects with an ileostomy who ingested *Lactobacillus acidophilus* and a *bifidobacterium*, the two microorganisms significantly converted primary bile acids into unbound secondary bile acids in the small intestine. Excessive degradation of the intestinal mucus may also be a side effect of certain probiotics. Ruseler van Embden studied the effects of three probiotic strains *in vitro* and *in vivo* in gnotobiotic rats. In this study, three strains of *Lactobacillus acidophilus*, *bifidobacterium*, and *Lactobacillus rhamnosus* did not break down the mucus [55].

Immunologic side effects

Parenteral administration of the bacterial wall components such as peptidoglycans can induce fever, arthritis, and auto-immune diseases [24]. These effects are mediated by cytokines; it is now well established that cytokine excretion is induced by many probiotics. Oral administration of high doses of probiotics did not induce any immunological side effects in mice, but increased systemic passage of bacterial wall polymers was observed in rats with colonic lesions or in cases of chronic bacterial colonization of the small intestine. To our knowledge, a single immunological side effect was observed in humans in the form of an anecdotal and non-detailed case of auto-immune hepatitis which may have been aggravated by the ingestion of very high quantities of yogurt. Potential modulation of auto-immune diseases by the ingestion of probiotics should lead to more extensive studies.

Gene transfer

Some microbial genes, especially plasmid-coded genes for antibiotic resistance, may be transferred between microorganisms. The probability of gene transfer depends on the nature of the genetic material to be transferred (plasmids, transposons, etc.), the type of donor and receiver strains, their respective concentrations, and the screening pressure in the medium (in particular the presence of antibiotics) promoting the growth of transconjugants. Probiotic resistance to antibiotics is not in itself a risk, unless this resistance renders the probiotic untreatable in cases of systemic infection by the probiotic, or if the resistance can be transmitted to pathogens. Infections caused by vancomycin-resistant enterococci pose a serious clinical problem. Consequently, the safety of *Enterococcus faecium* strains used as probiotics must be the subject of very careful studies.

Prebiotics and symbiotics

Definitions, composition

Prebiotics have been defined as "non-digestible food ingredients that beneficially affect the host by selectively stimulating the growth, activity or both, of one or a limited number of bacterial species already resident in the colon" [56-58]. To date, the bacterial groups involved are mainly bifidobacteria (hence referred to as bifidogenic effect) and other lactic bacteria. The level of evidence that these groups are indicators of a beneficial microflora is debatable, because it is based mainly on experts' opinion. Their arguments are that bifidobacteria are predominant in the microflora of breast-fed infants, that there are found in smaller quantities in the elderly, and that randomised, controlled studies using bifidobacteria or lactobacilli as probiotics have reported beneficial effects on health [56-61]. The best known and widely used prebiotics are fructanes—fructo-oligosaccharides (FOS), oligofructose, inuline—and other galactose and transgalactose oligosides (GOS and TOS). Many other carbohydrates could be considered as prebiotics (xylo-oligosaccharides, isomalto-oligosaccharides, glucooligosaccharides, etc.). Alcohol sugars can also have prebiotic properties. Lactulose is also a prebiotic and even lactose in lactase-deficient subjects (i.e., more than 50% of adults in France) [60]. Certain prebiotics are naturally present in foods and others are added to foods for functional purposes or to dietary supplements [59].

Symbiotics are defined as the combination of a probiotic and a prebiotic whose concomitant ingestion could promote the multiplication of the former in the GI tract (e.g. a combination of bifidobacteria or lactobacilli and fructo-oligosaccharides) [57]. The demonstration of a synergistic effect of pre- and probiotics is not required by the definition, and consequently to date it is generally lacking. The simultaneous consumption of inuline and bifidobacteria does not increase the faecal excretion of bifidobacteria observed with the ingestion of bifidobacteria alone [62].

Demonstrated or postulated mechanisms of action of prebiotics

Most prebiotics increase the faecal concentrations of bifidobacteria [56-61]. Dose-response studies have suggested that a minimum dose of 5 g/day of fructooligosaccharides is required to obtain a bifidogenic effect and that this effect was all the more pronounced when faecal concentrations of bifidobacteria were initially low in the subject [60]. But the ecological changes induced by prebiotics have a broad range and are not limited to a stimulation effect on one group of bacteria or another which metabolize them. The significant decrease in intracolonic pH, due to the stimulation of lactic bacteria, has a negative effect on other bacterial groups such as *Bacteroides*. Acidification of pH is also responsible for inhibiting certain enzymatic activities such as 7-α-dehydroxylase. Short-chain fatty acids have many physiological effects in the colon (in particular butyrate) and in the body (propionate and acetate). The main effects are summarized in Figure 5. Since fermentation profile varies based on substrate, some prebiotics such as FOS and some resistant starches seem to be more "butyrogenic" than others.

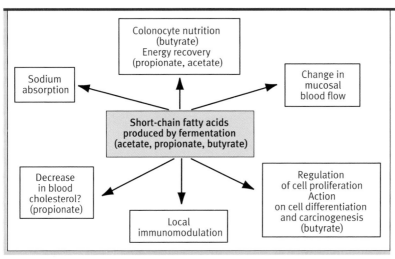

Figure 5.
Physiological effects of short-chain fatty acids produced during colonic fermentation

Clinical effects

Prebiotics are the subject of clinical studies in different therapeutic fields including constipation, various other functional gastrointestinal disorders, hepatic encephalopathy and the prevention of colorectal cancer [62, 63]. The level of evidence for clinical efficacy is satisfactory for lactulose and lactitol for the treatment of constipation and hepatic encephalopathy, and the level of evidence is increasing as studies are conducted on other topics. The metabolic effects of prebiotics are thus opening pathways for research on the increase of calcium absorption in the small intestine or the colon (and consequently the maintenance of bone stores) and the decrease of hypercholesterolemia; however, the level of evidence to date is relatively low due to the lack of controlled, randomised studies [64, 65].

Observed or theoretical side effects of prebiotics

Prebiotics are usually well tolerated but may also have side effects. These are related to the dose and consist primarily of excessive rectal gas and borborygmi, abdominal pains, and diarrhoea. Symptoms of intolerance can be due to the osmotic effect or to fermentation and originate in the small intestine or the colon (Figure 6).

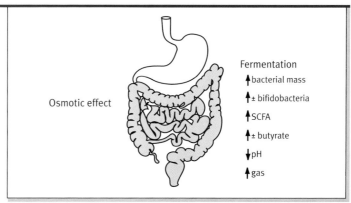

Figure 6.
Prebiotics: pathophysiology of side effects

Osmotic effect

Fermentation
↑ bacterial mass
↑ ± bifidobacteria
↑ SCFA
↑ ± butyrate
↓ pH
↑ gas

As long as they have not been metabolized, prebiotics produce an osmotic effect in the intestinal lumen, which is negatively correlated with their molecular mass. This effect increases the water flow through the intestine and may induce borborygmi, abdominal pain, and possibly diarrhoea if the capacity for colonic reabsorption of water and electrolytes is exceeded [13].

Fermentation produces gases which can also induce borborygmi, abdominal pains, and excessive expulsion of rectal gases. On the other hand, it decreases and may even eliminate diarrhoea through a decrease in the osmotic effect. The protective function of colonic microflora in reducing the severity of prebiotic-induced diarrhoea has been demonstrated in studies comparing faecal output after a dose of fermentable undigested sugars, to faecal output observed in response to non-fermentable osmotic substances such as polyethylene-glycol or magnesium sulphate. Hammer *et al.* [13] thus compared diarrhoea resulting from rising iso-osmolar doses of polyethylene-glycol and lactulose. Lactulose induced less diarrhoea than polyethylene-glycol at doses of less than 45 g/day. Saunders and Wiggins [13] showed that increasing the doses of magnesium sulphate increased faecal output, even at small doses, which was not the case with lactulose or other undigested sugars (mannitol, raffinose). The authors also showed that diarrhoea was observed only when sugar appeared in the stool, a finding which indicates the saturated colonic capacity for fermentation of doses up to 40-80 g of prebiotics. In another study [13], high doses of lactulose induced diarrhoea of variable intensity from one subject to another. Thus, after ingesting 80 g of lactulose, four subjects out of twelve had a stool volume exceeding one liter per day, while four others had a stool weight of less than 280 g/day. It is likely that inter-individual variations are related to differences in the ability to ferment carbohydrates, since gas production varied by a factor of ten when faecal samples from different subjects were incubated with the same sugar [66].

The risk of intolerance and the severity of symptoms, in a given subject and in a population, appears more or less dose-dependent [13]. A threshold was found in all cases regarding diarrhoea, but not always regarding borborygmi and excessive rectal gases insofar as these symptoms are more frequent in the control population (Figure 7).

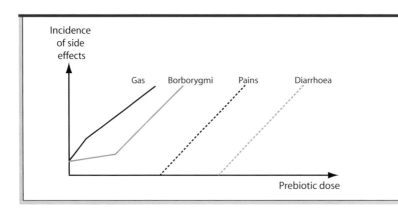

Figure 7.
Side effects
of prebiotics.
Intolerance depends on:
- the dose,
- the method
* of consumption,*
- the subject (irritable
* bowel syndrome...),*
- adaptation of
* the microflora?*

The existence of irritable bowel syndrome increases the risk of intolerance to prebiotics [13, 67-69]. Furthermore, the method of ingestion of sugars may affect their intestinal absorption and therefore modulate their arrival in the colon and their diarrhoea-inducing effect. For example, lactose absorption in a subject with decreased lactase activity is increased when this sugar is ingested in the form of whole milk, compared to its ingestion in the form of skim milk, as fats slow gastric emptying. Absorption is also increased if lactose is ingested at the same time as fibers, a meal, cocoa, or loperamide which slows gastric and/or intestinal motility [13].

Lastly, regular intake of certain prebiotics such as lactose or lactulose induces changes in the metabolic activity of intestinal microflora (bacterial adaptation), which increases its ability to ferment undigested sugar and decreases the excretion of hydrogen [70, 71]. One may expect lower diarrhoea-inducing effect and less flatulence when undigested sugars are consumed regularly (clinical adaptation). This was confirmed in some studies conducted recently in healthy volunteers who ingested a small dose of lactulose on a regular basis [72]. However, Briet *et al*. [73] reported that symptoms and the laxative threshold were similar regardless of whether the dose of fructooligosaccharides was administered occasionally or regularly. Lastly, a recent study demonstrated that the consumption of 6.6 g of fructooligosaccharides three times a day increased transient relaxation of the lower sphincter of the oesophagus and gastroesophageal reflux in subjects presenting with this disorder [74].

Conclusion

The knowledge acquired over the past twenty years on the pharmacokinetics, clinical spectrum and in some cases, the mechanism of action of probiotics, is such that the skepticism surrounding them in scientific circles has disappeared and has given way to genuine enthusiasm.

For their part, prebiotics have been the subject of fewer studies, and the price to be paid for the more or less targeted stimulation of endogenous colonic bacterial species is the side effects related to their fermentation and their osmotic activity.

Key points

- In a given subject, the microflora in the descending colon is very stable, while the microflora in the ascending colon, which receives many substrates, has proven to be more variable over time.

- Abiotic factors for controlling intestinal microflora are pH, redox potential, bile salts and, perhaps, pancreatic enzymes, mucus, defensins, immune cells and cytokines associated with mucosa and motility determining the GI motility.

- The use of antibiotics to modify the intestinal microflora is indicated in non-infectious disease in humans only in rare cases.

- Probiotics pass through the GI tract as live microorganisms, without colonizing it. They can exert direct effects in its lumen, such as providing digestive enzymes. Studies are underway to evaluate the possible delivery of vaccinal epitopes or anti-inflammatory substances after genetic manipulation. Probiotics modulate the mucosal and systemic immune system and the properties of epithelial cells through toll-like receptors. Their influence on endogenous intestinal microflora is poorly understood; they may interfere with the production of enzymes which activate procarcinogenes.

- Prebiotics can more or less selectively stimulate components of the colonic microflora, such as bifidobacteria. Their action is dose-dependent, but overly high doses produce osmotic diarrhoea.

References

1. Marteau P, Pochart P, Doré J, *et al*. Comparative study of bacterial groups within the human cecal and fecal microbiota. *Appl Environ Microbiol* 2001 ; 67 : 4939-42.

2. Chaslus-Dancla E. Les antibiotiques en élevage : état des lieux et problèmes posés http://www.tours.inra.fr/tours/pap/articles/antibio.htm.

3. Simon GL, Gorbach SL. Intestinal flora and gastrointestinal function. In : Johnson LR, ed. *Physiology of the gastrointestinal tract*. New York : Raven Press, 1987 : 1729-47.

4. Cook GC. Hypochlorhydria and vulnerability to intestinal infection. *Eur J Gastroenterol Hepatol* 1994 ; 6 : 693-5.

5. Marteau P, Minekus M, Havenaar R, *et al*. Survival of lactic acid bacteria in a dynamic model of the stomach and small intestine: validation and the effects of bile. *J Dairy Sci* 1997 ; 80 : 1031-7.

6. Drouault S, Corthier G, Ehrlich SD, *et al*. Survival, physiology, and lysis of *Lactococcus lactis* in the digestive tract. *Appl Environ Microbiol* 1999 ; 65 : 4881-6.

7. Pasquier MC, Vatier J. Mucus gastro-intestinal : une barrière protectrice complexe. Première partie. Structure et propriétés physicochimiques. *Gastroenterol Clin Biol* 1990 ; 14 : 352-8.

8. Khan J, Iiboshi Y, Cui L, *et al*. Alanyl-glutamine-supplemented parenteral nutrition increases luminal mucus gel and decreases permeability in the rat small intestine. *J Parenter Enteral Nutr* 1999 ; 23 : 24-31.

9. Hooper LV, Wong MH, Thelin A, *et al*. Molecular analysis of commensal host-microbial relationships in the intestine. *Science* 2001 ; 291 : 881-4.

10. Ganz T. Defensins: antimicrobial peptides of innate immunity. *Nat Rev Immunol* 2003 ; 3 : 710-20.

11. Coffin B. Troubles moteurs intestinaux. In : Rambaud JC, ed. *Traité de gastro-entérologie*. Paris : Flammarion, 2000 : 483-93.

12. Flourié B. Colonisation bactérienne chronique du grêle. In : Rambaud JC, ed. *Traité de Gastro-entérologie*. Paris : Flammarion, 2000 : 459-66.

13. Marteau P, Flourié B. Tolerance to low-digestible carbohydrates: symptomatology and methods. *Br J Nutr* 2001 ; 85, Suppl 1 : S17-21.

14. de Smet PA, Hellmuth NM. A multidisciplinary approach to ritual enema scenes on ancient Maya pottery. *J Ethnopharmacol* 1986 ; 16 : 213-62.

15. Greff M. Recommandations de la Société Française d'Endoscopie Digestive : prophylaxie antibiotique en endoscopie digestive. *Endoscopy* 1998 ; 30 : 873-5.

16. Lilly DM, Stillwell RH. Probiotics: growth promoting factors produced by microorganisms. *Science* 1965 ; 147 : 747-8.

17. Parker RB. Probiotics, the other half of the antibiotic story. *Anim Nutr Health* 1974 ; 29 : 4-8.

18. Fuller R. Probiotics in human medicine. *Gut* 1991 ; 32 : 439-42.

19. Marteau P. *Survie et effets de micro-organismes alimentaires non pathogènes dans le tube digestif de l'homme*. Thèse de Doctorat de l'Université Paris Sud, 1994.

20. Elmer GW, Surawicz CM, McFarland LV. Biotherapeutic agents: a neglected modality for the treatment and prevention of selected intestinal and vaginal infections. *JAMA* 1996 ; 275 : 870-6.

21. FAO/WHO. Health and nutritional properties of probiotics in food including powder milk with live lactic acid bacteria. Argentina, October 2001. http://www.fao.org/es/esn/Probio/report.pdf

22. Fasoli S, Marzotto M, Rizzotti L, *et al*. Bacterial composition of commercial probiotic products as evaluated by PCR-DGGE analysis. *Int J Food Microbiol* 2003 ; 82 : 59-70.

23. Marteau P, Flourié B, Pochart P, *et al*. Role of the microbial lactase (EC 3.2.123) activity from yogurt on the intestinal absorption of lactose: an *in vivo* study in lactase deficient humans. *Br J Nutr* 1990 ; 64 : 71-9.

24. Marteau P, Shanahan F. Basic aspects and pharmacology of probiotics – an overview on pharmacokinetics, mechanisms of action and side effects. *Best Pract Res Clin Gastroenterol* 2003 ; 17 (5) : 725-40.

25. Pochart P, Dewit O, Desjeux JF, *et al*. Viable starter culture, β-galactosidase activity and lactose in duodenum after yogurt ingestion in lactase-deficient humans. *Am J Clin Nutr* 1989 ; 49 : 828-31.

26. Drouault S, Juste C, Marteau P, *et al*. Oral treatment with *Lactococcus lactis* expressing *Staphylococcus hyicus* lipase enhances lipid digestion in pigs with induced pancreatic insufficiency. *Appl Environment Microbiol* 2002 ; 68 : 3166-8.

27. Blehaut H, Massot J, Elmer G, *et al*. Disposition kinetics of *Saccharomyces boulardii* in man and rat. *Biopharm Drug Dispos* 1989 ; 10 : 353-64.

28. Goldin BR, Gorbach S, Saxelin M, *et al*. Survival of *Lactobacillus species* (strain GG) in human gastrointestinal tract. *Dig Dis Sci* 1992 ; 37 : 121-8.

29. Johansson M., Molin G, Jeppsson B, *et al*. Administration of different Lactobacillus strains in fermented oatmeal soup: *in vivo* colonization of human intestinal mucosa and effect on the indigenous flora. *Appl Environment Microbiol* 1993 ; 59 : 15-20.

30. Alander M, Satokari R, Korpela R, *et al*. Persistence of colonization of human colonic mucosa by a probiotic strain, *Lactobacillus rhamnosus* GG, after oral consumption. *Appl Environment Microbiol* 1999 ; 65 : 351-4.

31. Harms HK, Bertele-Harms RM, Bruer-Kleis D. Enzyme substitution therapy with the yeast *Saccharomyces cerevisiae* in congenital sucrase-isomaltase deficiency. *N Engl J Med* 1987 ; 316 : 1306-9.

32. Sidhu H, Allison MJ, Chow JM, *et al*. Rapid reversal of hyperoxaluria in a rat model after probiotic administration of *Oxalobacter formigenes*. *J Urol* 2001 ; 166 : 1487-91.

33. Steidler L, Hans W, Schotte L, *et al*. Treatment of murine colitis by *Lactococcus lactis* secreting interleukin-10. *Science* 2000 ; 289 : 1352-5.

34. Buts JP, De Keyser N, De Raedemaeker L. *Saccharomyces boulardii* enhances rat intestinal enzyme expression by endoluminal release of polyamines. *Pediatr Res* 1994 ; 36 : 522-7.

35. Jahn HU, Ullrich R, Schneider T, *et al*. Immunological and trophical effects of *Saccharomyces boulardii* on the small intestine in healthy human volunteers. *Digestion* 1996 ; 57 : 95-104.

36. Isolauri E, Sutas Y, Kankaanpaa P, *et al*. Probiotics : effects on immunity. *Am J Clin Nutr* 2001 ; 73 (2 Suppl) : 444S-50S.

37. Isolauri E, Juntunen M, Rautanen T, *et al*. A human Lactobacillus strain (*Lactobacillus casei* sp strain GG) promotes recovery from acute diarrhea in children. *Pediatrics* 1991 ; 88 : 90-7.

38. Isolauri E, Joensuu J, Suomalainen H, *et al*. Improved immunogenicity of oral D x RRV reassortant rotavirus vaccine by *Lactobacillus casei* GG. *Vaccine* 1995 ; 13 : 310-2.

39. Blum S, Haller D, Pfeifer A, *et al*. Probiotics and immune response. *Clin Rev Allerg Immunol* 2002 ; 22 : 287-309.

40. Underhill DM. Toll-like receptors: networking for success. *Eur J Immunol* 2003 ; 33 : 1767-75.

41. Krieg AM. CpG motifs: the active ingredient in bacterial extracts? *Nature Med* 2003 ; 9 : 831-5.

42. Rachmilewitz D, Karmeli F, Takabayashi K, *et al*. Immunostimulatory DNA ameliorates experimental and spontaneous murine colitis. *Gastroenterology* 2002 ; 122 : 1428-41.

43. Rachmilewitz D, Karmeli F, Takabayashi K, *et al*. Amelioration of experimental colitis by probiotics is due to the immunostimulatory effect of its DNA. *Gastroenterology* 2002 ; 122 : T1004 abstract.

44. Haller D, Bode C, Hammes WP, *et al*. Non-pathogenic bacteria elicit a differential cytokine response by intestinal epithelial cell/leucocyte co-cultures. *Gut* 2000 ; 47 : 79-87.

45. Borruel N, Carol M, Casellas F, *et al*. Increased mucosal tumour necrosis factor a production in Crohn's disease can be downregulated *ex vivo* by probiotic bacteria. *Gut* 2002 ; 51 : 659-64.

46. Hennequin C, Kauffmann-Lacroix C, Jobert A, *et al*. Possible role of catheters in *Saccharomyces boulardii* fungemia. *Eur J Clin Microbiol Infect Dis* 2000 ; 19 : 16-20.

47. Lherm T, Monet C, Nougiere B, *et al*. Seven cases of fungemia with *Saccharomyces boulardii* in critically ill patients. *Intens Care Med* 2002 ; 28 : 797-801.

48. Riquelme AJ, Calvo MA, Guzman AM, *et al*. *Saccharomyces cerevisiae* fungemia after *Saccharomyces boulardii* treatment in immunocompromised patients. *J Clin Gastroenterol* 2003 ; 36 : 41-4.

49. Rautio M, Jousimies-Somer H, Kauma H, *et al*. Liver abscess due to a *Lactobacillus rhamnosus* strain indistinguishable from *L. rhamnosus* strain GG. *Clin Infect Dis* 1999 ; 28 : 1159-60.

50. MacKay A, Taylor M, Kibbler C, Hamilton Miller J. *Lactobacillus endocarditis* caused by a probiotic microorganism. *Clin Microbiol Infect* 1999 ; 5 : 290-2.

51. Peret Filho LA, Penna FJ, Bambirra EA, *et al*. Dose effect of oral *Saccharomyces boulardii* treatments on morbidity and mortality in immunosuppressed mice. *J Med Microbiol* 1998 ; 47 : 111-6.

52. Farina C, Arosio M, Mangia M, *et al. Lactobacillus casei subsp. rhamnosus* sepsis in a patient with ulcerative colitis. *J Clin Gastroenterol* 2001 ; 33 : 251-2.

53. Salminen MK, Tynkkynen S, Rautelin H, *et al*. Lactobacillus bacteremia during a rapid increase in probiotic use of *Lactobacillus rhamnosus* GG in Finland. *Clin Infect Dis* 2002 ; 35 : 1155-60.

54. Marteau P, Gerhardt MF, Myara A, *et al*. Metabolism of bile salts by alimentary bacteria during transit in human small intestine. *Microbiol Ecol Health Dis* 1995 ; 8 : 151-7.

55. Ruseler-van Embden JG, van Lieshout LM, Gosselink MJ, *et al*. Inability of *Lactobacillus casei* strain GG, *L. acidophilus*, and *Bifidobacterium bifidum* to degrade intestinal mucus glycoproteins. *Scand J Gastroenterol* 1995 ; 30 : 675-80.

56. Gibson GR, Roberfroid MB. Dietary modulation of the human colonic microbiota: introducing the concept of prebiotics. *J Nutr* 1995 ; 125 : 1401-12.

57. Schrezenmeir J, de Vrese M. Probiotics, prebiotics and synbiotics – approaching a definition. *Am J Clin Nutr* 2001 ; 73 (2 Suppl) : 361s-4s.

58. MacFarlane GT, Cummings JH. Probioties and prebiotics: can regulating the activities of intestinal bacteria benefit health? *Br Med J* 1999 ; 318 : 999-1003.

59. Van Loo J, Cummings J, Delzenne N, *et al*. Functional food properties of non-digestible oligosaccharides : a consensus report from the ENDO project (DGXII AIRII-CT94-1095). *Brit J Nutr* 1999 ; 81 : 121-32.

60. Szilagyi A. Lactose - a potential prebiotic. *Aliment Pharmacol Ther* 2002 ; 16 : 1591-602.

61. Bouhnik Y, Vahedi K, Achour L, *et al*. Short-chain fructo-oligosaccharide administration dose-dependently increases fecal bifidobacteria in healthy humans. *J Nutr* 1999 ; 129 : 113-6.

62. Bouhnik Y, Flourié B, Andrieux C. Effects of *Bifidobacterium sp* fermented milk ingested with or without inulin on colonic bifidobacteria and enzymatic activities in healthy humans. *Eur J Clin Nutr* 1996 ; 50 : 269-73.

63. Cummings JH, Macfarlane GT. Gastrointestinal effects of prebiotics. *Br J Nutr* 2002 ; 87 Suppl 2 : S145-51.

64. Nyman M. Fermentation and bulking capacity of indigestible carbohydrates: the case of inulin and oligofructose. *Br J Nutr* 2002 ; 87 Suppl 2 : S163-8.

65. Scholz-Ahrens KE, Schrezenmeir J. Inulin, oligofructose and mineral metabolism - experimental data and mechanism. *Br J Nutr* 2002 ; 87 Suppl 2 : S179-86.

66. Williams CM, Jackson KG. Inulin and oligofructose: effects on lipid metabolism from human studies. *Br J Nutr* 2002 ; 87 Suppl 2 : S261-4.

67. Hartemink R, Alles MS, Rombouts FM. Fermentation of selected carbohydrates by faecal inocula from volunteers on a controlled diet low in fibre. In : Hartemink R, ed. *Prebiotic effects of non-digestible oligo- and polysaccharides*. Thesis. Landbouwuniversiteit Wageningen, 1999.

68. Rumessen JJ, Gudmand-Hoyer E. Functional bowel disease: malabsorption and abdominal distress after ingestion of fructose, sorbitol, and fructose-sorbitol mixtures. *Gastroenterology* 1988 ; 95 : 694-700.

69. Vesa TH, Seppo LM, Marteau PR, *et al*. Role of irritable bowel syndrome in subjective lactose intolerance. *Am J Clin Nutr* 1998 ; 67 : 710-5.

70. Florent C, Flourié B, Leblond A, *et al*. Influence of chronic lactulose ingestion on the colonic metabolism of lactulose in man (an *in vivo* study). *J Clin Invest* 1985 ; 75 : 608-13.

71. Briet F, Pochart P, Marteau P, *et al*. Improved clinical tolerance to chronic lactose ingestion in subjects with lactose intolerance: a placebo effect? *Gut* 1997 ; 41 : 632-5.

72. Flourié B, Briet F, Florent C, *et al*. Can diarrhea induced by lactulose be reduced by prolonged ingestion of lactulose? *Am J Clin Nutr* 1993 ; 58 : 369-75.

73. Briet F, Achour L, Flourié B, *et al*. Symptomatic response to varying levels of fructo-oligosaccharides consumed occasionally or regularly. *Eur J Clin Nutr* 1995 ; 49 : 501-7.

74. Piche T, Bruley des Varannes S, Sacher-Huvelin S, *et al*. Colonic fermentation influences lower esophageal sphincter function in gastroesophageal reflux disease. *Gastroenterology* 2003 ; 124 : 894-902.

Gut Microflora
in Physiology
and Pathogenesis

Main Metabolic Functions of the Human Intestinal Microflora

Annick Bernalier-Donadille

Unité de Microbiologie,
INRA,
Centre de Recherches de
Clermont-Ferrand/Theix,
Saint-Genès-Champanelle,
France.

The human colon is a complex anaerobic ecosystem composed of an extremely dense flora comprising mainly strictly anaerobic microorganisms. The main carbon and energy sources of this microflora are undigested carbohydrates and proteins that have escaped digestion in the upper part of the gastrointestinal (GI) tract, as well as endogenous secretions (mucopolysaccharides, , desquamated cellules, enzymes, etc.). A large variety of substrates is therefore available for the colonic microflora, but the type and quantity of the different carbon-containing sources vary for a large part depending on the subject's diet. The total quantity of fermentable carbohydrates ranges from 10 to 60 grams per day, while that of nitrogen-containing compounds, of which 1 to 2 grams come from ileal effluent [1], is estimated at 6 to 18 grams per day [2]. Thus, carbohydrate metabolism is quantitatively more extensive than that of proteins, in particular in the proximal colon where a large amount of fermentable substrates is available.

The metabolic activities of the colonic microflora are thus numerous and diverse. Complex polymers are degraded by a wide variety of hydrolases (polysaccharidases, glycosidases, proteases, peptidases) into smaller fragments (oligosaccharides, sugars, amino acids) that can be digested by bacteria. Fermentation of these substrates by the microflora further leads to the production of different metabolites such as short-chain fatty acids (SCFAs), gas and ammonia. All of these fermentation reactions enable bacteria to obtain energy necessary for their growth and the maintenance of their cellular functions. These microbial activities are also important for the host because the metabolites formed are mainly absorbed and used in the body.

Substrates available for the colonic microflora

The variety of carbon and energy sources available for microorganisms in the colon may explain, for a large part, the important microbial diversity encountered within the ecosystem. Substrates fermented by the colonic microflora are both exogenous (provided by food) and endogenous (synthesized by the host) (Figure 1).

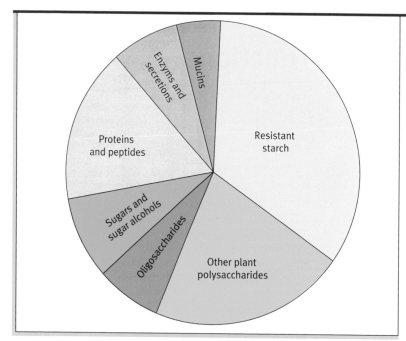

Figure 1.
The different exogenous and endogenous substrates available for the colonic microflora

Within the pie chart:
- Mucins
- Enzyms and secretions
- Proteins and peptides
- Resistant starch
- Sugars and sugar alcohols
- Oligosaccharides
- Other plant polysaccharides

Exogenous substrates

Food-derived substrates are mainly composed of carbohydrates not digested in the upper part of the digestive tract, ingested lipids and proteins being almost totally absorbed in the small intestine [3]. Such carbohydrates mainly consist of resistant starch, plant polysaccharides (plant cell wall and reserves) and some oligosaccharides and sugars. The fraction of starch resistant to pancreatic amylases as well as polysaccharides constituting plant cell walls are quantitatively predominant carbohydrates (Figure 1). Approximately 10% of ingested starch escapes digestion in the small intestine and represents the major exogenous substrate reaching the colon (8-40 grams per day). Plant cell wall polysaccharides are mainly represented by insoluble carbohydrates such as cellulose and hemicelluloses as well as pectins. Other plant polysaccharides such as inulin, gums or mucilages are also fermentable. Since some of these polymers are used as emulsifiers or texture-forming agents by food industry, the total exogenous supply of such plant polysaccharides is estimated at 8 and 20 grams per day. Lastly, some sugars, oligosaccharides and non-digestible sugar alcohols such as raffinose and stachyose contained in beans or fructo-oligosaccharides which are found in artichokes or onions also reach the colon.

Endogenous substrates

Endogenous substrates come from the small intestine (pancreatic enzymes, bile sterols, desquamated epithelial cells, mucins, etc.) as well as from the colonic epithelium (mucopolysaccharides, mucins, etc.).

Mucins, which are secreted throughout the GI tract, are glycoproteins composed of a peptide structure with branched chains containing variable amounts of fucose, galactose, hexosamines, sialic acid and uronic acids [3]. The mucopolysaccharides, such as hyaluronic acid and chondroitin sulphate, are constituted by a linear chain of glucuronic acids with branched chains of N-acetylglucosamine or N-acetylgalactosamine. In addition, chondroitins possess sulphate groups substituted on N-acetylgalactosamine residues. Desquamated epithelial cells are also a major endogenous substrate, since renewal capacity of the small bowel and colonic epithelium is very rapid. Pancreatic secretions, which contain a wide variety of hydrolytic enzymes, are important sources of organic nitrogen for the colonic microflora. Lastly, various sterols (cholesterol, bile acids, etc.) and bilirubin from bile secretions also reach the colon.

Carbohydrate metabolism

The trophic chain of carbohydrate fermentation

The anaerobic degradation of polysaccharides in the colon is a complex process involving several functional groups of microorganisms with complementary metabolic activities (Figure 2).

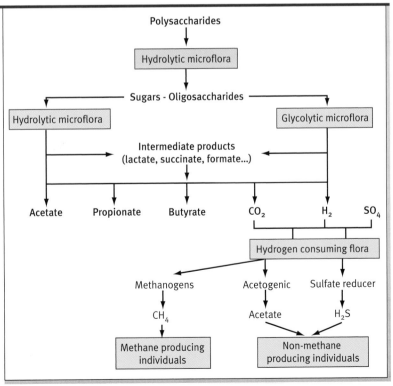

Figure 2. Trophic chain of carbohydrate degradation and fermentation by colonic microflora

The different microorganisms interact to form a trophic chain, ensuring the conversion of macromolecules into SCFAs (mainly acetate, propionate and butyrate) and gases (hydrogen, carbon dioxide and methane in some individuals). The first step of this chain consists of polysaccharide hydrolysis by hydrolytic bacteria, resulting in the release of smaller oligosaccharide fractions. The products of sugar fermentation by hydrolytic and glycolytic microorganisms include intermediate metabolites such as formate, ethanol, succinate and lactate which do not accumulate in the ecosystem but are further metabolized by other bacterial species into end products. Hydrogen formed during the fermentation process is mainly re-utilized *in situ* by hydrogen-consuming micro-organisms [4]. The hydrogen-consuming microflora thus plays a fundamental role in the ecosystem by maintaining hydrogen partial pressure at a low level, ensuring efficiency of organic matter degradation in the colon (more complete oxidation of substrates and increased of total ATP gain for the microflora). Production of methane (CH_4) from H_2 metabolism by methanogenic archaea in the colon is only observed in a fraction of individuals. Thus, the human population can be separated into two groups, depending on their capacity to excrete CH_4 or not (methane-producing subjects and non-methane producing subjects).

Degradation of polysaccharides

The human colonic microflora is well adapted to utilization of different complex polysaccharides. The main bacterial species for which hydrolytic activity has been demonstrated belong to the genera *Bacteroides, Bifidobacterium* and *Ruminococcus* as well as few species of the genera *Clostridium* and *Eubacterium*. These bacteria can synthesize different types of polysaccharidases and/or glycosidases, enzymes not produced by the host, which enable them to hydrolyze polysaccharides and to use released fragments as carbon and energy source. The activities of these hydrolases are mainly found associated with the bacterial fraction in faecal samples, particularly the hydrolytic activities involved in degradation of insoluble polysaccharides such as cellulose or hemicelluloses [5]. In this case, the highest hydrolylase activities are measured in the bacterial fraction associated with food particles.

Since *Bacteroides* is an anaerobic microorganism relatively easy to cultivate, these species are, to date, the hydrolytic bacteria most widely studied. These *Bacteroides* species present large hydrolytic capacity, in particular *Bacteroides ovatus* and *Bacteroides thetaiotaomicron*. These species can break down a wide variety of exogenous and endogenous polysaccharides [6]. However, they appear to be specialized in the breakdown of soluble polysaccharides. The different hydrolases that they synthesize are inducible and, in addition, are always associated with the bacterial cell [6].

Amylolytic species

Most of the predominant bacterial species from the human colon are able to use starch as an energy source. However, *Bacteroides* is considered the predominant amylolytic bacteria. *Bacteroides thetaiotaomicron* has the ability to bind starch polymer to the surface of the cells in order to digest it more efficiently. The glucan fragments are then transported across the outer membrane to the periplasm [7]. In addition to *Bacteroides*, other species belonging to the genera *Bifidobacterium*, *Eubacterium* and *Clostridium* are also able to degrade starch. The contribution of these Gram-positive bacteria to hydrolysis of this polymer is still considered minor as compared to that of *Bacteroides*. However, high amylase and polygalacturonase activities, which differ from those expressed by *Bacteroides*, have been measured in the bacterial fraction of human faeces [8].

Hydrolytic species

Although plant cell wall polysaccharides (cellulose, hemicelluloses, etc.) are largely degraded in the colon, the hydrolytic microflora involved in the breakdown of these insoluble polysaccharides has not been extensively studied.

The microflora that can hydrolyse cellulose has been detected in only a limited number of subjects [9]. The majority of cellulolytic species isolated to date are Gram-positive organisms and may be related to the genera *Ruminococcus* (Figure 3A), *Clostridium* and *Eubacterium*, except for that identified by Betian *et al.* [10] assimilated to *Bacteroides* sp. (Figure 3B). More recently, Robert and Bernalier-Donadille [11] have demonstrated that only methane-producing subjects possess a cellulolytic microflora able to hydrolyze crystalline cellulose to a population level of approximately 10^7 to 10^8 bacteria per gram of faeces. Among the predominant cellulolytic species isolated, some correspond to new species of the genus *Ruminococcus* and are closely related to *Ruminococcus flavefaciens*, a major cellulolytic bacterium from the rumen. Other isolates have been identified as species of the genera *Enterococcus* (Figure 3C) and *Propionibacterium* [11].

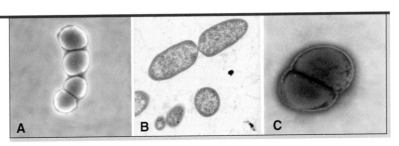

Figure 3.
Cellulolytic species isolated from the human colon observed by electron transmission microscopy (sections by B. Gaillard-Martinie, Microscopy Workshop, INRA Clermont-Ferrand/Theix).
A : *Ruminococcus* sp. nov (negative staining, magnified 25,000 times)
B : *Bacteroides* sp. (positive staining, magnified 25,000 times)
C : *Enterococcus* sp. (negative staining, magnified 43,000 times)

The utilization of less crystalline cellulose and of a non-purified cellulose fraction extracted from spinach has allowed the presence of cellulolytic microflora in all subjects to be demonstrated, whatever their methane status. The cellulolytic microflora of non-methane producing subjects was shown to be composed of new species of the genus *Bacteroides* (Figure 3B) (unpublished results). The structure of the microflora involved in the breakdown of cellulose seems thus to depend on the presence or absence of methanogenic archaea in the gut.

The population level of hemicellulolytic microflora appears to be higher than that of the cellulolytic microflora [9]. Xylanolytic species isolated are related to the genera *Clostridium*, *Butyrivibrio* and *Bacteroides*. In addition, the hydrolytic activity of *Bacteroides sp.* against xylanes and soluble arabinogalactans, has been widely studied [6, 12].

The pectinolytic microflora is also composed of species from the genus *Bacteroides.*, in particular *Bacteroides thetaiotaomicron* [13], pectin being also degraded by some *Bifidobacterium*, *Eubacterium* and *Clostridium* species.

Among the plant storage polysaccharides, gums (gum Arabic, guar gum), are broken down by *Bacteroides ovatus* and some species of *Ruminococcus* and *Bifidobacterium*. *Bifidobacterium sp.* also use inulin.

Degradation of plant polysaccharides thus involves many different enzymatic activities. Some bacterial species can produce different types of hydrolases. However, degradation of a complex structure such as plant cell wall probably requires the contribution of several bacterial species with complementary activities.

Mucolytic species

The bacterial species involved in degradation of mucins and mucopolysaccharides belong to the genera *Bacteroides*, *Bifidobacterium* and *Ruminococcus*. Mucin degradation requires contribution of different enzymes such as a sialidase, a specific α-glucosidase, as well as a β-D-galactosidase. Some *Ruminococcus* species express all of these enzymes and thus can degrade almost all gastric mucins. Other species of *Bifidobacterium* only produce some of these enzymes. Mucopolysaccharides such as chondroitin sulphates and hyaluronic acids are mainly degraded by *Bacteroides* [14], in particular *Bacteroides thetaiotaomicron*, which acts on these substrates through synthesis of different categories of hydrolases such as lyases, sulphates and β-glucuronidases.

Degradation of oligosaccharides

The glycolytic microflora of the human colon contains a large number of bacterial species that are unable to hydrolyze complex polysaccharides but use oligosaccharide fragments released by hydrolytic species. Therefore, growth of these glycolytic organisms is, to a large extent, controlled by the activity of hydrolytic species and by competition between these different species for utilization of the substrates released. The wide variety of polysaccharides broken down in the colon generates a large number of sugars of different types, contributing to the maintenance of the microbial diversity within the functional group formed by the glycolytic microorganisms.

Carbohydrate fermentation

Despite the large variety of carbohydrates available and the wide number of species able to ferment them, these substrates are catabolized by the microflora according to a relatively limited number of metabolic pathways (Figure 4).

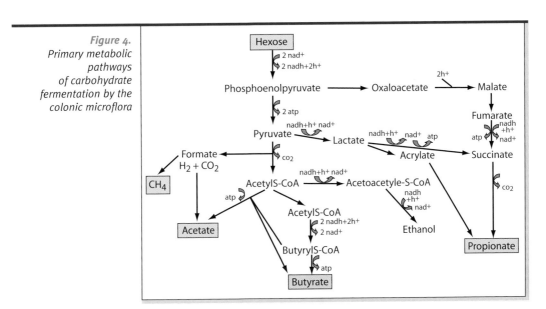

Figure 4.
Primary metabolic pathways of carbohydrate fermentation by the colonic microflora

The majority of bacterial species, except bifidobacteria, use glycolysis, also known as the Embden-Meyerhof-Parnas pathway, to convert carbohydrates into pyruvate. The pentose phosphate pathway, also used by some colonic bacteria, in particular during pentose metabolism, also leads to pyruvate synthesis. Pyruvate is thus the central metabolite of these fermentation processes, that is further converted through different pathways into end products of fermentation which represent the final electron acceptors. The main metabolites formed are acetate, propionate and butyrate. However, some bacterial species also produce intermediate metabolites such as succinate, lactate, acrylate, ethanol, formate as well as H_2 and CO_2 in order to re-oxidize reduced cofactors such as NADH + H$^+$ produced during glycolysis. These intermediate products do not accumulate in the ecosystem since they are quickly metabolized *in situ* by other bacterial species into main metabolites. Synthesis of these intermediate compounds also contributes to maintain diversity within the colonic microflora.

The majority of the bacterial species present in the colon are characterized *in vitro* by a mixed acid fermentation and therefore produce several metabolites from substrate utilization. Acetate is synthesized during carbohydrate fermentation by the majority of the predominant species in the colon (*Bacteroides, Clostridium, Bifidobacterium, Ruminococcus, Eubacterium, Fusobacterium*, etc.). The main pathway of acetate biosynthesis is the oxidative decarboxylation of pyruvate, leading to ATP molecule (Figure 4).

Propionate is mainly synthesized by the predominant *Bacteroides* species as well as by *Propionibacterium* and *Veillonella*. In the human colon, the two possible pathways for propionate biosynthesis (succinate pathway and acrylate pathway) could exist (Figure 4). Formation of propionate through decarboxylation of succinate may be the major pathway used, in particular in predominant *Bacteroides* species [15]. However, the acrylate pathway, corresponding to synthesis of propionate from lactate, may also be significant in particular in the case of diets containing high amounts of indigestible oligosaccharides.

Butyrate-producing species in the colon have been little studied and identified until very recently [16]. Although this metabolite is one of the main fermentative endproducts in the gut, only a few species of this ecosystem (*Clostridium*, *Eubacterium*, *Fusobacterium* and *Butyrivibrio*) are able to form butyrate *in vitro* from carbohydrate fermentation. Pryde *et al.* [16] showed that the butyrate-producing microflora is composed of new species belonging to the genera *Eubacterium* and *Coprococcus* as well as to the recently identified genera *Roseburia* and *Faecalibacterium*. The main pathway of butyrate biosynthesis involves condensation of two molecules of acetylS-CoA and is accompanied by the synthesis of one molecule of ATP (Figure 4).

The bacterial species that mainly produce lactate from sugar fermentation are commonly known as lactic acid bacteria. In the human colon, lactic acid bacteria mainly belong to *Bifidobacterium* and *Lactobacillus* as well as *Streptococcus* and *Enterococcus*. The pathway of lactate formation corresponds to oxidation of pyruvate by the lactate dehydrogenase (Figure 4).

Lactate, produced from sugar fermentation in the colon, is, to a large extent, re-utilized *in situ*. Colonic bacterial species belonging to *Veillonella* and *Propionibacterium* have the capacity to metabolize lactate into propionate *in vitro*, *via* the pathway of succinate decarboxylation. However, some species of *Clostridium* as well as *Megasphaera elsdenii* present in the GI tract of herbivores use the acrylate pathway to metabolize lactate into propionate [17]. This pathway of propionate synthesis may exist in the human colon, but the species involved remain poorly identified.

Metabolism of gases by hydrogen-consuming microorganisms

Although large quantities of H_2 are produced in the colon daily [1, 2, 21] (about 300 ml per gram of fermented substrate), the microflora involved in the production of this gas remains poorly identified. Microbial species that produce H_2 *in vitro* during fermentation of sugars or polysaccharides mainly belong to *Clostridium*, *Ruminococcus* and *Eubacterium*. The H_2 produced is partly excreted in breath and flatus, but the majority is re-utilized *in situ* by hydrogen-consuming microorganisms [4] (Figure 5).

Three hydrogen-consuming mechanisms have been described in the human colon: methanogenesis, sulphate reduction and reductive acetogenesis.

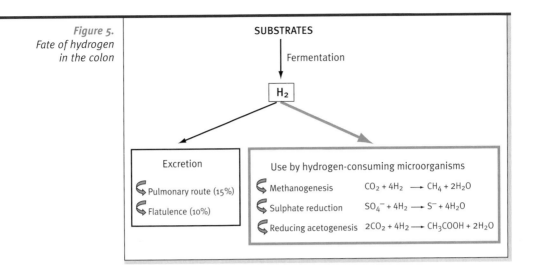

Figure 5.
Fate of hydrogen
in the colon

SUBSTRATES

Fermentation

H_2

Excretion

Pulmonary route (15%)

Flatulence (10%)

Use by hydrogen-consuming microorganisms

Methanogenesis $CO_2 + 4H_2 \longrightarrow CH_4 + 2H_2O$

Sulphate reduction $SO_4^- + 4H_2 \longrightarrow S^- + 4H_2O$

Reducing acetogenesis $2CO_2 + 4H_2 \longrightarrow CH_3COOH + 2H_2O$

Methanogenesis

Methanogenesis leads to the formation of another gas, CH_4, from H_2 and CO_2 (Figure 5). Only two methanogenic archaea have been described in the human colon. The predominant methanogenic species, *Methanobrevibacter smithii*, derives its energy from the production of CH_4 by reduction of CO_2 by H_2. The other species *Methanosphaera stadmaniae*, present at lower population levels than *Methanobrevibacter smithii*, produces CH_4 only from reduction of methanol by H_2. This specific metabolism is probably associated with pectin hydrolysis by pectinolytic microorganisms that release methanol [18]. CH_4 produced is totally excreted in breath and flatus. Miller & Wolin [18] have demonstrated that a threshold concentration of 10^8 methanogens per gram of faeces is necessary in order to produce sufficient quantity of CH_4 to be detected in the expired gases. The level of the methanogenic population thus varies from undetectable to 10^7 per gram faeces in nonmethane-producing individuals and is superior to 10^7 per gram faeces in methane-producing individuals. The percentage of methane-producing subjects in occidental populations ranges from 30 to 50% [19].

Sulphate reduction

Sulphate reduction corresponds to the reduction of sulphate into H_2S, this reaction being coupled with the generation of ATP (Figure 5). In addition to H_2 and formate, the other electron donors that can be used by sulphate-reducing bacteria are mainly lactate, pyruvate and ethanol, which are converted into acetate. Sulphate reduction by H_2 leads to the formation of sulphides which are potentially toxic for eukaryotic cells [20]. Sulphate-reducing species in the human colon belong to different bacterial genera, the predominant genus being *Desulfovibrio* [21]. The genera *Desulfobacter, Desulfomonas, Desulfobulbus* and *Desulfatomaculum* are also observed at lower population levels. The genus *Desulfovibrio*, like *Desulfobulbus*, can use H_2 produced from sugar fermentation and therefore represents one of the important components of this hydrogen-consuming microflora. Activity of the hydrogen-consuming sulphate-reducing bacteria is dependent on the amount of sulphate available in the ecosystem. Sulphate sources in the gut are sulphated dietary substrates and endogenous secretions. As availability of sulphate is likely to differ greatly according to the diet and mucus secretions, the sulphate-reducing microflora should therefore be able to adapt to important variations in sulphate concentrations in the ecosystem.

Reductive acetogenesis

Reductive acetogenesis is a specific pathway of acetate biosynthesis occurring through reduction of two moles of CO_2 by four molecules of H_2 [22] (Figures 4 and 5). One of the two moles of CO_2 undergoes a series of reductions through tetrahydrofolate derivatives and forms the methyl group of acetate. The second mole of CO_2 is reduced to CO *via* the carbon monoxide dehydrogenase and will form the carboxyl group of acetate. The two groups are then condensed into acetylS-CoA and the final synthesis of acetate occurs with production of ATP. Therefore, hydrogen-consuming acetogenic microorganisms are able to grow autotrophically using H_2 and CO_2, but this metabolic pathway also occurs during the heterotrophic growth of these species. In this case, one mole of hexose is metabolized into three moles of acetate. Two moles of acetate are formed by oxidative decarboxylation of pyruvate, releasing two moles of CO_2. The hydrogen-consuming acetogenic bacteria have the capacity to reutilize these two moles of CO_2 to form a third mole of acetate *via* the reductive pathway. The contribution of reducing acetogenesis to H_2 elimination is especially significant in nonmethane-producing subjects who harbor little or no methanogenic archaea. In such individuals, 35% of the acetate produced in the colon would be synthesized by the reductive pathway. Conversely, the acetogenic microflora does not appear able to express its hydrogenotrophic potential in the presence of methanogenic archaea [23]. Hydrogen-consuming acetogenic bacteria isolated from faeces of nonmethane-producing subjects belong to different genera such as *Clostridium*, *Ruminococcus* and *Streptococcus* [24-26] (Figure 6).

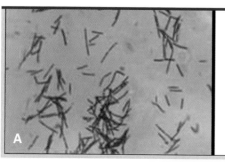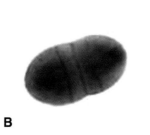

Figure 6.
Microscopic observation of hydrogen-consuming acetogenic species isolated from human faeces (slide provided by B. Gaillard-Martinie, Microscopy Workshop, INRA Clermont Ferrand/ Theix).

A: *Clostridium sp. nov., photon microscopy (Gram staining, magnification 2,000 times)*
B: *Hydrogen-consuming Ruminococcus, electron microscopy (negative staining, magnification 34,000 times)*

All acetogenic species have a large nutritional capacity [27, 28], allowing them to adapt to variations of nutritional conditions in the ecosystem. The capacity of some of these species to co-metabolize an organic substrate and H_2 also confers them an ecological advantage compared to other hydrogen-consuming microorganisms. Indeed, this metabolic characteristic allows these bacteria to obtain more energy per time unit and per mole of H_2 consumed.

Protein metabolism

Unlike carbohydrate fermentation, degradation of proteins in the colon generates many metabolites that are potentially toxic for the host (phenols, indoles, ammonia, amines).

Proteolysis

Since proteins and peptides are the main nitrogen source in the colon, gut bacteria hydrolyze these polymers in order to allow carbon and nitrogen to enter their composition. Proteolysis is thus a fundamental process in the colon. The mechanisms that regulate this process are still poorly understood [1]. The structure and solubility of proteins as well as their transit time are probably important factors. Intraluminal pH also plays a role since proteases have optimum pH close to neutrality. Factors influencing colonic pH, such as production of acids during carbohydrates fermentation, are thus able to modulate proteolytic activity within the ecosystem. Therefore, bacterial proteases would be particularly active in the distal colon where the pH is close to 7.0 [21].

Protein hydrolysis by proteolytic enzymes (proteases) results in the release of peptides (Figure 7).

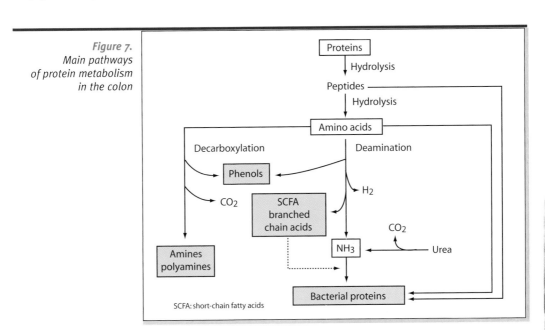

Figure 7.
Main pathways
of protein metabolism
in the colon

SCFA: short-chain fatty acids

Some bacterial species can assimilate peptide nitrogen while others only assimilate unbound amino acids resulting from the breakdown of peptides [1]. Bacterial proteases are serine-, cystine- or metallo-proteases [21].

A large number of bacterial species in the human colon have proteolytic activity. Predominant proteolytic bacteria belong to *Bacteroides*, *Clostridium*, *Propionibacterium*, *Fusobacterium*, *Streptococcus* and *Lactobacillus* [1]. Bacterial proteases are either extracellular (*Clostridium* and *Propionibacterium*) or associated with the cell (*Lactobacillus*), the mechanisms that regulate this activity varying considerably from one species to another.

Metabolism of peptides and amino acids

Although they have been little studied, peptides play an important role in the colonic ecosystem. Indeed, they can stimulate *in vitro* growth of many intestinal bacterial species. Their utilization is frequently accompanied by excretion of amino acids that are not necessary for bacterial growth (Figure 7). These amino acids then become potentially available for other bacterial species in the colon that do not digest peptides [21].

A large number of species in the colon can use amino acids. Among them, some species of *Veillonella*, *Peptococcus*, *Fusobacterium*, *Acidaminococcus*, *Clostridium* and *Eubacterium* use amino acids as their main source of energy, since these bacteria do not ferment carbohydrates. However, many glycolytic species also use amino acids and peptides as nitrogen source [1]. Fermentation of amino acids involves a variety of oxidation and reduction reactions, with diverse final electron acceptors (unsaturated fatty acids, other amino acids, H_2, etc.). Among these different reactions (deaminations, Stickland reaction, etc.), deamination of amino acids, leading to formation of SCFAs and ammonia, appears as the main pathway used by bacterial species in the colon [21]. Acetate, propionate and butyrate are the major metabolites produced. Some *Clostridium* species ferment threonine into propionate, *Fusobacterium nucleatum* produces acetate and butyrate from lysine, and *Bacteroides sp.* metabolize aspartate into acetate and succinate. However, a variety of other compounds are also formed during amino acid metabolism, such as phenols, dicarboxylic acids, and branched-chain fatty acids (isobutyrate, 2-methylbutyrate, isovalerate formed from valine, isoleucine and leucine respectively). Branched-chain fatty acids could be considered as markers of proteolysis in the colon, since these compounds are only formed from amino acids metabolism. The concentration of such metabolites increases significantly from the proximal colon to the distal colon [1]. Phenol and indole are released from the breakdown of aromatic amino acids (tyrosine, tryptophan and phenylalanine) by certain *Clostridium*, *Lactobacillus*, *Bifidobacterium* species as well as *Enterobacteriaceae*. These metabolites are absorbed and detoxified by the colonic mucosa and then excreted in urine. However, an increase in phenol and indole formation has been found associated with different pathologies in humans, particularly in the case of colon cancer [21].

Lastly, fermentation of some amino acids (valine, alanine, glutamate, leucine) can also contribute to production of H_2 in the ecosystem. Hydrogen-consuming microorganisms (methanogens, acetogens or sulfate-reducing bacteria) could thus potentially affect the metabolism of amino acids through interspecies H_2 transfers.

Ammonia

The majority of ammonia produced in the colon comes from deamination of amino acids, with minor contribution of urea to this production [1, 21] (Figure 7). Ammonia formed by the intestinal microflora is absorbed by the colonic mucosa and transported to the liver by the portal vein where it is converted into urea, which is excreted in urine. Ammonia is also the main source of nitrogen for a large number of bacterial species in the colon. These species assimilate ammonia *via* two metabolic pathways: one involving the glutamine synthetase and the other, the glutamate dehydrogenase. The relative importance of these two pathways in the colon is poorly understood. Inside the bacterial cell, amino transferases allow synthesis of amino acids necessary for the bacterium by transfer of ammonia on carbon-skeletons [1, 21].

Ammonia is a potentially toxic compound for the host. At low concentrations (5-10 mM), this metabolite can deteriorate the morphology and intermediate metabolism of intestinal cells and increase DNA synthesis [21]. Ammonia may thus be involved in the mechanisms of initiation of colon cancer. Ammonia concentrations in the colon result from a balance between deamination of amino acids by bacteria and its utilization by the cells for their biosynthesis. Fermentation of carbohydrates, by stimulating protein synthesis, contributes to decrease ammonia concentration in the colonic lumen, together with absorption by the mucosa.

Amines and polyamines

Amines are major products of the metabolism of amino acids by the colonic microflora. They are produced mainly by decarboxylation of amino acids (Figure 7) and, to a small extent, dealkylations and transamination reactions. They are also produced by the degradation of polyamines [21]. A large variety of amines is produced in the colon, such as histamine, tyramine, piperidine, etc., as well as polyamines such as cadaverine or putrescine (Table I). Different bacterial species from the human colon have the ability to produce amines. They belong to *Bacteroides, Clostridium, Lactobacillus, Eubacterium, Streptococcus* and also include some *Enterobacteriaceae* [21]. Polyamine synthesis (diamines to hexamines and branched-chain tertiary and quaternary amines) depend, to a major extent, on the presence of specific bacterial decarboxylases: arginine decarboxylase, ornithine decarboxylase, lysine decarboxylase and diaminobutyric acid decarboxylase. [29]. The precursors of these compounds include arginine, lysine, phenylalanine, etc. (Table 1). Many species (*Bacteroides, Prevotella, Veillonella*) require the presence of polyamines in the culture medium for optimal growth, but the physiological mechanisms involved are still poorly understood.

Amines	Precursors	Reactions involved
Methylamine	Glycine	Decarboxylation
Dimethylamine	Choline	N-Dealkylation
Propylamine	Aminobutyric acid	Decarboxylation
Pyrrolidine	Putrescine	Oxidative deamination
Piperidine	Cadaverine	Oxidative deamination
2-methylbutylamine	Valine	Decarboxylation
Putrescine	Ornithine	Decarboxylation
	Arginine	Decarboxylation and hydrolysis
Cadaverine	L-lysine	Decarboxylation
Agmatine	Arginine	Decarboxylation
Phenylethylamine	Phenylalanine	Decarboxylation
Tyramine	Tyrosine	Decarboxylation
Ethylamine	Alanine	Decarboxylation

Table I.
Main amines formed by the colonic microflora [1]

Amines are probably quickly absorbed and oxidized in the colonic mucosa. Some of them are excreted in urine and are markers of bacterial digestion of proteins. Amines produced by the colonic microflora are recognized as harmful compounds for the host and may play an important role in different disorders (migraines, schizophrenia, pediatric gastroenteritis, etc.) [1, 21]. Indeed, amines can affect a large number of functions in humans. Despite this potentially harmful role, the bacterial species and metabolic pathways of amine production in the colon have not been extensively explored. The role of polyamines in the physiology of the colonic epithelium and in colonic carcinogenesis is discussed in the chapter entitled "Gut Microflora and the Colonic Epithelium".

Metabolism of sterols

Endogenous sterols reach the colon mainly through the bile and, in addition to exogenous sterols, represent a potential source of substrates for the bacterial microflora. Bile sterols are mainly (composition in g/g dry weight): bile acid (67%), cholesterol (4%) and steroid hormones [30]. The metabolism of these different substances by the colonic microflora is now recognized and some bacterial species which are able to metabolize them have been identified. However, enzymatic pathways involved in these bio-transformations are still poorly understood. Similarly, the physiological importance of the microbial conversion of these substrates on human health has not been completely clarified.

Microbial metabolism of cholesterol

Although the majority of cholesterol is absorbed in the small intestine, a fraction (about 1 gram per day) reaches the colon that comes from diet, bile or gastrointestinal mucosa.

Cholesterol metabolism by the colonic microflora mainly leads to the synthesis of coprostanol and small quantities of coprostanone (Figure 8).

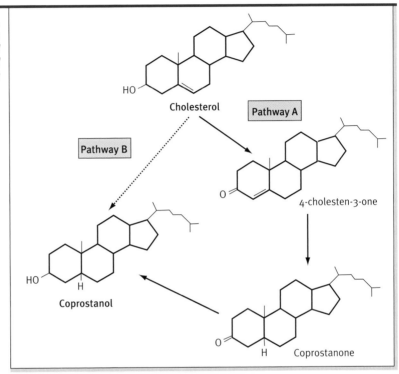

Figure 8.
Metabolism
of cholesterol
by the intestinal
microflora

These products of cholesterol biotransformation are found in faeces. In rats, bacterial transformation of cholesterol appears to be mainly confined to the caecum [30]. In humans, the conversion of cholesterol into coprostanol and/or coprostanone in the colon is observed only in a fraction of the population with large inter-individual variations. Thus, Wilkins and Hackman [31] demonstrated that excretion of these metabolites in faeces was observed in only twenty-three North American subjects out of thirty-one studied.

Several bacterial species that can metabolize cholesterol have been isolated from human or animal faeces. The majority of these species belong to the genus *Eubacterium,* the ability to reduce cholesterol into coprostanol having also been observed in different strains of *Clostridium, Bifidobacterium* and *Bacteroides* [30]. More recently, Pereira & Gibson [32] showed that *Lactobacillus fermentum* KC5b, isolated from human faeces, can metabolize a large quantity of cholesterol. The enzymatic mechanisms involved in the reduction of cholesterol in such microbial species in the colon have been very little studied. Few studies have concerned one species of *Eubacterium* isolated from rat faeces [30]. The reaction may consist of a series of oxidations of the 3β-hydroxide group and isomerisation resulting in formation of 4-cholesten-3-one.

Coprostanone would then be formed by reduction of 4-cholesten-3-one. Lastly, reduction of the 3-oxo group in coprostanone would enable the synthesis of coprostanol. However, a second pathway of coprostanol synthesis through reduction of cholesterol would also be possible (Figure 8).

Microbial metabolism of bile acids

Bile acids are synthesized in liver from cholesterol and are conjugated with glycine or taurine by an amide bond. In humans, the major bile acids are cholic acid and chenodeoxycholic acid. Bile acids are actively absorbed in the terminal ileum and are transported *via* the portal vein to the liver where they are again excreted in bile (enterohepatic cycle). About 5% of the bile salts (0.2-0.3 gram per day) escape this cycle and reach the colon where they are deconjugated and metabolized by the microflora. The majority of products resulting from these conversions are excreted in the faeces. The remainder is absorbed, transported to the liver by the portal vein, reconjugated and re-excreted in the bile, constituting secondary bile salts. More than twenty different secondary bile acids have been found in faeces, demonstrating the large variety of metabolic pathways of primary bile salts transformation by the intestinal microflora [30] (Table II).

Reactions	Bacterial genera
Hydrolysis of glycine and taurine	*Bacteroides, Bifidobacterium, Fusobacterium Clostridium, Lactobacillus, Streptococcus, etc.*
Oxidation and epimerisation	*Clostridium, Eubacterium, Fusobacterium, Ruminococcus (R. productus)*
7-dehydroxylation	*Clostridium, Eubacterium*
Esterification	*Bacteroides, Eubacterium, Citrobacter, Lactobacillus, Ruminococcus (R. productus)*
Desulphatation	*Clostridium, Fusobacterium, Peptococcus*

Table II.
Metabolism of bile acids by the colonic microflora [30]

Hydrolysis of the amide bond between glycine or taurine and bile acids is catalyzed by a specific hydrolase, found in species belonging to different bacterial genera (Table II). The contribution of each of these species appears to depend on the host. Tannock *et al.* [33] have demonstrated that this conversion is mainly carried out, in mice, by *Lactobacillus*. Other possible transformation of bile acids by the intestinal microflora include oxidation of different hydroxyl groups present on the molecule into oxo groups, and epimerisation of α-hydroxyl groups into β-hydroxyl ones [30]. Such reactions involve a specific dehydrogenase that exits in some species of *Clostridium, Eubacterium, Fusobacterium* and *Ruminococcus*. Physiologically, the most significant bacterial biotransformation in humans is 7-dehydroxylation of cholic acid and chenodeoxycholic, into deoxycholic and lithocholic acids respectively.

Deoxycholic acid is absorbed by colonic mucosa and accounts for 25% of the pool of circulating bile acids in humans [30]. By contrast, lithocholic acid is strongly insoluble and thus mainly excreted in faeces. The microflora responsible for 7-dehydroxylation of bile acids was only detected at low population levels in human faeces (10^3-10^5 per gram of stools), and is mainly composed of *Clostridium* and *Eubacterium* species [30, 34]. The presence of bile acid esters has also been detected in human faeces, but the metabolic pathways for production of these metabolites are poorly understood. Some bacterial species from the colonic microflora (*Bacteroides, Eubacterium, Lactobacillus* and *Ruminococcus*) were, however, shown to be capable of saponification of cholic acid or chenodeoxycholic acid *in vitro*. Desulphatation of bile acids through a specific sulphatase has also been described. This reaction is only observed for the sulphate group in position C-3 of molecules and is stereospecific. The α or β configuration of this group determines the type of compound synthesized. Some *Clostridium, Fusobacterium* and *Peptococcus* species have the ability to desulphate bile acids.

Microbial metabolism of steroid hormones

Steroid hormones in bile secretions are present in conjugate form (glucuronide or sulphate). The total concentration of these compounds in the bile remains low, but major variations are observed depending on gender (approximately 13 milligrams per day in men *versus* 6 milligrams per day in women). Part of these steroid hormones (2 milligrams per day), after undergoing deconjugation, may be metabolized by the intestinal microflora. The metabolites formed are mainly reabsorbed and transported to the liver where they are again conjugated and excreted in bile [30].

Different pathways for biotransformation of steroid hormones by the colonic microflora have been described. Hydrolysis of sulphate and/or glucuronide groups in these structures, through bacterial sulphatases and/or glucuronidases, has been demonstrated [30]. These enzymatic activities have been detected in some *Clostridium, Lactobacillus, Eubacterium, Bacteroides* and *Peptococcus* species [35]. Different bacterial biotransformations have been demonstrated, mainly in *Eubacterium* and *Clostridium* species [30]. *Eubacterium lentum* is also able to dehydroxylate the group in position 21 in corticosteroid molecules. Two species isolated from human faecal samples, *Eubacterium desmolans* and *Clostridium scindens*, possess desmolase activity, enabling side-chain cleavage of glucocorticoids. Reductase activities that allow reduction of the first cycle (A) of the structure of steroid hormones have also been found in other species of *Clostridium* and *Eubacterium* species, as well as in *Bacteroides fragilis* and *Bifidobacterium adolescentis*. These biotransformations imply that the bacterial species possess specific enzymes to catalyze such reactions, such as reductases, dehydratases and/or dehydrogenases.

Conclusion

The large variety of carbon- and nitrogen-containing substrates available in the colon mainly contributes to maintain diversity of bacterial species and of metabolic activities in this ecosystem. The various metabolic functions of the colonic microflora generate a wide range of metabolites that have major impacts on human physiology and health.

Key points

- There are many different and diverse metabolic functions of the intestinal microflora. These microbial activities have a major impact on the health of the host, with the metabolites produced by the microflora being mainly absorbed and metabolized in the body.

- The nature of the substrates available for the intestinal microflora is extremely varied (indigestible dietary carbohydrates, endogenous secretions rich in proteins and sterols, desquamated cells, etc.) which accounts for the wide variety of bacterial species and the metabolic activities observed within the colonic ecosystem.

- The primary products of carbohydrate fermentation in the colon are short-chain fatty acids (primarily acetate, propionate and butyrate) and gases (H_2, CO_2 and, in 30-50% of cases, CH_4). Short-chain fatty acids are quickly absorbed while the gases are either excreted (*via* the lungs or the anus), or re-utilized *in situ* (H_2 and CO_2) by the hydrogen-consuming bacterial microflora.

- The degradation of proteins by the intestinal generates many metabolites, which are potentially toxic for the host organism (ammonia, phenols, indoles, etc.). However, the fermentation of carbohydrates by stimulating microbial proteosynthesis contributes greatly to decreasing the availability of these compounds.

- The intestinal microflora metabolizes the sterols that reach the colon into different compounds. These compounds are mainly absorbed and then are either re-excreted in the intestine or excreted in the urine. They can also be eliminated in the stools. The pathways for biotransformation of sterols used by bacteria continue to be poorly understood.

References

1. Macfarlane GT, Cummings JH. The colonic flora, fermentation and large bowel digestive function. In : Phillips SF, Pemberton JH, Shorter RG, eds. *The large intestine: physiology, pathophysiology and disease*. New York : Raven Press, 1991 : 51-92.

2. Cummings JH, Macfarlane GT. The control and consequence of bacterial fermentation in the human colon. *J Appl Bacteriol* 1991 ; 70 : 443-59.

3. Flourié B, Florent C, Etanchaud F. Fonction digestive du caecum chez l'homme normal. *Cah Nut Diét* 1988 ; 23 : 111-5.

4. Christl SU, Murgatroyd PR, Gibson GR, *et al*. Production, metabolism and excretion of H_2 in the large intestine. *Gastroenterology* 1992 ; 102 : 1269-77.

5. Englyst HN, Hay S, Macfarlane GT. Polysaccharides breakdown by mixed populations of human faecal bacteria. *FEMS Microbiol Ecol* 1987 ; 95 : 163-71.

6. Salyers AA. Fermentation of polysaccharides by human colonic anaerobes. In : Cherbut C, Barry JL, Lairon D, Durand M, eds. *Dietary fibre*. Paris : John Libbey Eurotext, 1995 : 29-35.

7. Tancula E, Feldhaus MJ, Bedzyk LA, *et al*. Location and characterization of genes involved in binding of starch to the surface of *Bacteroides thetaiotaomicron*. *J Bacteriol* 1992 ; 174 : 5609-16.

8. McCarthy RE, Salyers AA. Evidence that polygalacturonic acid is not an important substrate for *Bacteroides* species in the colon. *Appl Environ Microbiol* 1986 ; 52 : 9-16.

9. Wedeking KJ, Mansfield HR, Montgomery L. Enumeration and isolation of cellulolytic and hemicellulolytic bacteria from human feces. *Appl Environ Microbiol* 1988 ; 54 : 1530-5.

10. Betian HG, Linehan BA, Bryant MP, *et al*. Isolation of a cellulolytic *Bacteroides sp.* from human feces. *Appl Environ Microbiol* 1977 ; 33 : 1009-10.

11. Robert C, Bernalier-Donadille A. The cellulolytic microflora of the human colon: evidence of microcrystalline cellulose-degrading bacteria in methane-excreting subjects. *FEMS Microbiol Ecol* 2003 ; 46 : 81-9.

12. Salyers AA, Gherardini F, O'Brien M. Utilization of xylan by two species of human colonic *Bacteroides*. *Appl Environ Microbiol* 1981 ; 41 : 1065-8.

13. McCarthy RE, Kotarski SF, Salyers AA. Location and characteristics of enzymes involved in the breakdown of polygalacturonic acid by *Bacteroides thetaiotaomicron*. *J Bacteriol* 1985 ; 161 : 493-9.

14. Salyers AA, O'Brien M, Kotarski SF. Utilization of chondroitin sulfate by *Bacteroides thetaiotaomicron* growing in carbohydrate-limited continuous culture. *J Bacteriol* 1982 ; 150 : 1008-15.

15. Miller TL, Wolin MJ. Fermentation by saccharolytic intestinal bacteria. *Am J Clin Nutr* 1979 ; 32 : 164-72.

16. Pryde SE, Ducan SH, Hold GL, *et al*. The microbiology of butyrate formation in the human colon. *FEMS Microbiol Lett* 2002 ; 217 : 133-9.

17. Counotte GH, Prins RA, Janssen RHA, *et al*. Role of *Megasphaera elsdenii* in the fermentation of DL- [2-13C] lactate in the rumen of dairy cattle. *Appl Environ Microbiol* 1981 ; 42 : 649-55.

18. Miller TL, Wolin MJ. Methanogens in human and animal intestinal tracts. *System Appl Microbiol* 1986 ; 7 : 223-9.

19. Colombel JF, Flourié B, Neut C, *et al*. La méthanogenèse chez l'homme. *Gastroenterol Clin Biol* 1987 ; 11 : 694-700.

20. Roediger WEW, Duncan A, Kapaniris O, *et al*. Reducing sulfur compounds of the colon impair colonocyte nutrition: implication for ulcerative colitis. *Gastroenterology* 1993 ; 104 : 802-9.

21. Macfarlane GT, Gibson GR. Metabolic activities of the normal colonic flora. In : Gibson SAW, ed. *Human health. The contribution of microorganisms*. Londres : Springer-Verlag, 1994 : 17-52.

22. Wood HG, Ljungdahl LG. Autotrophic character of the acetogenic bacteria. In : Shively JM, Barton LL, eds. *Variations in aurotrophic life*. San Diego : Academic Press, 1991 : 201-50.

23. Bernalier A, Lelait M, Rochet V, *et al*. Acetogenesis from H_2 and CO_2 by methane- and non-methane-producing human colonic bacterial communities. *FEMS Microbiol Ecol* 1996 ; 19 : 193-202.

24. Bernalier A, Rochet V, Leclerc M, *et al*. Diversity of H_2/CO_2-utilizing acetogenic bacteria from feces of non-methane-producing humans. *Curr Microbiol* 1996 ; 33 : 94-9.

25. Bernalier A, Willems A, Leclerc M, *et al*. *Ruminococcus hydrogenotrophicus* sp. nov, a new H_2/CO_2-utilizing acetogenic bacterium isolated from human feces. *Arch Microbiol* 1996 ; 166 : 176-83.

26. Kamlage B, Gruhl B, Blaut M. Isolation and characterization of two new homoacetogenic hydrogen-utilizing bacteria from the human intestinal tract that are closely related to *Clostridium coccoides*. *Appl Environ Microbiol* 1997 ; 63 : 1732-8.

27. Leclerc M, Bernalier A, Donadille G, *et al*. H_2/CO_2 metabolism in acetogenic bacteria isolated from the human colon. *Anaerobe* 1997 ; 3 : 307-15.

28. Leclerc M, Bernalier A, Lelait M, *et al*. ^{13}C-NMR study of glucose and pyruvate catabolism in four acetogenic species isolated from the human colon. *FEMS Microbiol Lett* 1997 ; 146 : 199-204.

29. Morrison M, Mackie RI. Biosynthesis of nitrogen-containing compounds. In : Mackie RI, White BA, eds. *Gastrointestinal microbiology, gastrointestinal ecosystems and fermentations*. New York : Chapman & Hall, 1997 : 424-69.

30. Baron SF, Hylemon PB. Biotransformation of bile acids, cholesterol and steroid hormones. In : Mackie RI, White BA, eds. *Gastrointestinal microbiology, gastrointestinal ecosystems and fermentations*. New York : Chapman & Hall, 1997 : 470-510.

31. Wilkins TD, Hackman AS. Two patterns of neutral steroid conversion in the feces of North Americans. *Cancer Res* 1974 ; 34 : 2250-4.

32. Pereira DIA, Gibson GR. Cholesterol assimilation by lactic acid bacteria and bifidobacteria isolated from the human gut. *Appl Environ Microbiol* 2002 ; 68 : 4689-93.

33. Tannock GW, Dashkeviez MP, Feighner SD. Lactobacilli and bile salt hydrolase in the murine intestinal tract. *Appl Environ Microbiol* 1989 ; 55 : 1848-51.

34. White BA, Lipsky RL, Fricke RJ, *et al*. Bile acid induction specificity of 7 α – dehydroxylase activity in an intestinal *Eubacterium sp*. *Steroids* 1980 ; 35 : 103-9.

35. Van Eldere J, Robben J, De Prauw G, *et al*. Isolation and identification of intestinal steroid-desulfating bacteria from rats and humans. *Appl Environ Microbiol* 1988 ; 54 : 2112-7.

Fernando Azpiroz

Servicio de
Aparato Digestivo,
Hospital General
Vall d'Hebron,
Universidad Autónoma
de Barcelona,
Barcelona, España.

Intestinal Microflora and Intraluminal Gas

Colonic bacteria produce and consume large quantities of gases in the gut lumen. Hence, intestinal microflora plays a major role in intestinal gas homeostasis, but many aspects of this relationship are still unknown. This chapter will review the physiology of intestinal microflora and gas, and their role in two pathophysiological conditions: gas and pneumatosis intestinalis. Excellent reviews on this topic can be found in references [1, 2].

Physiology

Little is known about intestinal gas homeostasis; however, it seems a finely regulated process, because different studies with different techniques and on different populations have shown that despite the very large capacity of the entire gastrointestinal tract, the total volume of intraluminal gas amounts to only 100-200 mL [3-5]. This fairly constant and relatively low volume is even more surprising considering the dynamic and complicated processes of digestive tract gas input and gas output [1, 2]. Gas input results from swallowing, chemical reactions, diffusion from blood, and bacterial fermentation. Gas output is achieved by absorption, bacterial consumption, and anal evacuation (Figures 1 & 2).

Gas metabolism

Swallowing introduces a small amount of air into the stomach, which is obviously much greater with gaseous beverages. In contrast to other species, for instance dogs, humans invariably have a small chamber of air in the stomach of about 20 mL. It is not known whether or not this gastric gas bubble accomplishes a physiological function, for instance as a cushion during the gastric accommodation process. Excess air is eliminated from the stomach by belching, absorption or emptying into the intestine. Chemical reactions, particularly in the upper gut, resulting from neutralization of acids and alcalis, produce enormous quantities of gas [6]. Intraluminal gases tend to equilibrate with the gases in venous blood, depending on three factors: the partial pressure of each gas at both sides of the gut-blood barrier, its diffusibility, and the time of exposure of the gas to the diffusible surface, that is the speed of gas transit [1, 7, 8]. Hence, highly diffusible gases in large quantities within the gut, such as as CO_2, are readily absorbed. Oxygen (O_2), coming from swallowed air, is also absorbed from the small intestine to equilibrate with its partial pressure in blood. However, the diffusibility of nitrogen, also coming from swallowed air, is much lower.

Whereas most of the above processes are predictable, the role of microflora on gas metabolism exhibits tremendous interindividual variations, and is the factor that by and large determines the metabolism of intraluminal gas. From a flatological point of view, two types of microflora are important: gas-producing and gas-consuming microorganisms [1, 2]. The amount and composition of the gases produced and consumed by the microflora depend on the combination of microorganisms in each subject and in each colonic segment.

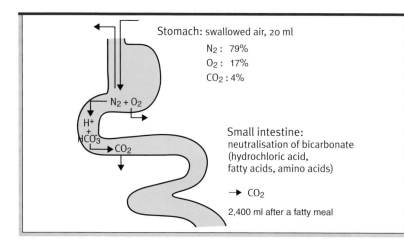

Figure 1.
Source and outcome of gas in the upper digestive tract

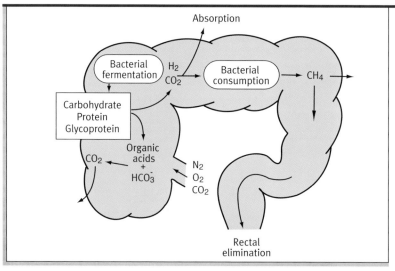

Figure 2.
Source and outcome of gas in the colon

The composition of colonic microflora is highly individual and seems to be related to early environmental conditions in life. There seems to be also and adaptive component to the alimentary habits later on life [9, 10]. Hence, with the same types of substrates the quantity and composition of net gas production varies tremendously among individuals. About 90% of the general western population have bacteria that ferment different substrates, particularly carbohydrates, and release hydrogen and CO_2 [11-13]. Most individuals also have a pool of sulphate-reducing bacteria that may be present throughout the colon [13]. These bacteria produce very small amounts of sulphur-containing gases (H_2S, methanethiol, and dimethyl-sulfide) that are highly odoriferous. About 30 to 50% of the population also has a pool of methanogenic bacteria, which exist in high concentrations only in the left colon [13-16]. Methanogens and sulphate-reducing bacteria are mutually exclusive, and hence, in subjects with methanogenic microflora, the sulphate-reducing bacteria are just circumscribed to the right colon [13].

Part of the colonic microflora consumes intraluminal gases, and this may account for a considerable proportion of intraluminal gas disposal [13, 14, 17]. Indeed, part of the oxygen reaching the colon is consumed by aerobic bacteria, thereby reducing the intraluminal content of oxygen in the colon and maintaining anaerobiosis. Hydrogen and also CO_2 are consumed in large quantities. The pools of methanogenic and sulphate-reducing bacteria compete for hydrogen [18]. Part of the gases produced by colonic bacteria diffuse into the blood and are excreted by breath, where they can be detected by gas chromatography [1]. This is the basis for the hydrogen and methane breath tests (Figure 3). The remaining gases are eliminated by the anus. The composition of intraluminal gas varies greatly along the gut, and that of anal outflow reflects the net balance of the multiple processes within the gut lumen. To note, the study of the composition of flatus may provide an interesting insight into the physiology of colonic microflora at the different levels of the gut [13].

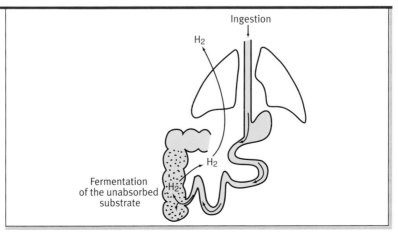

Figure 3.
Hydrogen
breath testing

Ingestion

H₂

H₂

Fermentation
of the unabsorbed
substrate

Gas-producing substrates

The total amount of gas within the gut is fairly constant, but only represents a small fraction of the volumes really handled by the gut. Gas homeostasis is finely regulated by the transit and the anal evacuation of the gases in excess. Evacuation of gas by different subjects on the same diet depends on the different composition of colonic microflora. However, intraindividual differences depend on the diet, and specifically on the residues of the diet arriving into the colon that serve as gas producing substrate to the colonic microflora. It is amazing the paucity of information about diet-related gas metabolism and evacuation. Some relatively old studies [19, 20] measured anal evacuation of gas after consumption of different types of meals, and showed that evacuation was 15 mL per hour with a low fiber diet, 93 mL per hour with a normal diet, 140 mL per hour after eating Brussels sprouts, and 176 mL per hour with a pork and beans diet. A more recent study measured 24 hour gas evacuation, showing that with a normal diet containing 200 g of beans, 705 mL were evacuated and 50% of this volume was hydrogen, whereas with a fiber free diet, 214 mL gas were eliminated containing very low hydrogen proportion [21].

Based on systematic and methodical observations of a patient that produced large amounts of flatus, a classification of foodstuffs depending on their gas-producing capacity was elaborated [22]. Very few controlled studies on specific foodstuffs have been later added to complement this information [23-25]. Extremely flatulogenic foodstuffs include beans, Brussels sprouts, onions, celery, carrots, raisins, bananas, prune juice, apricots, wheat germ and bagels. Moderately flatulogenic foodstuffs include potatoes, eggplant, citrus fruit, apples, pastries and bread. Low producing foodstuffs include meat, fowl, fish, eggs, some vegetables, such as lettuce, tomato, avocado broccoli, cauliflower, asparagus, some fruits, such as cherries, grapes, cantaloupe, carbohydrates including rice, corn chips, popcorn, and finally, nuts and chocolate.

Another system to investigate the gas producing capacity of foodstuffs is to analyse the content of hydrogen in breath. Breath hydrogen remains extremely stable during fasting, but increases when colonic microflora ferments substrates releasing hydrogen, which is readily absorbed and excreted by breath. Using gas chromatography analysis, increments in hydrogen concentration of parts per million can be detected. With this method it has been shown that normally there is an incomplete absorption of some food components that pass into the colon and are fermented, the volume of gas produced depending on the individuals microflora [26-28].

Gas-producing food components include the following:

- some types of dietary fiber, such as xylan and pectin are fermentable and produce gas, whereas nonfermentable fiber, such as cellulose and corn bran, does not [24, 29];
- a significant proportion (10-30%) of the starch ingested escapes small intestinal absorption and contributes to the production of gas in the colon; for instance, starch in macaroni and white wheat bread is incompletely absorbed, whereas absorption of low-gluten wheat bread and rice bread is complete in the small intestine [26];
- some oligosaccharides, such as raffinose and stachyose, seem the most important source of gas in beans, because they are not absorbed in the small intestine [20, 25, 30];
- also some monosaccharides, such as sorbitol and fructose, are incompletely absorbed and are fermented in the colon [31, 32];
- other components of normal meals exert a modulatory role on absorption; for instance, beans contain a protein that inhibits pancreatic amylase, and thus, contributes to carbohydrate malabsorption [33-36].

Furthermore, interactions between different components of the meals have been described, for instance, fiber increases starch malabsorption [37].

Intestinal gas transit and tolerance

Despite inter and intraindividual variations in gas production, the total amount of gas in the gut remains constant, due to a regulated process of gas propulsion and evacuation. It is important to keep in mind that gas transit determines the time of exposure for diffusion of intraluminal gases across the gut-blood barrier, as well as for bacterial consumption, and hence, may influence the final composition of gas in flatus [38]. Intestinal gas transit and tolerance has been measured using a gas challenge test. The test consists of an infusion of a mixture of gases, in venous proportions to minimize absorption, into the jejunum while measuring anal gas evacuation [39] (Figure 4).

A dose-response study demonstrated that most healthy subjects propulse and evacuate as much gas as infused, up to 30 mL/min, without discomfort [39]. Hence, gas transit is finely adapted to any intestinal gas load. Obviously, gas transit is produced by the motor activity of the gut. Glucagon, which inhibits motor activity, produces gas retention [40], whereas neostigmine, with potent prokinetic effects, has been shown to clear gas in patients with retention [41]. However, the type of motor activity that determines gas transit is not known. Gas infusion does not induce detectable changes in small bowel intestinal motility recorded by manometry [42]. By contrast, preliminary experiments using the barostat suggest that gas infusion induces tonic changes: a contraction upstream to the infusion site and a relaxation downstream to it [43]. Conceivably, movement and displacement of large masses of low-resistance gas are produced by changes in tonic activity and capacitance of the gut.

Gas transit is regulated by various intestinal reflexes [44]. Intraluminal lipids dose-dependently delay gas transit and induce retention of exogenous gas loads [45]. Lipids seem more effective when infused into the ileum than in the duodenum, in consonance with the ileal brake mechanism that regulates the transit of solid/liquid chyme [46]. By contrast, other reflexes speed gas transit. For instance, gastric distension produces an immediate evacuation of the endogenous gas present in the gut, and accelerates transit of exogenous gas loads, suggesting the release of gastrocolic reflexes [44]. However, this seems to be a more generalized phenomenon, because distension at various levels of the gut, such as the duodenum or the rectum, produces the same stimulatory effect [43]. Furthermore, focal gut distension prevents the inhibitory effect of lipids [43]. Conceivably, under physiological conditions, different types of reflexes interact to produce a net final effect. Colonic microflora may play an important role in this regulation, because its potential effects on gut motility (*see chapter entitled* "Microflora and Colonic Motility"), but to date the effect of microflora on gas propulsion remains unknown.

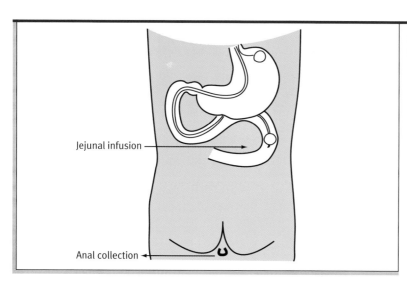

Jejunal infusion

Anal collection

Figure 4.
Gas challenge testing

Gas symptoms

Gas symptoms may be associated with different diseases, such as malabsorption, where excessive amounts of substrates escape small bowel absorption and are fermented in the colon, or bacterial overgrowth with bacterial colonization of territories where normally the nutrients are digested, e.g. the small bowel. In these conditions gas symptoms constitute only a side manifestation, and hence, are of limited interest in this context. The real challenge in clinical practice are the patients without detectable abnormalities by conventional testing, that complain of gas symptoms.

These patients fall into the category of functional gastrointestinal disorders and will be the focus of this section [47].

Clinical manifestations

Gas symptoms may allude to different situations, in which the patient interprets that his or her complaints are related to gas.

Belching

In the upper gut, gas complaints are usually related to dyspeptic symptoms that are alleviated by belching. The problem here is that during repetitive attempted belching, the patient swallows air, thereby increasing the discomfort, which is finally alleviated by belching, and this confirms the false impression of the patient that his or her symptoms are related to gas in the stomach [1, 48]. Usually these patients can be the retrained to control air swallowing, but their basal dyspeptic symptoms may remain. Nevertheless, this type of gas symptom has nothing to do with colonic microflora.

Excessive or odoriferous gas evacuation

Symptoms putatively related to microflora-produced gas are usually related to the lower gut. Some patients complain of bad smell of flatus, which may become socially disabling. As described before, odour depends on trace elements, such has sulphur-containing gases and other yet non identified components [13, 49]. Other patients complain of excessive gas evacuation. The normal number of evacuations per day in healthy subjects varies depending on the factors reviewed above, but is usually around twenty evacuations per day [50]. Using the gas challenge test, it has been shown that the number of evacuations depends on the rate of gas outflow, whereas the volume per evacuation remains fairly constant around 50 mL [40]. Excessive gas evacuation may or may not be associated with bad smell, but both problems are related to the interaction of the substrates arriving into the colon and the composition of the microflora. Excessive gas evacuation could be also related to impaired absorption of gas into the blood [22, 51].

Patients complaining of bad smell and/or excessive gas evacuation usually benefit from a diet excluding gas-producing foodstuffs. After one week on a "gas free diet" usually they experience frank symptom relief. By an orderly reintroduction of other foodstuffs, they should then learn to identify their offending meal components. Basically, these patients need to learn the price they have to pay for each type of meal, and decide whether or not the occasion deserves the try. At the same time, it is important in this context not to forget the possibility of phobia—which is actually far more common than any real, organic problem—in which case, prescribing a highly restrictive diet would be ill-advised.

Gas retention, bloating and distension

This is a more complicated problem of obscure origin, but probably related to gut motility and intestinal perception. The complaint of gas retention, bloating and abdominal distension is usually associated with irritable bowel syndrome (IBS) or functional bloating [47]. Two potential pathophysiological mechanisms have been considered to explain the symptoms in these patients: increased gas production, either due to malabsorption or abnormal colonic fermentation, and impaired gas handling.

Increased gas production

The role of malabsorption in this context remains dubious, because whereas some studies indicate that IBS patients may have reduced small bowel absorption capacity of some substrates [52-54], other studies did not replicate these results [55, 56]. Since the definition of malabsorption is *per se* difficult, the effect of exclusion diets has been also investigated. Again in this area the results are not the least uniform [57]. Furthermore, the exclusion of offending foodstuffs may not necessarily be related to their fermentation, but rather to other possible pathophysiological mechanisms, such as allergic or atopic reactions. A clinically relevant point in this context is the effect of dietary fiber. Some IBS patients have a large dietary fiber intake, which may increase colonic fermentation and gas production. Indeed it has been demonstrated that fiber may have deleterious effects on IBS symptoms [58]. Actually, many patients with fiber overload experience a frank benefit from removing the extra fiber load. An interesting study showed that, exposed to the same non-absorbable substrates, IBS patients had more colonic gas production than healthy subjects, suggesting that patients may have colonic disbacteriosis [59]. However, increased intestinal gas production, whether due to malabsorption or disbacteriosis, would not explain the symptoms, because most healthy subjects propulse and evacuate very large gas loads without perception [39].

Impaired handling

The data reviewed above suggest that impaired gas handling and tolerance is a key underlying mechanism in the origin of abdominal gas-related symptoms. This mechanism could be associated, or not, to increased gas production. It is interesting to note that a small proportion of the healthy population exhibits impaired handling and increased perception of intestinal gas [39]. If this fraction of the otherwise healthy population would be challenged with a gas overload, they would then experience symptoms [39]. Increased colonic gas formation, experimentally induced by direct infusion of starch into the colon, produces abdominal symptoms only in a fraction of healthy subjects [60]. A similar effect can be observed in case of experimental malabsorption induced by amylase inhibitors [34].

Using the gas challenge test it has been shown that patients complaining of unexplained abdominal bloating, either with IBS or functional bloating, have impaired transit and tolerance of intestinal gas [4, 41, 45]. These patients retain gas and/or experience abdominal discomfort in response to intestinal gas loads that are well tolerated by healthy subjects. Furthermore, the gas challenge reproduces their customary symptoms. In these experiments, patients also developed objective abdominal distension that correlated with the volume of gas retention. Nevertheless, the mechanism of distension is not clear, and although not demonstrated, it may be mediated *via* viscero-somatic reflexes [61, 62].

Mechanism of gas retention

In healthy subjects the anus has been shown to effectively retain gas. However, in most patients complaining of gas symptom, gas retention and symptoms during the gas challenge test were similar when gas was collected by an external cannula or by an intrarectal cannula that by-passed the anal gate [4]. Nevertheless, there is probably a small fraction of patients in which the anus plays a major role in gas retention. Normally rectal evacuation is achieved by a mild abdominal compression associated with an anal relaxation. In some patients this coordination fails and the anus does not relax [63]. Some of these patients complain of abdominal symptoms, that are conceivably related to faecal retention with an increased time for fermentation, and possibly also, to impaired gas evacuation. This anal incoordination can be resolved with biofeedback treatment, and sometimes, by resolving retention, the abdominal symptoms fade.

The mechanism of gas retention in patients is not known, but in healthy subjects two mechanisms have been shown to be potentially involved in intestinal gas retention: increased resistance to gas flow, modelled by self-restraint anal gas evacuation, and impaired intestinal propulsion, produced by glucagon-induced motor inhibition [40]. Using the gas challenge test it has been shown that gas retention induced by impaired propulsion was well tolerated and did not induce symptoms, but the same volume of retention produced by increased resistance to flow was associated with significant abdominal symptoms. Hence, symptomatic gas retention in patients may be related to incoordinated motility rather than to weak propulsion.

Further data indicate that impaired gas transit in patients with unexplained bloating is the result of abnormal reflex control. It has been shown that the slowing effect of lipids is up-regulated in these patients, whereas the stimulatory effect of distension is markedly impaired [43, 45]. The gas challenge test, in conjunction with intraluminal lipid infusion, provides a clear-cut distinction between patients and healthy subjects: patients retain large volumes of gas and or report symptoms, indicating that gas propulsion may be ineffective and/or symptomatic [45]. Gas symptoms in functional patients have been traditionally treated by means of spasmolytic drugs with inconsistent results. Neostigmine has been recently used as a proof of concept to test the potential effects of prokinetic stimulation on intestinal gas retention and symptoms in IBS. Using the gas challenge test it was shown that retention of gas loads in patients with IBS and functional bloating was effectively cleared by neostigmine administration, and reduced gas retention was associated with improvement of both abdominal distension and symptom perception [41].

Intestinal gas distribution

In apparent conflict with the data presented above, it has been previously shown by a series of the studies in the seventies by Levitt et al. that the amount and composition of gas in IBS patients is similar than that in healthy subjects [64]. In these studies, gas was measured by means of a wash-out technique, infusing argon into the intestine at a relatively high flow rate and recovering rectal gas. Studies using imaging techniques also failed to show marked intestinal gas pooling in IBS patients [62, 65, 66]. However, some of these studies were performed during fasting, whereas IBS patients usually complain of abdominal bloating and distension as the day progresses and they eat meals. Furthermore, studies with the gas challenge test suggest that the amount of gas required to produce symptoms in these patients may be relatively small, and hence, undetected by those techniques [4]. Indeed it may not be too much gas, but an abnormal gas distribution which causes abdominal bloating.

Recent studies have shown that the same volumes of gas induce significant symptoms in the small bowel, but not in the colon [67]. Furthermore, IBS patients develop gas retention when gas loads are delivered into the jejunum, but not into the ileum or the cecum, pointing towards the small intestine as the site of retention [68]. Ineffective propulsion and retention of jejunal gas are associated with symptoms, but interestingly, similar perception is produced by distal gas infusion, despite the lack of retention, suggesting an uncoordinated, symptomatic propulsion [68]. Conceivably, small gas bubbles pushed against high resistance barriers may increase intestinal wall tension and produce symptoms. Furthermore, if several bubbles are trapped at different levels, perception may increase by spatial summation phenomena [69]. Alternatively, the triggering factor of bloating may not be gas, but another element of gut contents [70]. Nevertheless, gas transit studies in patients with unexplained bloating have evidenced a motility failure associated with increased perception, which, by some way or another, conceivably play a pathophysiological role in their abdominal symptoms.

Pneumatosis intestinalis

Pneumatosis cystoides intestinalis is characterized by the presence of gas bubbles within the gut wall [71, 72] (Figure 5). This condition may affect different territories of the small bowel and the colon. Usually the patients are asymptomatic, but not infrequently a cyst ruptures and produces a spontaneous pneumoperitoneum, which usually follows an uneventful course.

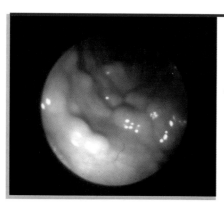

Figure 5.
Endoscopic image of pneumatosis cystoides intestinalis.
(photograph A. Bitoun, Hôpital Lariboisière, Paris.
Traité de Gastro-entérologie, 2000,
J.C. Rambaud, ed. Médecine-Sciences Flammarion)

The initiating factor of this condition is the development of small gas bubbles within the gut wall. Different mechanisms have been postulated, such as bacterial infiltration of the gut wall or gas dissection of mucosal rents [73]. In otherwise healthy subjects, once the initiating mechanism disappears, gases within the cyst are slowly absorbed into the blood by equilibration of their partial pressures. However, in patients with pneumatosis intestinalis another factor causes the persistence and enlargement of these bubbles.

A frequently observed feature in patients with pneumatosis intestinalis is increased hydrogen in the gut lumen, detected by breath test [74]. The cause of this hydrogen excess is a dysbalance between hydrogen-producing and hydrogen-consuming microflora in the region affected. For instance, in patients with colonic pneumatosis cystoides, a decrease of hydrogen-consuming bacteria, either methanogenic or sulphate-reducing pools, has been reported [75]. In other patients with small bowel pneumatosis cystoides it has been demonstrated a colonization of the small bowel by hydrogen-producing microflora without the consuming component, in the presence of normal hydrogen-consuming methanogenic bacteria in the colon [73].

The mechanism by which increased intraluminal hydrogen results in pneumatosis cystoides remains unclear, but a very suggestive hypothesis has been recently proposed [73]. If hydrogen in the gut lumen is high, the partial pressure of hydrogen in the mucosa would be also high, and thus, would prevent reabsorption of hydrogen from the cyst. To equilibrate the partial pressures of gases in blood and cysts, nitrogen, CO_2 and oxygen will diffuse from the blood into the cyst, producing a several fold increase in intracyst volume, ever if the initiating factor has disappeared. Disappearance of the cysts has been reported using measures that reduce intraluminal hydrogen, such as low residue diets or antibiotics [71, 72]. An alternative approach is the inhalation of oxygen-enriched air, that is air with higher partial pressure of oxygen and lower partial pressure of nitrogen [71, 72]. In the presence of the decreased partial pressure of nitrogen in blood, nitrogen, the largest gaseous component within the cysts, is reabsorbed and the cysts progressively shrink and disappear over a period of several days.

Key points

- A major source of intestinal gas production is the fermentation of meal residues in the colon by colonic bacteria. The gases produced are either absorbed into the blood or consumed by colonic bacteria, and the remainder evacuated by the anus.

- Excessive or odoriferous gas evacuation depends on the meal residues arriving into the colon and on the composition of colonic microflora. Since the latter is highly individual, treatment of these symptoms benefits of a poorly flatulogenic diet.

- Some patients complaining of abdominal bloating and distension produce a defective anal relaxation during attempted evacuation, which may result in gas retention. Faecal retention in these patients may also contribute to increased gas production due to prolonged fermentation time.

- Recent data indicate that a large proportion of these patients with bloating have impaired transit and tolerance of intestinal gas. Some data indicate that these dysfunctions may be related to a sensory-motor disorder of the gut.

- Pneumatosis cystoides is characterized by gas bubbles within the gut wall. This disorder seems related to altered dynamics of gas diffusion between the gut lumen and the blood. Cyst reabsorption may be achieved either by dietary manipulations to reduce intestinal hydrogen or by a diet which reduces intestinal hydrogen or by inhalation of oxygen-rich air to reduce the partial pressure of nitrogen in the blood.

References

1. Strocchi A, Levitt MD. Intestinal gas. In : Feldman M, Scharschmidt BF, Sleisenger MH, eds. *Sleisenger & Fordtran's gastrointestinal and liver disease: pathophysiology/diagnosis/management*, 6th ed. Philadelphia, PA : WB Saunders, 1998 : 153-60.

2. Cloarec D, Flourié B, Marteau P, *et al*. Les gaz digestifs : aspects physiopathologiques et thérapeutiques au cours des troubles fonctionnels. *Gastroenterol Clin Biol* 1990 ; 14 : 641-50.

3. Levitt MD. Volume and composition of human intestinal gas determined by means of an intestinal washout technic. *N Engl J Med* 1971 ; 284 : 1394-8.

4. Serra J, Azpiroz F, Malagelada JR. Impaired transit and tolerance of intestinal gas in the irritable bowel syndrome. *Gut* 2001 ; 48 : 14-9.

5. Bedell GN, Marshall R, Dubois AB, *et al*. Measurement of the volume of gas in the gastro-intestinal tract: values in normal subjects and ambulatory patients. *J Clin Invest* 1956 ; 35 : 336-45.

6. Fordtran JS, Morawski SG, Santa Ana CA, *et al*. Gas production after reaction of sodium bicarbonate and hypochloric acid. *Gastroenterology* 1984 ; 87 : 1014-21.

7. Foster RE. Physiological basis of gas exchange in the gut. *Ann N Y Acad Sci* 1968 ; 150 : 4-12.

8. Pogrund RS, Steggerda FR. Influence of gaseous transfer between the colon and blood stream on percentage gas compositions of intestinal flatus in man. *Am J Physiol* 1948 ; 153 : 475-82.

9. Scheppach W, Fabian C, Ahrens F. Effect of starch malabsorption on colonic function and metabolism in humans. *Gastroenterology* 1988 ; 1549-55.

10. Stephen AM, Cummings JH. Mechanism of action of dietary fibre in the human colon. *Nature* 1980 ; 284 : 283-4.

11. Levitt MD, Bond JH. Volume, composition, and source of intestinal gas. *Gastroenterology* 1970 ; 59 : 921-9.

12. Levitt MD. Intestinal gas production - recent advances in flatology. *N Engl J Med* 1980 ; 302 : 1474-5.

13. Suarez F, Furne J, Springfield J, *et al*. Insights into human colonic physiology obtained from the study of flatus composition. *Am J Physiol* 1997 ; G1028-33.

14. Strocchi A, Levitt MD. Factors affecting hydrogen production and consumption by human fecal flora. The critical roles of hydrogen tension and methanogenesis. *J Clin Invest* 1992 ; 89 : 1304-11.

15. Flourié B, Pellier P, Florent C, *et al*. Site and substrates for methane production in human colon. *Am J Physiol* 1991 ; 260 : G752-7.

16. Kajs TM, Fitzgerald JA, Buckner RY, *et al*. Influence of a methanogenic flora on the breath H_2 and symptom response to ingestion of sorbitol or oat fiber. *Am J Gastroenterol* 1997 ; 92 : 89-94.

17. Gibson GR, Cummings JH, Macfarlane GT, *et al*. Alternative pathways for hydrogen disposal during fermentation in the human colon. *Gut* 1990 ; 31 : 679-83.

18. Strocchi A, Furne J, Ellis C, *et al*. Methanogens outcompete sulphate reducing bacteria for H_2 in the human colon. *Gut* 1994 ; 35 : 1098-101.

19. Kirk E. The quantity and composition of human colonic flatus. *Gastroenterology* 1949 ; 12 : 782-94.

20. Steggerda FR. Gastrointestinal gas following food consumption. *Ann N Y Acad Sci* 1968 ; 150 : 57-66.

21. Tomlin J, Lowis C, Read NW. Investigation of normal flatus production in healthy volunteers. *Gut* 1991 ; 32 : 665-9.

22. Sutalf LO, Levitt MD. Follow-up of a flatulent patient. *Dig Dis Sci* 1979 ; 24 : 652-4.

23. Hickey C, Calloway D, Murphy E. Intestinal gas production following ingestion of fruits and fruit juice. *Am J Dig Dis* 1972 ; 17 : 383-9.

24. Wolever TM, Robb PA. Effect of guar, pectin, psyllium, soy polysaccharide, and cellulose on breath hydrogen and methane in healthy subjects. *Am J Gastroenterol* 1992 ; 87 : 305-10.

25. Wagner JR, Carson JF, Becker R, *et al*. Comparative flatulence activity of beans and bean fractions for man and the rat. *J Nutr* 1977 ; 107 : 680-9.

26. Anderson IH, Levine AS, Levitt MD. Incomplete absorption of the carbohydrate in all-purpose wheat flour. *N Engl J Med* 1981 ; 304 : 891-2.

27. Levitt MD, Hirsh P, Fetzer CA, *et al*. H$_2$ excretion after ingestion of complex carbohydrates. *Gastroenterology* 1987 ; 92 : 383-9.

28. Flourie B, Leblond A, Florent C, *et al*. Starch malabsorption and breath gas excretion in healthy humans consuming low- and high-starch diets. *Gastroenterology* 1988 ; 95 : 356-63.

29. Grimble G. Fibre, fermentation, flora, and flatus. *Gut* 1989 ; 30 : 6-13.

30. Steggerda FR, Dimmick JF. Effects of bean diets on concentration of carbon dioxide in flatus. *Am J Clin Nutr* 1966 ; 19 : 120-4.

31. Stone-Dorshow T, Levitt MD. Gaseous response to ingestion of a poorly absorbed fructo-oligosaccharide sweetener. *Am J Clin Nutr* 1987 ; 46 : 61-5.

32. Wursch P, Koellreutter B, Schweizer TF. Hydrogen excretion after ingestion of five different sugar alcohols and lactulose. *Eur J Clin Nutr* 1989 ; 43 : 819-25.

33. Brugge WR, Rosenfeld MS. Impairment of starch absorption by a potent amylase inhibitor. *Am J Gastroenterol* 1987 ; 82 : 718-22.

34. Boibin M, Flourié B, Rizza RA, *et al*. Gastrointestinal and metabolic effects of amylase inhibition in diabetics. *Gastroenterology* 1998 ; 1988 :387-94.

35. Taylor RH, Barker HM, Bowey EA, *et al*. Regulation of the absorption of dietary carbohydrate in man by two new glycosidase inhibitors. *Gut* 1986 ; 27 : 1471-8.

36. Layer P, Zinsmeister AR, DiMagno EP. Effects of decreasing intraluminal amylase activity on starch digestion and postprandial gastrointestinal function in humans. *Gastroenterology* 1986 ; 91 : 41-8.

37. Hamberg O, Rumessen JJ, Gudmand-Hoyer E. Inhibition of starch absorption by dietary fibre. A comparative study of wheat bran, sugar-beet fibre, and pea fibre. *Scand J Gastroenterol* 1989 ; 24 : 103-9.

38. El Oufir L, Flourie B, Bruley des Varannes S, *et al*. Relations between transit time, fermentation products, and hydrogen consuming flora in healthy humans. *Gut* 1996 ; 30 : 870-7.

39. Serra J, Azpiroz F, Malagelada JR. Intestinal gas dynamics and tolerance in humans. *Gastroenterology* 1998 ; 115 : 542-50.

40. Serra J, Azpiroz F, Malagelada JR. Mechanisms of intestinal gas retention in humans: impaired propulsion *versus* obstructed evacuation. *Am J Physiol Gastrointest Liver Physiol* 2001 ; 281 : G138-43.

41. Caldarella MP, Serra J, Azpiroz F, Malagelada JR. Prokinetic effects of neostigmine in patients with intestinal gas retention. *Gastroenterology* 2002 ; 122 : 1748-55.

42. Galati JS, McKee DP, Quigley EM. Response to intraluminal gas in irritable bowel syndrome. Motility *versus* perception. *Dig Dis Sci* 1995 ; 40 : 1381-7.

43. Harder H, Serra J, Azpiroz F, *et al*. Reflex control of intestinal gas dynamics and tolerance. *Gastroenterology* 2000 ; 118 : A689.

44. Serra J, Azpiroz F, Malagelada JR. Gastric distension and duodenal lipid infusion modulate intestinal gas transit and tolerance in humans. *Am J Gastroenterol* 2002 ; 97 : 2225-30.

45. Serra J, Salvioli B, Azpiroz F, *et al*. Lipid-induced intestinal gas retention in the irritable bowel syndrome. *Gastroenterology* 2002 ; 123 : 700-6.

46. Passos MC, Serra J, Azpiroz F, *et al*. Impaired reflex control of intestinal gas propulsion in patients with abdominal bloating. *Gastroenterology* 2002 ; 122 : A549.

47. Thompson WG, Longstreth G, Drossman DA, *et al*. Functional bowel disorders. Functional abdominal pain. In : Drossman DA, Corazziari E, Talley NJ, Thompson WG, Whitehead WE, eds. *The functional gastrointestinal disorders*. 2nd ed. Mc Lean, VA : Degnon Associates, 2000 : 351-432.

48. Bond JH, Levitt MD. Gaseousness and intestinal gas. *Med Clin North Am* 1978 ; 62 : 155-64.

49. Suarez FL, Springfield J, Levitt MD. Identification of gases responsible for the odour of human flatus and evaluation of a device purported to reduce this odour. *Gut* 1998 ; 43 : 100-4.

50. Furne JK, Levitt MD. Factors influencing frequency of flatus emission by healthy subjects. *Dig Dis Sci* 1996 ; 41 : 1631-5.

51. Levitt MD, Lasser RB, Schwartz JS, *et al*. Studies of a flatulent patient. *N Engl J Med* 1976 ; 295 : 260-2.

52. Rumessen JJ, Gudmand-Hoyer E. Functional bowel disease: malabsorption and abdominal distress after ingestion of fructose, sorbitol, and fructose-sorbitol mixtures. *Gastroenterology* 1988 ; 95 : 694-700.

53. Fernandez-Banares F, Esteve-Pardo M, de Leon R, *et al*. Sugar malabsorption in functional bowel disease: clinical implications. *Am J Gastroenterol* 1993 ; 88 : 2044-50.

54. Symons P, Jones MP, Kellow JE. Symptom provocation in irritable bowel syndrome. Effects of differing doses of fructose-sorbitol. *Scand J Gastroenterol* 1992 ; 27 : 940-4.

55. Afdhal NH, Piggott C, Long AA, *et al*. Carbohydrate handling by colonic flora - is it pathogenic in the irritable bowel syndrome? *Ir J Med Sci* 1986 ; 155 : 197-201.

56. Nelis GF, Vermeeren MA, Jansen W. Role of fructose-sorbitol malabsorption in the irritable bowel syndrome. *Gastroenterology* 1990 ; 99 : 1016-20.

57. McKee AM, Prior A, Whorwell PJ. Exclusion diets in irritable bowel syndrome: are they worthwhile? *J Clin Gastroenterol* 1987 ; 9 : 526-8.

58. Francis CY, Whorwell PJ. Bran and irritable bowel syndrome: time for reappraisal. *Lancet* 1994 ; 344 : 39-40.

59. King TS, Elia M, Hunter JO. Abnormal colonic fermentation in irritable bowel syndrome. *Lancet* 1998 ; 352 : 1187-9.

60. Flourie B, Florent C, Jouany JP, *et al*. Colonic metabolism of wheat starch in healthy humans. Effects on fecal outputs and clinical symptoms. *Gastroenterology* 1986 ; 90 : 111-9.

61. McManis PG, Newall D, Talley NJ. Abdominal wall muscle activity in irritable bowel syndrome with bloating. *Am J Gastroenterol* 2001 ; 96 : 1139-42.

62. Maxton DG, Martin DF, Whorwell P, *et al*. Abdominal distension in female patients with irritable bowel syndrome: exploration of possible mechanisms. *Gut* 1991 ; 32 : 662-4.

63. Azpiroz F, Enck P, Whitehead WE. Anorectal functional testing. Review of a collective experience. *Am J Gastroenterol* 2002 ; 97 : 232-40.

64. Lasser RB, Bond JH, Levitt MD. The role of intestinal gas in functional abdominal pain. *N Engl J Med* 1975 ; 293 : 524-6.

65. Chami TN, Schuster MM, Bohlman ME, *et al*. A simple radiologic method to estimate the quantity of bowel gas. *Am J Gastroenterol* 1991 ; 86 : 599-602.

66. Poynard T, Hernandez M, Xu P, *et al*. Visible abdominal distension and gas surface: description of an automatic method of evaluation and application to patients with irritable bowel syndrome and dyspepsia. *Eur J Gastroenterol Hepatol* 1992 ; 4 : 831-6.

67. Harder H, Serra J, Azpiroz F, *et al*. Intestinal gas distribution determines abdominal symptoms. *Gastroenterology* 2001 ; 120 : A72.

68. Salvioli B, Serra J, Azpiroz F, *et al*. Tolerance of ileal and colonic gas loads in patients with irritable bowel syndrome and functional bloating. *Gastroenterology* 2001 ; 120 : A755.

69. Serra J, Azpiroz F, Malagelada JR. Modulation of gut perception in humans by spatial summation phenomena. *J Physiol* 1998 ; 506 : 579-87.

70. Levitt MD, Furne J, Olsson S. The relation of passage of gas an abdominal bloating to colonic gas production. *Ann Intern Med* 1996 ; 124 : 422-4.

71. Jouët P, Marteau P. Pneumatose kystique intestinale. *Hepato-Gastro* 1994 ; 1 : 563-8.

72. Heng Y, Schuffler MD, Rodger MD HMRC. Pneumatosis intestinalis: a review. *Am J Gastroenterol* 1995 ; 90 : 1747-58.

73. Levitt M, Olsson S. Pneumatosis cystoides intestinalis and high breath H_2 excretion: insights into the role of H_2 in this condition. *Gastroenterology* 1995 ; 108 : 1560-5.

74. Gillon J, Tadesse K, Logan RFA, *et al*. Breath hydrogen in pneumatosis cystoides intestinalis. *Gut* 1979 ; 20 : 1008-11.

75. Christi SU, Gibson GR, Murgatroyd PR, *et al*. Impaired hydrogen metabolism in pneumatosis cystoides intestinalis. *Gastroenterology* 1993 ; 104 : 392-7.

Microflora and Colonic Motility. Physiological Data and Irritable Bowel Syndrome

Benoît Coffin, Jean-Marc Sabaté

Service d'Hépato-Gastro-entérologie, Hôpital Louis-Mourier, Colombes, France.

In the fasting state, normal gastrointestinal motility is characterized by cyclic, propagated activity, the migrating motor complex, the presumed functions of which are to propel the indigestible residues of a meal on the one hand, and to counter bacterial proliferation in the gut lumen on the other. In contrast, normal colonic motility is low except during certain moments of the nyctohemeral cycle; this promotes mixing and the slow progression of the colonic contents. Because of this special motility, a rich and polymorphic microflora colonizes the colon in the first few days of life, then develops and fulfils various essential functions, notably the fermentation of carbohydrate and proteinaceous residues from both exogenous sources (food) and endogenous ones. In return, the presence of the microflora, with its various functions, influences motility. Relationships between fermentation and colonic motility are therefore very close but as yet poorly understood because of a lack of animal studies and the difficulties of performing experiments in humans.

Normal parietal colonic motility in humans

Smooth muscle cells in the colonic wall—as in other segments of the digestive tract—generate two types of motor activity. Phasic activity is measured by electromyography or manometry using the perfused catheter method [1]. In healthy volunteers, 24-hour electromyographic and manometric recordings have shown that the major part of colonic motor activity is irregular, of low amplitude (contractions < 60 mm Hg) and not propagated [2]. During fasting and sleep, this activity is weak promoting stagnation and admixture of the colonic contents. Waking up in the morning and the consumption of food induce increased phasic activity, more marked in the distal colon than the proximal colon [2-4]. High-amplitude phasic contractions (HAPC) ($\geq$ 100 mm Hg in manometry, or Long Spike Bursts in electromyography), rapidly propagated over long distances in an oral anal direction, are usually recorded on waking or in the post-prandial period (Figure 1) [2, 4]. Tonic activity is measured by the electronic barostat method [1]. Colonic tone is little understood. It has essentially been shown that eating also induces diffuse tonic contraction [3] and that, at night, tone diminishes.

Similarly, the relationships between motor activity and intraluminal movements are poorly understood. HAPCs could explain certain mass movements. Variations in colonic tone could explain the reservoir function of the proximal colon and certain displacements of the contents which are not explained by variations in phasic activity [1].

In any case, motor activity is weaker in the proximal colon than in the distal colon. These local variations are multifactorial and probably arise from an embryological source and differential innervation, but also perhaps from local effects of the luminal contents. Cause or consequence, it should be noted that the right and left bacterial microfloras are not superimposable, e.g. almost all the methanogenic microflora are found in the left colon [5].

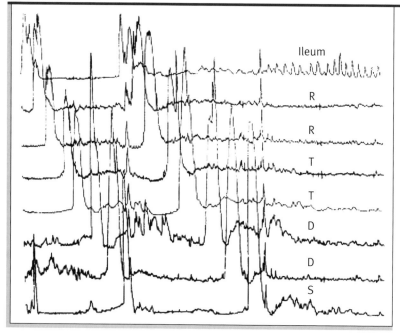

Figure 1.
Manometric measurements of colonic contractions which are of high amplitude and are rapidly propagated through the colon.
R : right colon,
T : transverse colon,
D : descending colon,
S : sigmoid
(taken from [4])

In humans, most of the electromyographic and manometric data were obtained in relatively non-physiological conditions which do not make it possible to study relationships with the colonic microflora correctly; the recording probe is implanted during colonoscopy after colonic preparation which temporarily but drastically changes the colonic microflora. In recent years, in our previous research group at the Hôpital Saint-Lazare (Paris) we have developed a novel method for measuring colonic motility which does not affect colonic contents. The probe is introduced *via* the mouth and slowly directed down through the digestive tract until its distal end comes out through the anus. By various technical manipulations, it is possible either to preferentially explore the tonic and phasic activity in different segments (e.g. the proximal or distal colon [3, 6]), or to study overall colonic motility [4, 7]. Although each experiment necessitates immobilization of the volunteer for four or five days and the failure rate is significant, this method has allowed us to study various aspects of colonic motility in healthy subjects, without damaging the physiological colonic microflora. We have been able therefore to study certain relationships between the microflora and colonic motility, in particular in the course of fermentation reactions. Given its limitations, this method cannot be used in patients. On the other hand, it makes it possible to measure intra-colonic movements using various techniques such as the progression of radiopaque pellets or segmental scintigraphy, without disturbing the colonic microflora.

Effects of colonic motility on the microflora

No study has shown that pharmacological modification of parietal colonic motility (as measured using conventional methods) could result in modification of the microflora. However, slowing down digestive transit with loperamide or speeding it up with cisapride changes the bacterial ecosystem in healthy volunteers, although the focus and the types of modification of parietal motility responsible for these changes are unknown [8]. Compared with the control period, although the absolute number of anaerobic bacteria may not be increased, the acceleration of transit by cisapride results in a reduced faecal density of methane-producing bacteria and an increase in that of sulphate-reducing bacteria; exactly the contrary is observed following the administration of loperamide (Figure 2). Moreover, cisapride significantly increases the faecal concentrations of propionate and butyrate, reduces faecal pH, and increases hydrogen excretion in the breath. The effects of loperamide on these parameters are again exactly the opposite [8].

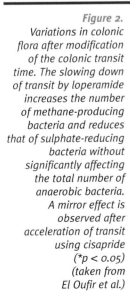

Figure 2.
Variations in colonic flora after modification of the colonic transit time. The slowing down of transit by loperamide increases the number of methane-producing bacteria and reduces that of sulphate-reducing bacteria without significantly affecting the total number of anaerobic bacteria. A mirror effect is observed after acceleration of transit using cisapride (*p < 0.05) (taken from El Oufir et al.)

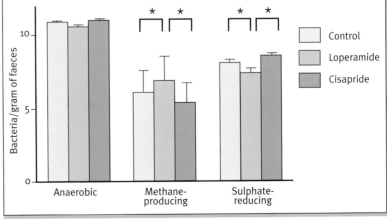

Effects of the colonic microflora on parietal motility and colonic transit

Possible effects of the colonic bacterial microflora on parietal motility are particularly difficult to investigate in humans because of, on the one hand the diversity of the microflora and the difficulty in identifying the bacterial species present and, on the other hand, the quasi-impossibility of durably implanting an easily identified bacterial strain. Nevertheless, Lémann et al. [4] have shown in healthy volunteers that colonic preparation with polyethylene glycol (PEG), which temporarily diminishes the colonic microflora, modifies certain parameters of phasic parietal motility. Analysis of the results showed that motor indices (which reflect global motor activity) or the motor response to eating were not affected by the administration of PEG. On the other hand, the number of HAPCs was significantly increased after the PEG compared with the period without preparation (8.6 ± 2.8 versus 5.4 ± 1.8/subject/9 h, respectively; $p < 0.05$). These data suggest that the colonic microflora could be directly or indirectly involved in colonic motility, following fermentation reactions. Numerous experiments have shown that probiotics such as lactobacilli and bifidobacteria arrive in a viable state in the colon and proliferate there [9] but do not manage to establish themselves on a durable basis because they are no longer detectable in the days following administration [10]. Findings concerning the effects of probiotics on the time of colonic transit are contradictory. In one study, it was shown that the consumption of yogurt containing *Bifidobacterium longum* did not affect oro-anal transit time [11]. Another experiment showed that taking *Propionibacterium freudenreichii*, a bacterium found in certain types of cheese, modified neither the overall colonic transit time nor the right colonic transit time but significantly increased the transit time in the left colon compared with placebo (respectively 11.9 ± 9.4 h versus 7.0 ± 5.0 h, $p < 0.05$) [12]. Finally, a more recent study showed that, compared with the control period, the DN-173 010 strain of *Bifidobacterium animalis* reduced both the overall colonic transit time (51.5 ± 30.2 h versus 60.7 ± 27.1, respectively, $p < 0.05$) and the sigmoid transit time (21.6 ± 14.9 versus 26.8 ± 14.2, respectively, $p < 0.05$) [13]. This effect was more marked in women with a long baseline transit time (over 40 hours). The weight of faeces, the faecal pH, the bacterial faecal mass, and faecal bile acids were not different between the two periods. Even if they are significant, these variations in colonic transit remain moderate and without obvious repercussions on the treatment of patients with slow transit. Taking small doses of a prebiotic such as oligofructose or inulin, the arrival of which in the colon should promote the growth of bifidobacteria, does not affect colonic transit time [14].

Indigestible or completely digestible forms of fibre such as cellulose or mucilages like ispaghula, have long been used for their laxative properties in the treatment of chronic idiopathic constipation. They act, on the one hand, by a bulk effect and, on the other hand, by increasing the faecal bacterial mass which represents nearly one-half of the weight of the normal stool. In healthy volunteers, fibre supplementation does not affect phasic colonic motility whatever its fermentable properties [15]. Fibre from peas (relatively unfermentable) or carrots (more fermentable and more soluble) does not affect any of these motor parameters.

The study of the motor effects of lactulose, a fermentable, non-absorbable sugar used for many years in the treatment of chronic idiopathic constipation, suggests that the bacterial metabolites released in the course of fermentation reactions participate in the regulation of colonic motility. In practice, once arrived in the colon, lactulose is rapidly fermented, releasing mainly lactate and short-chain fatty acids (SCFA). Lactulose accelerates colonic transit measured by scintigraphy, mainly by accelerating emptying of the right colon [16, 17]. Concerning the motor activity, the administration of 15 grams of lactulose induces, on the one hand, tonic contraction of the right colon [18] and, on the other hand, the appearance of waves of irregular contraction which are little or not at all propagated [7]. This motor effect could have been linked to the osmolarity of the product but this hypothesis can be ruled out because the administration of macrogol, the osmolarity of which is the same but which is not fermentable, has no effect on colonic motility [19]. In contrast, the rapidity of the appearance of motor events (which are observed as soon as fermentation begins as shown by concomitant hydrogen breath testing) strongly suggests the role of metabolites of fermentation in the regulation of colonic motility. In addition, the intracolonic infusion of 15 grams of starch, a quantity which is physiologically poorly absorbed after 24 hours in the small intestine (resistant starch), does not significantly affect colonic tone but significantly increases the number of HAPCs [20]. This differential motor effect of starch could be explained by a fermentation profile which is distinct from that of lactulose, preferentially leading to the formation of propionate and butyrate.

The mechanisms underlying these effects on motility and the colonic transit of fermentable carbohydrates remain incompletely understood. In healthy volunteers, the intracolonic infusion of a quantity of SCFAs equivalent to that produced by the fermentation of 15 grams of starch modifies neither tone nor phasic activity [21]. Acidification of the colonic contents using a solution of pH 4.5, as during rapid fermentation, modified neither phasic colonic motility nor colonic tone. However, in rats, the intracolonic infusion of large doses of SCFAs reduced colonic motility, accelerated transit time, and induced an increase in the concentration of circulating neuropeptide YY [22]. This effect is abolished by preliminary local anaesthesia which points to the presence of sensory receptors which are sensitive to variations in SCFA concentrations.

SCFAs are also involved in the regulation of oesogastrointestinal motility. Infusion of a mixture of SCFAs into the terminal ileum induces tonic and phasic contraction [23]. This motor effect could counter bacterial colonization of the terminal intestine in the context of physiological caeco-ileal reflux. In contrast, colonic fermentation of lactulose induces tonic relaxation at the level of the proximal stomach [24]. This regulatory mechanism, referred to as colonic brake, probably results from hormone release. It could play a role in certain pathological situations, notably in patients suffering from short bowel syndrome [25]. Finally, in healthy volunteers, the colonic fermentation of lactulose induces the appearance of transient relaxations of the lower oesophageal sphincter, the role of which in the pathophysiology of gastro-oesophageal reflux no longer needs demonstration [26]. This effect was recently confirmed in patients suffering from gastro-oesophageal reflux [27].

Microflora and irritable bowel syndrome

In the course of irritable bowel syndrome (IBS), a range of different abnormalities affecting colonic motility and sensitivity has been reported in recent years [28]. The role of the digestive microflora in the pathophysiology of these abnormalities is ever more frequently evoked (Figure 3).

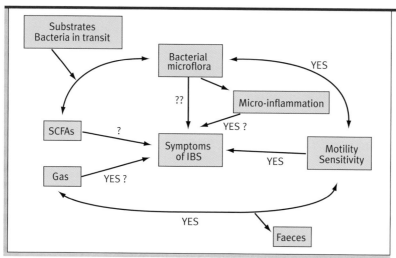

Figure 3. Relationships between the bacterial microflora, motility and colonic sensitivity in irritable bowel syndrome (IBS) SCFA = Short-chain fatty acid

Several epidemiological studies have shown that the typical symptoms of IBS (as stipulated in the Rome criteria) appear in 7-30 % of patients who have experienced an episode of acute digestive tract infection [28-30]. Predictive factors of the appearance of IBS were the duration of the acute diarrhoeal episode (> 5 days), female gender and the coexistence of stress during the acute episode. In these patients, it was shown that there exist abnormalities of colonic motility [28, 31], abnormalities of the functions of epithelial cells, and an increase in enterochromaffin cells of the rectal mucosa [32], but no qualitative abnormality of the microflora was reported. The relationship between these abnormalities and the symptoms of IBS has not been elucidated. On the physiopathological front, the increase in enterochromaffin cells and an infiltrate of the nervous plexus by T lymphocytes [33, 34] could entail up-regulation of neuro-immune reactions which could be sustained by the presence of the colonic microflora. However, this hypothesis of sub-acute inflammation without any macroscopic consequences triggered by an infectious phenomenon cannot be held responsible for symptoms in most IBS patients.

The role of the colonic microflora in the pathogenesis of the symptoms of IBS is not a new hypothesis. In 1983, Newcomer *et al.* showed that taking *Lactobacillus acidophilus* did not affect the various functional symptoms, including in the sub-group of lactase-deficient patients [35]. Other studies of this type have been carried out since, the results of which are discordant and inconsistently convincing. In twenty patients with IBS, defined on the basis of the Rome criteria, it has been shown, in a randomised, cross-over, placebo-controlled study, that taking the 299V strain of *Lactobacillus plantarum* did not affect any of the usual symptoms of IBS [36] whereas, in another placebo-controlled study using the same strain of *Lactobacillus plantarum*, a significant reduction was observed in the severity of abdominal pain [37]. A placebo-controlled study addressing the efficacy of a heat-stabilized strain of *Lactobacillus acidophilus* showed a positive effect on symptoms in more than half of the patients although only eighteen patients were included [38].

One placebo-controlled study showed a beneficial effect of the administration of *Saccharomyces boulardii* on intestinal transit in patients presenting an irritable bowel with diarrhoea predominant [39]. Finally, a strain of *Lactobacillus casei* GG did not induce any improvement in symptoms compared with placebo [40]. The same methodological problems as those encountered recently for the development of compounds with potential action in IBS, such as the size of the population, the inclusion criteria, the efficacy criteria and the extent of the response to placebo, may well arise in the context of the development of probiotics for the treatment of IBS.

As far as the metabolites of fermentation are concerned, SCFA production has not been studied in the course of IBS. The role of gases released in fermentation reactions is not perfectly clear in the pathophysiology of symptoms such as bloating, so common in IBS. For a long time, it was considered that gaseous productions were normal in these patients. Sensations of gas or abdominal bloating would therefore be secondary to impaired visceral sensitivity [41] or to an abnormality in motility [42]. A controlled study conducted in six patients complaining of bloating nevertheless showed that they produced abnormally high volumes of gas when consuming a standard diet, a problem which was resolved by switching them to a restrictive diet [43]. This study, well conducted in methodological terms, suggests that there exists a group of patients with IBS in whom some of the symptoms could be explained by an abnormality in microflora resulting in abnormal gas production. A clinical study in sixty IBS patients showed that the DSM9483 strain of *Lactobacillus plantarum* reduced the intensity of bloating [44]. This promising line of research aimed at correcting gas production could possibly lead to changes in the way IBS is managed. In contrast, for a long time, bran supplementation was recommended to regulate transit in IBS patients with constipation predominant. If the effects of bran on transit have been confirmed, it has unfortunately been clearly shown that consuming bran exacerbates the symptoms of bloating in these patients and therefore has a deleterious effect [45, 46].

Conclusion

The colonic microflora can develop because colonic motility permits it. The relationships between these two partners are certainly multiple, complex and probably indirect *via* fermentation reactions, but remain extremely poorly understood, essentially because of methodological difficulties (Figure 3). In certain pathological processes such as IBS, temporary modification of the microflora during an acute, infectious, intestinal episode could be involved in triggering the problems. Modifying the colonic microflora with antibiotics or intestinal antiseptics cannot be recommended in daily clinical practice in IBS patients, and antibiotics could even have an adverse effect. Several trials have demonstrated the value of certain probiotics on the symptoms of the irritable bowel (*see chapter entitled* "Probiotics and Digestive problems").

Key points

- In the fasting state and during sleep, colonic parietal motility is characterized by irregular phasic activity which is of low amplitude and is not propagated, promoting colonization by a rich saprophytic microflora. On waking and after eating, high amplitude phasic contractions (HAPC) appear, propagated in the aboral direction and propulsive. Eating also increases colonic tone.

- Cisapride, which accelerates colonic transit, increases the faecal concentrations of propionate and butyrate, and reduces the faecal pH and the amount of hydrogen excreted in the breath. Loperamide, which slows colonic transit down, has the opposite effects.

- Lavage of the colonic contents including the microflora increases the number of HAPCs. Several probiotics can accelerate overall and segmental colonic transit.

- The effect of unabsorbed, fermentable carbohydrates (lactulose, resistant starch) on phasic and tonic motor activity is well established, although the underlying mechanisms remain unelucidated.

- In irritable bowel syndrome, the role of the colonic microflora, notably through excess gas production, is very probable in certain patients, and certain probiotics have proven effective against all or some of the symptoms.

References

1. Jouet P, Coffin B, Cuillerier E, *et al*. Colonic motility in humans. Recent physiological, pathophysiological and pharmacological data. *Gastroenterol Clin Biol* 2000; 24 : 284-98.

2. Narducci F, Bassotti G, Gaburri M, *et al*. Twenty four hour manometric recording of colonic motor activity in healthy man. *Gut* 1987 ; 28 : 17-25.

3. Jouet P, Coffin B, Lemann M, *et al*. Tonic and phasic motor activity in the proximal and distal colon of healthy humans. *Am J Physiol* 1998; 274 : G459-64.

4. Lemann M, Flourie B, Picon L, *et al*. Motor activity recorded in the unprepared colon of healthy humans. *Gut* 1995; 37 : 649-53.

5. Flourie B, Pellier P, Florent C, *et al*. Site and substrates for methane production in human colon. *Am J Physiol* 1991 ; 260 : G752-7.

6. Coffin B, Fossati S, Flourie B, *et al*. Regional effects of cholecystokinin octapeptide on colonic phasic and tonic motility in healthy humans. *Am J Physiol* 1999 ; 276 : G767-72.

7. Jouet P, Sabate JM, Coffin B, *et al*. Sugar intolerance: origin and mechanisms of symptoms? *Dig Dis Sci* 2002 ; 47 : 886-93.

8. El Oufir L, Flourie B, Bruley des Varannes S, *et al*. Relations between transit time, fermentation products, and hydrogen consuming flora in healthy humans. *Gut* 1996 ; 38 : 870-7.

9. Rambaud JC, Bouhnik Y, Marteau P, *et al*. Manipulation of the human gut microflora. *Proc Nutr Soc* 1993 ; 52 : 357-66.

10. Bouhnik Y, Pochart P, Marteau P, *et al*. Fecal recovery in humans of viable *Bifidobacterium sp* ingested in fermented milk. *Gastroenterology* 1992; 102 : 875-8.

11. Bartram HP, Scheppach W, Gerlach S, *et al*. Does yogurt enriched with Bifidobacterium longum affect colonic microbiology and fecal metabolites in health subjects? *Am J Clin Nutr* 1994 ; 59 : 428-32.

12. Bougle D, Roland N, Lebeurrier F, *et al*. Effect of propionibacteria supplementation on fecal bifidobacteria and segmental colonic transit time in healthy human subjects. *Scand J Gastroenterol* 1999 ; 34 :144-8.

13. Marteau P, Cuillerier E, Meance S, *et al*. Bifidobacterium animalis strain DN-173 010 shortens the colonic transit time in healthy women: a double-blind, randomized, controlled study. *Aliment Pharmacol Ther* 2002 ; 16 : 587-93.

14. Gibson GR, Beatty ER, Wang X, *et al*. Selective stimulation of bifidobacteria in the human colon by oligofructose and inulin. *Gastroenterology* 1995 ; 108 : 975-82.

15. Guedon C, Ducrotte P, Antoine JM, *et al*. Does chronic supplementation of the diet with dietary fibre extracted from pea or carrot affect colonic motility in man? *Br J Nutr* 1996 ; 76 : 51-61.

16. Barrow L, Steed KP, Spiller RC, *et al*. Scintigraphic demonstration of lactulose-induced accelerated proximal colon transit. *Gastroenterology* 1992 ; 103 : 1167-73.

17. Cuillerier E, Coffin B, Lémann M, *et al*. Comparaison de l'effet du lactulose et du polyéthylène glycol sur le transit colique isotopique. *Gastroenterol Clin Biol* 1999, 23 : A157.

18. Jouët P, Gorbatchef C, Flourié B, *et al*. Colonic fermentation of lactulose produces a tonic contraction in the human colon. *Gastroenterology* 1998, 114 : A 773.

19. Herve S, Leroi AM, Mathiex-Fortunet H, *et al*. Effects of polyethylene glycol 4000 on 24-h manometric recordings of left colonic motor activity. *Eur J Gastroenterol Hepatol* 2001 ; 13(6) : 647-54.

20. Jouët P, Gorbatchef C, Flourié B, *et al*. Colonic fermentation of starch increases propulsive activity in the human colon. *Gastroenterology* 1997 ; 112 : A756 (resumen).

21. Gorbatchef C, Jouët P, Flourié B, *et al*. Effects of short-chain fatty acids on the phasic and tonic motor activity in the unprepared colon of healthy humans. *Gastroenterology* 1998, 114 : A 756 (resumen).

22. Cherbut C, Ferrier L, Roze C, *et al*. Short-chain fatty acids modify colonic motility through nerves and polypeptide YY release in the rat. *Am J Physiol* 1998 ; 275 : G1415-22.

23. Coffin B, Lemann M, Flourie B, *et al*. Local regulation of ileal tone in healthy humans. *Am J Physiol* 1997 ; 272 : G147-53.

24. Ropert A, Cherbut C, Roze C, *et al*. Colonic fermentation and proximal gastric tone in humans. *Gastroenterology* 1996 ; 111 : 289-96.

25. Nightingale JM, Kamm MA, van der Sijp Jr, *et al.* Disturbed gastric emptying in the short bowel syndrome. Evidence for a « colonic brake ». *Gut* 1993 ; 34 : 1171-6.

26. Piche T, Zerbib F, Bruley des Varannes S, *et al.* Modulation by colonic fermentation of LES function in humans. *Am J Physiol Gastrointest Liver Physiol* 2000 ; 278 : G578-84.

27. Piche T, Bruley des Varannes S, Sacher-Huvelin S, *et al.* Colonic fermentation influences lower esophageal sphincter function in gastroesophageal reflux disease.*Gastroenterology.* 2003 ;124 : 894-902.

28. Drossman DA, Camilleri M, Mayer EA, *et al.* AGA technical review on irritable bowel syndrome. *Gastroenterology* 2002 ; 123 : 2108-31.

29. Neal KR, Hebden J, Spiller R. Prevalence of gastrointestinal symptoms six months after bacterial gastroenteritis and risk factors for development of the irritable bowel syndrome: postal survey of patients. *Br Med J* 1997 ; 314 : 779-82.

30. Rodriguez LA, Ruigomez A. Increased risk of irritable bowel syndrome after bacterial gastroenteritis: cohort study. *Br Med J* 1999 ; 318 : 565-6.

31. Bergin AJ, Donnelly TC, McKendrick MW, *et al.* Changes in anorectal function in persistent bowel disturbances following salmonella gastroenteritis. *Eur J Gastroenterol Hepatol* 1993 ; 5 : 617-20.

32. Spiller RC, Jenkins D, Thornley JP, *et al.* Increased rectal mucosal enteroendocrine cells, T lymphocytes, and increased gut permeability following acute *Campylobacter* enteritis and in post-dysenteric irritable bowel syndrome. *Gut* 2000 ; 47 : 804-11.

33. O'Sullivan M, Clayton N, Breslin NP, *et al.* Increased mast cells in the irritable bowel syndrome. *Neurogastroenterol Motil* 2000 ; 12 : 449-57.

34. Tornblom H, Lindberg G, Nyberg B, *et al.* Full-thickness biopsy of the jejunum reveals inflammation and enteric neuropathy in irritable bowel syndrome. *Gastroenterology* 2002; 123 : 1972-9.

35. Newcomer AD, Park HS, O'Brien PC, *et al.* Response of patients with irritable bowel syndrome and lactase deficiency using unfermented acidophilus milk. *Am J Clin Nutr* 1983; 38 : 257-63.

36. Di Baise JK, Lof J, Taylor K, *et al. Lactobacillus plantarum* 299v in the irritable bowel syndrome: a randomized, double-blind, placebo-controlled crossover study. *Gastroenterology* 2000 ; 118 : A615 (résumé).

37. Niedzielin K, Kordecki H, Birkenfeld B. A controlled, double-blind, randomized study on the efficacy of *Lactobacillus plantarum* 299V in patients with irritable bowel syndrome. *Eur J Gastroenterol Hepatol* 2001 ; 13 : 1143-7.

38. Halpern GM, Prindiville T, Blankenburg M, *et al.* Treatment of irritable bowel syndrome with Lacteol Fort: a randomized, double-blind, cross-over trial. *Am J Gastroenterol* 1996; 91 : 1579-85.

39. Maupas JL, Champemont P, Delforge M. Traitement des colopathies fonctionnelles. Essais en double aveugle de l'Ultra-levure. *Méd Chir Dig* 1983 : 77-9.

40. O'Sullivan MA, O'Morain CA. Bacterial supplementation in the irritable bowel syndrome. A randomised double-blind placebo-controlled crossover study. *Dig Liver Dis* 2000; 32 : 294-301.

41. Lasser RB, Bond JH, Levitt MD. The role of intestinal gas in functional abdominal pain. *N Engl J Med* 1975 ; 293 : 524-6.

42. Serra J, Azpiroz F, Malagelada JR. Impaired transit and tolerance of intestinal gas in the irritable bowel syndrome. *Gut* 2001; 48 : 14-9.

43. King TS, Elia M, Hunter JO. Abnormal colonic fermentation in irritable bowel syndrome. *Lancet* 1998 ; 352 : 1187-9.

44. Nobaek S, Johansson ML, Molin G, *et al.* Alteration of intestinal microflora is associated with reduction in abdominal bloating and pain in patients with irritable bowel syndrome. *Am J Gastroenterol* 2000 ; 95 : 1231-8.

45. Hebden JM, Blackshaw E, D'Amato M, *et al.* Abnormalities of GI transit in bloated irritable bowel syndrome: effect of bran on transit and symptoms. *Am J Gastroenterol* 2002 ; 97 : 2315-20.

46. Francis CY, Whorwell PJ. Bran and irritable bowel syndrome: time for reappraisal. *Lancet* 1994 ; 344 : 39-40.

Gut Microflora and the Colonic Epithelium

Claire Cherbuy,
Hervé Blottière,
Pierre-Henri Duée

Institut National de la
Recherche Agronomique,
Unité de Nutrition
et Sécurité Alimentaire,
Domaine de Vilvert,
CRJ,
Jouy-en-Josas, France.

The colonic epithelium is a dynamic structure and its turnover rate is one of the highest in the body. The presence of a complex bacterial microflora in the large intestine is a key determinant of its environment. In practice, one of the microflora's main functions is to break down food which has escaped digestion in the small intestine and endogenous substrates; these bacterial fermentation processes generate many metabolites, including butyrate, one of the short-chain fatty acids (SCFA), which represents the main energy substrate of the colonic epithelium. By virtue of its diversity, largely linked to that of the substrates, the colonic microflora is a rich source of signals which affect the host's physiology; a relationship approaching symbiosis follows on from this, and compromise of this relationship could constitute a factor that promotes the installation of pathological situations.

Structure and turnover of the colonic epithelium

The organisation of the colonic epithelium is very structured and hierarchical:
- crypt epithelium, a sort of deep depression in which the epithelium sinks down into the underlying tissue (the *lamina propria*);
- surface epithelium which borders the flat part of the mucosa of the luminal side (Figure 1).

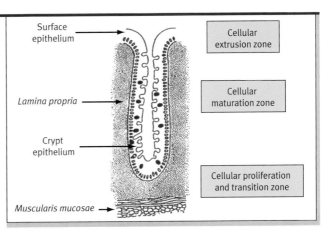

Figure 1.
Schematic drawing of a colonic crypt. The proliferative zone is localized in the basal part of the crypt. Dividing cells are derived from the proliferation of stem cells. The cells, which cease dividing in the upper part of the crypt, migrate towards the surface epithelium where they are shed. In the course of migration, the cell differentiates and acquires novel morphological and functional characteristics

Surface epithelium — Cellular extrusion zone

Lamina propria — Cellular maturation zone

Crypt epithelium

Cellular proliferation and transition zone

Muscularis mucosae

Studies based on labelling with tritiated thymidine (which becomes incorporated into proliferating cells) have shown that the lower part of the crypt is composed of dividing cells, derived from stem cells and multiplying for five to nine cycles. In mice, it has been estimated that each colonic crypt contains about one hundred dividing cells and produces about ten cells per hour.

The cells migrate rapidly from the base of the crypt towards the surface epithelium. They cease dividing in the upper part of the crypt and are exfoliated into the colonic lumen. This migration along the axis of the crypt is coupled with the process of cell differentiation, characterized by morphological and functional changes. In mice, the lifetime of mature absorbing cells is three days. Table I summarizes the dynamics of turnover of the colonic epithelium in mice and humans, showing that in these two species, the proliferative capacity is high [1].

	Mouse	Human	
			Table I.
Cells per crypt	300-450	2 250	Dynamics of cell turnover in the colonic
Duration of cell cycle	15-36 h	36-96 h	epithelium in humans
Number of stem cells per crypt	1-4	?	and mice (taken from [1])

In a healthy adult, maintenance of epithelial homeostasis depends on a finely regulated balance between the number of cells produced on the one hand and the number eliminated on the other. When this equilibrium is perturbed, the integrity of the colonic epithelium is lost.

Differentiated cells of the colonic epithelium

In the colonic epithelium, the following three main types of cells are present:

- absorbing cells or colonocytes: these are the most abundant (accounting for about 80% of the cells). These cells are mainly responsible for the transport of electrolytes and SCFAs generated by colonic fermentation. They are polarised cells. They have an asymmetrical, cellular organisation with distinct apical and basolateral membrane domains. The two poles differ, in particular with respect to their content in terms of specific proteins, such as ion transporters;
- mucous cells: these synthesize and secrete the mucus which lines the wall of the colon and protects the epithelium against physical and chemical insults;
- entero-endocrine cells: these represent less than 3% of epithelial cells. These cells specialize in the secretion of gastrointestinal peptides (somatostatin, enteroglucagon, peptide YY, etc.).

Colonic crypt stem cells

It is now established that the differentiated cell types of the colonic epithelium derive from a single cellular precursor, the colonic crypt stem cell [2, 3]. The absence of specific markers for these cells currently restricts their study. The localization of stem cells was determined by the team of Potten in Manchester (Great Britain) from the results of tritiated thymidine incorporation experiments [2]. According to the data obtained, stem cells would be confined to the base of the crypts. Stem cells correspond to a small population of cells, defined by the following set of criteria:
- undifferentiated cells with the capacity to proliferate;
- cells capable of maintaining themselves at a constant number;
- pluripotent cells which can give rise to different types of differentiated epithelial cells;
- cells which can regenerate tissue when the epithelium has been damaged.

The number of stem cells per crypt is not known (Table I). In a healthy epithelium, this number is kept stationary, probably by a process of asymmetric division, i.e., one of the daughter cells proceeds along the differentiation pathway while the other remains a stem cell. However, this capacity of cells to undergo asymmetric division (i.e. restore the stocks of stem cells) disappears soon after migration has begun towards the epithelial surface.

In any case, profound understanding of the cells which give rise to the crypt cell population is essential because any genetic damage affecting these cells is transmitted to the daughter cells.

In this context, the team of Gordon at the University of Saint Louis (United States) has worked in chimeric animals whose cells either contain or do not contain a gene encoding an easily identifiable marker (β-galactosidase) [4, 5]. After histochemical staining, the data obtained showed that the colonic crypts are exclusively composed of either cells that were positive for β-galactosidase expression, or negative cells. In no case were any colonic crypts "mosaics", i.e., composed of two different cell populations. These preliminary results suggested therefore that the entire cell population of the colonic crypt would be derived from a single stem cell [4, 5]. Nevertheless, this hypothesis is still controversial and others have been proposed, in particular one based on competition between stem cells [2].

Regulation of cell number by apoptosis

Cell loss is also a key factor in maintaining tissue homeostasis. Apoptosis is an active form of cell death which involves a set of mechanisms acting in a cascade and leading to the destruction of damaged cells.

Such a process, pre-programmed or triggered by specific factors, could be involved in the loss of surface epithelial cells. In practice, analysis of apoptotic cells by studying DNA fragmentation (the TUNEL method) shows that apoptosis does indeed occur at this site. Moreover, the expression of *bax*, a pro-apoptotic gene, in the region of the surface epithelium is also indicative of some form of apoptosis at this site (Figure 2) [2].

Nevertheless, these findings are not supported by electron microscopy in which only very rare apoptotic cells can be identified [2]. The mechanisms leading to the physiological elimination of surface cells remain therefore controversial.

A process of spontaneous apoptosis has also been reported in the basal part of crypts [6]. This could be associated with regulation of the number of cells in division. However, in this zone of cell proliferation, spontaneous apoptosis seems to be tightly controlled, in particular by the anti-apoptotic gene *bcl-2* (Figure 2). In practice, expression of this gene is high at this location. Moreover, in mice in which the *bcl-2* gene had been knocked out, a higher frequency of spontaneous apoptosis was observed than in wild-type mice [6]. Thus, the product of the *bcl-2* gene could contribute to protecting stem cells of the colon from excessive apoptosis induced, for example, by toxins present in this area of the gastrointestinal tract or derived from the bacterial microflora [2]. Nevertheless, it could allow the survival of cells in which certain genes are mutated, possibly leading, in this case, to a process of tumorigenesis.

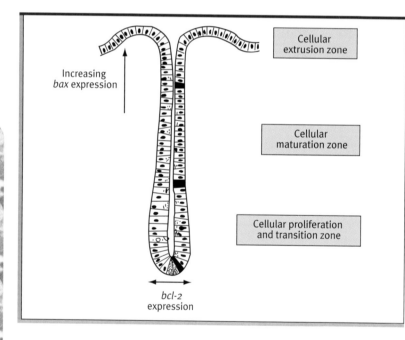

Increasing
bax expression

Cellular
extrusion zone

Cellular
maturation zone

Cellular proliferation
and transition zone

bcl-2
expression

Figure 2.
*Expression of pro-
and anti-apoptotic
genes along
the colonic epithelium.
The expression of bax
(a pro-apoptotic gene)
follows a gradient
increasing towards
the top of the crypts.
The expression of bcl-2
(an anti-apoptotic gene)
is high in the basal part
of the colonic crypts
(taken from [2])*

Differentiation of absorbing cells

One of the main functions of the large intestine is to regulate the volume and electrolyte composition of the faeces [7]. At this site, in practice, the reabsorption of water and electrolytes (sodium and chloride) is observed as well as the secretion of potassium and bicarbonate. Most of these ion movements involve energy-dependent, active transport systems [7] (Figure 3).

Gradually, as the cells migrate towards the surface epithelium, they commit to a process of cellular differentiation. This maturation results in changes, both morphological (presence of microvilli on the apical membrane, appearance of the rectangular shape of the cells, loss of the vacuoles seen in the crypt cells) and functional (expression of transporters which give rise to the transepithelial movement of electrolytes, cellular polarisation with distinct apical and basolateral domains). Thus, there is a spatial distribution of transporters along the axis of the crypt.

Na^+/H^+ exchangers (NHE) are proteins involved in transepithelial sodium absorption and also in the regulation of cell pH and volume [8]. Among the various isoforms identified, cloned and sequenced thus far, some (NHE1, NHE2 and NHE3) are expressed in the epithelial cells of the colon [8]. It should be noted that NHE3, which plays a major role in sodium absorption, is abundantly present in the apical membrane of surface epithelial cells. Nevertheless, recent results suggest that sodium absorption is not exclusively localized in the surface cells since a new member of the NHE family was just identified in cells deep down in the crypts.

Other transporters also have an expression pattern which follows the gradient of cell differentiation, whether they are expressed at the apical pole (the transporters responsible for the absorption of chloride or that for SCFAs) [9] or the basolateral pole (potassium transport) [7].

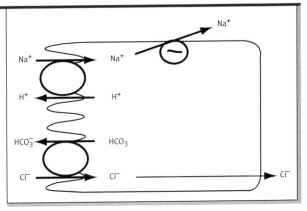

Figure 3.
Transport systems expressed in differentiated colon cells: example of transporters involved in Na^+ and Cl^- absorption. The absorption of Na^+ and Cl^- is coupled by virtue of two transporters: a Na^+/H^+ exchanger and a $Cl^-HCO_3^-$ exchanger. These two transporters are localized in the apical colonocyte membrane. The transport of electrolytes across the basolateral membrane involves other transporters (taken from [7])

Molecular and cellular mechanisms controlling turnover of the colonic epithelium

Homeostasis of the colonic epithelium is controlled by complex cellular and molecular mechanisms involving growth factors, transcription factors and molecules found in the extracellular matrix. Numerous interactions between these various proteins participate in the regulation of the population of cells in the crypt.

The complexity of the mechanisms involved, clearly illustrated by Hermiston *et al.* [10], could also lead to distinguishing specific factors varying according to the position occupied by the cell in the crypt. In particular, the factors controlling the fate of stem cells could be different from those identified in the regulation of daughter cells [2].

The consequence of abnormalities affecting these mechanisms is perturbation of the equilibrium existing between cell proliferation, differentiation and elimination. The loss of function conferred by key genes leads to disorganisation of the epithelium or, in more serious situations, to pathology. Thus, among these mechanisms, the "actors" involved in the transduction pathway of the Wnt signal play a key role: inactivation of effectors in this pathway, secondary to mutation of the corresponding genes, is an early event appearing in the development of colon cancer and notably in most hereditary cancers associated with familial adenomatous polyposis due to mutation of the *APC* gene [11].

This Wnt signal transduction pathway (which has been remarkably conserved through evolution) is involved in embryonic development in species from drosophila to the vertebrates. Activation of the Wnt signal transduction pathway leads to the formation of a transcription complex, including β-catenin and the Tcf-4 nuclear transcription factor (Figure 4), the target genes of which are involved in cell proliferation.

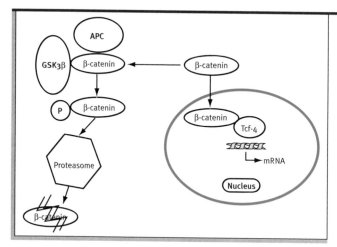

Figure 4.
Transduction pathway of the Wnt signal. The intracellular concentration of β-catenin, a partner of the transcription factor Tcf-4, is tightly controlled by a cytoplasmic protein complex including, in particular, the APC (adenomatous polyposis coli) protein and GSK3β (glycogen synthase kinase-3 β). Phosphorylation of β-catenin by GSK3β tags it for breakdown in the proteasome. Therefore, when the Wnt signal transduction pathway is turned on, this protein complex is destabilized and β-catenin then associates with the Tcf-4 transcription factor

Thus, in mice in which the gene encoding Tcf-4 has been knocked out, the intestinal epithelium has no proliferative compartment and is composed of only non-proliferating, differentiated cells [12]. These mice die soon after birth. The intracellular concentration of β-catenin, a partner of the Tcf-4 factor, is itself tightly regulated by a cytoplasmic, protein complex involving, in particular, the APC (adenomatous polyposis coli) protein and GSK3β (glycogen synthase kinase-3β). Phosphorylation by GSK3β of β-catenin directs it towards breakdown in the proteasome (Figure 4). By "sequestering" β-catenin in this complex and, in consequence, preventing the latter from binding Tcf-4, the APC protein acts as a negative regulator of cell proliferation.

The role of the β-catenin/Tcf-4 transcription complex has been elucidated in colon tumour cell lines in which the β-catenin/Tcf-4 complex is constitutively expressed [13]. The activity of the transcription complex (analysed by the expression and localization of genes under its control) can be inhibited by introducing negative dominants. In this case, the over-expressed genes reveal lifting of the inhibition by the β-catenin/Tcf-4 complex; in contrast, those whose expression is inhibited represent genes that are stimulated by the transcription complex. These elegant studies showed that the genes stimulated by the β-catenin/Tcf-4 complex are involved in cell proliferation, and are selectively expressed in the proliferative compartment of the epithelial crypt. Inversely, the genes that are repressed by the β-catenin/Tcf-4 complex are involved in cell differentiation and are expressed towards the top of the crypts. Thus, this β-catenin/Tcf-4 transcription complex orchestrates the transition of colonic epithelial cells from proliferation to differentiation.

In addition, the role of homeotic genes should also be remembered. In vertebrates, these genes which encode transcription factors are related to those which determine the establishment of the anteroposterior axis in the course of embryonic development in drosophila. They share a sequence encoding a DNA-binding region (homeodomain) and are involved in intestinal development in the embryo. The expression of certain homeotic genes in the intestine persists into adulthood, e.g. *cdx2* is expressed in the adult colon, mainly in the proximal part. The role of *cdx2* in the adult colon has not been clearly elucidated. It could play a role in the differentiation of intestinal epithelial cells [14]. In mice in which one of the alleles of the *cdx2* gene has been knocked out, the injection of azoxymethane induces, mainly in the distal part of the colon, a higher frequency of tumours than that observed in wild-type mice [15]: the *cdx2* gene could act therefore as a tumour-suppressor gene.

Effects of bacterial metabolites on the colonic epithelium

In the colon, residual food and constituents of endogenous origin represent the material available for bacterial fermentation (remembering that the bacterial mass rises to 10^{11} bacteria per gram of contents). What do these substrates represent in quantitative terms?

With a normal diet, it is accepted that the amount of lipids reaching the colon every day is small, of the order of a few grams. Concerning the protein fractions and especially the carbohydrate fractions of food, intestinal digestion is variable, in particular depending on the nature of the ingested food (composition, physicochemical structure, processing modalities, etc.).

Thus, protein-derived compounds can represent up to twenty-odd grams per day (half of which comes from food with the rest corresponding to pancreatic enzymes and gastrointestinal secretions). As to carbohydrate compounds, so-called "resistant" starch accounts for 10-40 grams per day, and cell wall material and other plant-derived polysaccharides another 10-20 grams. Although other compounds may be present in the caecum and colon such as minerals, vitamins, trace dietary ingredients, mucins (constitutive glycoproteins of the mucus) and shed epithelial cells, it appears that the bacterial mass draws most of the substrates necessary for its metabolic processes from dietary carbohydrate.

The fermentation of resistant starch and plant-derived polysaccharides leads to the production of gases and SCFAs (acetate, propionate, butyrate). In the distal part of the colon, proteins also give rise to the production of SCFAs as well as branched-chain fatty acids (isobutyrate, isovalerate) and nitrogen-containing compounds (ammonia, amines, polyamines, phenolic compounds). Few fatty acids reach the colon: a fraction is metabolized by the microflora to generate toxic metabolites (hydroxylated fatty acids).

It should be noted that the colonic microflora develops other metabolic pathways, including the metabolism of bile acids (leading to the generation of secondary bile acids after deconjugation and dehydroxylation), the conversion of xenobiotics and the production of mutagenic compounds, secondary to the conversion of nitrates into nitrites: the extent of these metabolic pathways also affects the integrity of the host's epithelium.

Definitively, the final concentration of bacterial metabolites will depend, to a large extent, on the composition of the diet and that of the colonic microflora. For example, the presence of a high content of unfermentable fibre increases the faecal volume and rate of transit, which will lower the concentration of metabolites, including that of toxic metabolites, thereby reducing exposure of the colonic epithelium to these products. In addition, deamination of amino acids leads, in particular, to the production of ammonia, the luminal concentration of which will depend on the equilibrium between synthesis by the microflora, sequestration by the mucosa, and the size of the bacterial mass which uses ammonia in protein synthesis. Finally, it should be remembered that regional differences exist in bacterial fermentation processes. The caecum, and the right or ascending colon house maximal activities associated with strong bacterial growth; the luminal pH here is low. The left, descending or sigmoid colon house fermenting activity of proteolytic nature with high rates of amine and phenol production; the luminal pH here is close to neutral.

Because of its rapid turnover and absorption functions, the energy requirement of the colonic epithelium is high. To cover their needs, colonic epithelial cells have access to SCFAs and nutrients derived from the plasma, such as glucose and glutamine.

Butyrate: a main energy substrate for colonic epithelial cells

At the pH of the colonic lumen, butyrate is found in a dissociated form and the anion does not readily cross cell membranes. Its transport requires, therefore a specific transporter, MCT1, a recently characterized member of the family of monocarboxylate transporters. MCT1 is abundantly present in surface epithelial cells but absent from cells at the base of crypts. Its expression is positively regulated by butyrate itself [16].

Studies conducted on isolated epithelial cells have evaluated the contribution of energy substrates to cellular metabolism. These have revealed a high capacity of colonocytes to metabolize SCFAs, in particular butyrate [17, 18]. Metabolism of this substrate accounts for 70-80% of the consumption of oxygen, suggesting that it might represent the major oxidative substrate for these cells. The remaining 20-30% are provided by other SCFAs as well as glucose and glutamine from the blood. The presence of butyrate inhibits the oxidation of glucose, glutamine and the other SCFAs [18]. In contrast, the production of $^{14}CO_2$ from [1-^{14}C] butyrate, as well as oxygen consumption due to metabolism of this substrate in colonocytes, is not affected by the presence of other nutrients [17, 18]. These findings indicate that butyrate is preferentially used for energy production by colonocytes.

In colonocytes, butyrate metabolism occurs in the mitochondrial compartment. The selective use of butyrate over the other two SCFAs could result from preferential activation in the mitochondria. In practice, there would exist, at this point, two enzymes activating SCFAs: a butyrate-specific enzyme and another enzyme common to all the main SCFAs.

Most of the carbons of butyrate are found in the form of CO_2, but some in the form of ketone bodies, acetoacetate and β-hydroxybutyrate [17]. In other words, butyrate is the main precursor for ketogenesis in colonocytes since this process is relatively low-level with other possible substrates such as long-chain fatty acids or other SCFAs.

The pathways involved in the colonic utilization of butyrate are summarized in Figure 5.

Mitochondrial activation of butyrate generates butyryl-CoA which joins the last steps of the β-oxidation pathway. Acetoacetyl-CoA produces acetyl-CoA which can be used in the Krebs cycle or the ketogenesis pathway. The metabolic pathway involved in the production of ketone bodies from butyrate seems to be the same as that in the liver, i.e., the pathway involving mitochondrial 3-hydroxy-3-methylglutaryl-coenzyme A (HMG-CoA) synthase [19].

The physiological significance of ketone body production from butyrate is not known, although molecules of this type can be used as precursors in the lipogenesis pathway.

Extensive research has addressed the role of SCFAs, and more specifically that of butyrate, in colonocyte proliferation [20]. Two broad sets of findings seem to contradict one another: on the one hand, butyrate exerts a trophic effect on the colonic mucosa *in vivo*; on the other hand, it inhibits the proliferation of tumoural colon cells. Thus, a fibre-depleted diet or parenteral alimentation leads to atrophy of the colonic mucosa in rats. In contrast, the intracolonic infusion of physiological or supra-physiological doses (20-100 mM) of butyrate or other SCFAs reverses atrophy of the colonic mucosa. Sakata & von Engelhardt [21] showed that increases in mitotic index and DNA synthesis in the colon involve not only the colonic epithelium exposed to infused SCFAs but also the unexposed part of the colon. In addition, they showed that the autonomous nervous system is involved. Subsequently, Hass et al. [22] showed that the absence of butyrate induced expression of the pro-apoptotic protein Bax and apoptosis in the colonic epithelium of the guinea pig; this effect was abolished in the presence of a physiological concentration of butyrate (10 mM). In contrast, other studies conducted *in vivo* have yielded contradictory results and it is now generally accepted that butyrate, the preferred energy source in the colonic epithelium, only enhances cell proliferation in situations in which energy sources are limiting. Otherwise, some experiments have indicated that butyrate can stimulate the release of gastrointestinal peptides or growth factors. It also increases the colonic expression of receptors for these trophic factors (as is the case for EGF receptors), and activates the pathways involved in their transduction (as is the case for G proteins). This indirect effect of butyrate can, in certain conditions, modulate turnover of the colonic epithelium.

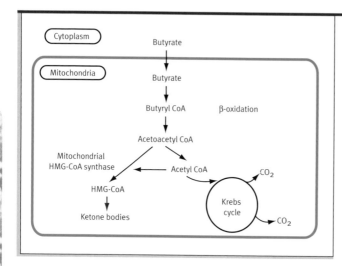

Figure 5.
Metabolic fate of butyrate
in colonocytes.
The mitochondrial activation
of butyrate generates butyryl-CoA
which rejoins the final steps in
the fatty acids β-oxidation pathway.
The acetyl CoA is used in the Krebs
cycle or in the ketogenesis pathway.
The metabolic pathway leading to the
production of ketone bodies involves
mitochondrial 3-hydroxy-3-
methylglutaryl-coenzyme A
(HMG-CoA) synthase

Definitively, in conditions in which the amount of energy available to the cell is not a limiting factor, the action of butyrate *in vivo* and *in vitro* is to inhibit cell proliferation [20]. This inhibition of proliferation has been studied in cell lines derived from human colonic tumours. It seems to be associated with the blockage of cells in the G1 phase of the cell cycle, the phase which is regulated by cyclins D and their cofactors, the cyclin-dependent kinases (cdk-4 and cdk-6) (Figure 6). These kinases phosphorylate the Rb protein, thereby releasing the E2F transcription factor which is involved in the cell cycle. Butyrate induces expression of p21[Cip1], an inhibitor of cyclin-cdk complexes, and strongly stimulates the expression of cyclin D3, a partner of cdk-4 and 6. The key role played by p21^{Cip1} has been demonstrated. Thus, in the absence of this protein (in cells in which p21^{Cip1} has been deleted by homologous recombination), the cells accumulate in G2/M (i.e., no longer in G1), and apoptosis is common. The mechanism leading to this apoptosis has been well characterized. It involves the mitochondrial pathway based on cytochrome c, and over-expression of the pro-apoptotic Bax protein [23, 24]. Butyrate, by inhibiting Class I and Class II histone deacetylases, stimulates the transcription of many genes, including p21^{Cip1}, *bax* and *c-fos*, by acting at their promoters, in particular in the guanosine/cytosine-rich region. The enzymes which modulate histone acetylation (histone acetyl transferase and deacetylase) play a role as factors regulating gene expression. The mechanisms involved are complex and would also involve the action of kinases and phosphatases [25]. Moreover, it seems that the acetylation of certain genes would be necessary to induce the binding of transcription factors. Thus, SCFAs and notably butyrate are molecules that are essential for colonic homeostasis: they act not only as energy sources for colonocytes but also as modulators of the expression of many genes.

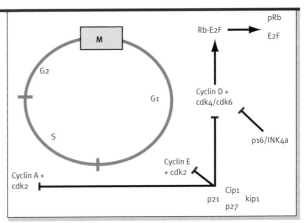

Figure 6.
Control of the transition between the G1 phase and the S phase of the cell cycle. Transition between G1 and S phases involves a whole set of regulatory proteins. It is regulated by the D cyclins and their partners, the cyclin-dependent kinases (cdk-4 and cdk-6). The kinases phosphorylate the Rb protein which releases the E2F transcription factor, involved in progress of the cell cycle. p21^{Cip1} is an inhibitor of cyclin-cdk complexes. Butyrate stimulates p21^{Cip1} expression thereby arresting the cell cycle in G1

Fate of bacterial ammonia

The concentration of ammonia, most of which is derived from the caecal and colonic fermentation of amino acids and nucleic acids, can reach high levels (up to 60-70 mM). Its absorption at the colonic epithelium is coupled to proton flow and it is converted to urea in the liver. Ammonia is a potential toxin for the colonic epithelium: it modifies DNA synthesis and reduces the half-life of cells. Research by Sakata and his team in Japan [26], conducted in rats, showed that the *in situ* infusion of ammonia increased cell proliferation without modifying crypt size, which suggests that ammonia would also stimulate the elimination of colonocytes.

In isolated colonocytes, the addition of ammonia at a concentration of 10 mM reduces cellular utilization of butyrate at a stage upstream of acetyl-CoA generation. At the same time, glycolysis is enhanced [27]. Can these metabolic changes be linked to those concerning turnover of the colonic epithelium? The available data do not make it possible to answer this question.

Hydrogen sulphide is potentially toxic

Hydrogen sulphide (H_2S) is a molecule that can be found at high concentrations in the colonic lumen (0.2-2 mM). It is generated by the reduction of sulphate by sulphate-reducing bacteria, a reaction which uses the hydrogen produced in carbohydrate fermentation. Sulphur-containing amino acids and certain additives can also give rise to H_2S production. Finally, the sulphur in mucins (a fraction of these mucins correspond to sulphated proteins) can become incorporated into H_2S which can be toxic for the colonic epithelium because it acts on cellular respiration (being a potent inhibitor of cytochrome c-oxidase, an enzyme in the electron transfer chain).

One of the metabolic consequences of this effect was illustrated by the team of Roediger in Australia, who detected inhibition of the mitochondrial β-oxidation pathway following the addition of H_2S. In consequence, the oxidation of butyrate is inhibited and, as a result, acyl-CoA derivatives build up [28]. In addition, although there are pathways which detoxify H_2S in the colonic epithelium (methylation of H_2S), Roediger's team defends the hypothesis that the metabolic effects mediated by H_2S would partly explain ulcerative colitis. However, attempts to treat this disease with butyrate enemas have been unsuccessful.

Polyamines and the colonic epithelium

Polyamines (putrescine, spermine, spermidine) play an essential role in the maintenance of colonic homeostasis [29]. In practice, the intracellular polyamine concentration is closely related to the state of growth of epithelial cells. A reduction in intracellular concentrations inhibits growth *in vivo* and *in vitro*. The intracellular polyamine concentration is dependent on dietary intake, bacterial input and patterns of endogenous synthesis. Thus, it has been demonstrated that, when dietary polyamine intake is low, the cytostatic effect of an inhibitor of polyamine synthesis, α-difluoromethylornithine (DFMO) depends on the activity of the colonic microflora. The presence of a colonic microflora, engaged in polyamine synthesis, abolished the DFMO effect [30]. Polyamines stimulate proliferation by acting on progress of the cell cycle. The intracellular polyamine concentration rises during the G1 and S phases of the cell cycle and depletion of polyamines induces blockage in the G1 phase. In addition, a high concentration of polyamines drives the cells towards apoptosis. In contrast, the likelihood of a cell to enter in apoptosis is modulated following a strong reduction in polyamine concentration. One of the underlying mechanisms would involve the transcription factor NFκB. Other molecular mechanisms can account for the effects of polyamines. In this respect, it has been shown that polyamines, *via* interactions with DNA, stabilize the latter and induce its condensation, allowing conformational changes in certain sequences. Polyamines can also modulate interactions between DNA and certain proteins, including polymerases and transcription factors [31]. Finally, polyamines would stabilize cell membranes by reducing their fluidity, and would therefore also act as antioxidants.

In conclusion, these various examples demonstrate that bacterial metabolites act on many targets in the colonic epithelium, sometimes mediating opposing effects. This observation suggests that the interrelationships which exist between these various bacterial metabolites must be taken into account in the analysis of parameters which modulate turnover of the colonic epithelium.

Microbial microflora: effects on the colonic epithelium

Can the effect of modulation of the microbial microflora on metabolism and turnover of the colonic epithelium be studied? This line of research needs the development and control of experimental models for directly investigating the interactions between the host and a complex or simplified microflora.

Models for the study of interactions between the host and the bacterial microflora: animals raised in sterile isolators

Animal models with defined microflora, raised in sterile isolators, provide relevant models for studying interactions between microflora and host (Figure 7).

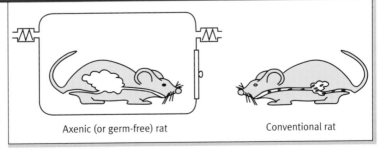

Figure 7. Animal models with defined microflora. The raising process begins with the removal of the uterus from a gravid female and its introduction into a sterile isolator. The germ-free progeny (devoid of microflora) is raised in the isolator for several generations. These environmentally controlled conditions mean that the microflora can be manipulated by inoculating one or more bacterial strains

Axenic (or germ-free) rat   Conventional rat

The raising process begins with the removal of a gravid female uterus and its introduction into a sterile isolator. The germ-free (i.e., devoid of microflora) progeny is raised in the isolator for several generations. These breeding conditions, under environmentally controlled conditions, also make it possible to manipulate the microflora by inoculating one or more bacterial strains (gnotoxenic animals). Axenic animals can also be inoculated with a microflora from conventionally raised counterparts, thereby making them conventional.

This strategy, based on studying animals with a defined microflora, has allowed us to gain a better understanding of the interactions between the bacterial microflora and the host's intestinal epithelium, as well as of some of the underlying mechanisms.

Adaptations of the colonic epithelium in the absence of microflora and the role of short-chain fatty acids

Colonic epithelial structure and turnover are different in axenic animals (Figure 8).

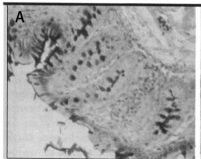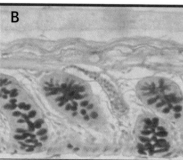

Figure 8.
Transverse sections of the colonic mucosa: a conventional rat (A) and an axenic rat (B) (photographed by J.-C. Meslin, INRA, Jouy-en-Josas)

In the absence of microflora, there is marked hypoplasia of the colonic mucosa [32]. The number of cells per crypt is reduced by about 20% in the axenic animal compared with the conventional animal. The rate of cell production per crypt is slower and this can lead to a daily differential corresponding to about fifty cells. Finally, the duration of the cell cycle is longer in axenic animals (66 *versus* 50 hours in conventional animals) and the number of crypt cells in axenic animals is smaller [32]. Epithelial turnover appears therefore to be slower in the absence of microflora. Studies in which three SCFAs were administered have been performed in axenic animals [33] and the results indicate that SCFAs stimulate the proliferation of colonic crypt cells. The effect of butyrate dominated those of the other two SCFAs. As discussed above, this SCFA activity reflects the effect of adequate energy intake, essential for renewal of the colonic epithelium.

Modifications in the metabolic capacities of colonocytes are also observed in the absence of microflora [19]. Metabolic capacities have been studied in isolated colonocytes from axenic or conventional animals incubated *in vitro* in the presence of various substrates. These results demonstrate that the capacity to metabolize butyrate is conserved in colonocytes from axenic animals. However, the production of ketone bodies is reduced in these cells (Figure 9A). This reduced ketogenic capacity is accompanied by lower expression of mitochondrial HMG-CoA synthase, an enzyme involved in colonic ketogenesis (Figure 9B). In contrast, the capacity to utilize glutamine is increased in colonocytes from axenic animals (Figure 9C) which could be explained by elevated glutaminase activity (the first enzyme involved in glutamine utilization) in these cells. Recent results suggest that the enhancement of glutaminase activity in colonocytes from axenic animals could be linked to an increase in the number of messenger RNA molecules encoding this enzyme [34].

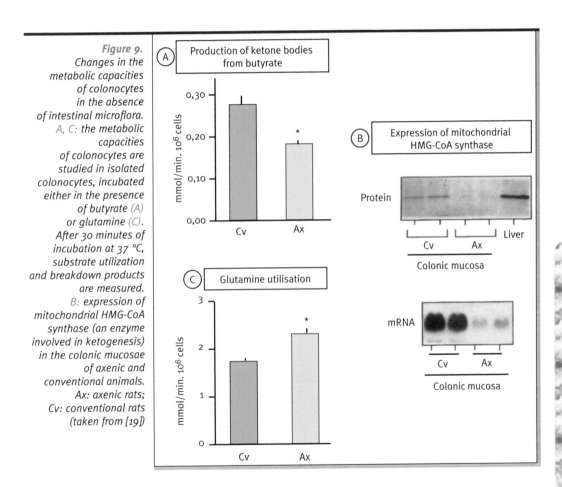

Figure 9. Changes in the metabolic capacities of colonocytes in the absence of intestinal microflora. A, C: the metabolic capacities of colonocytes are studied in isolated colonocytes, incubated either in the presence of butyrate (A) or glutamine (C). After 30 minutes of incubation at 37 °C, substrate utilization and breakdown products are measured. B: expression of mitochondrial HMG-CoA synthase (an enzyme involved in ketogenesis) in the colonic mucosae of axenic and conventional animals. Ax: axenic rats; Cv: conventional rats (taken from [19])

These findings show that, in the absence of microflora and as a result, in the absence of bacterial metabolites, one of the butyrate utilization pathways is reduced. In contrast, the capacity to utilize glutamine, a nutrient of vascular origin, is increased. These changes in the capacities of colonocytes to utilize these two molecules would involve regulation of the expression of the two enzymes which are crucial for their metabolism. It should be noted that these results also suggest that glutamine might represent an energy substrate for the colonocyte, compensating for the absence of SCFAs. However, despite this enhanced capacity to utilize glutamine, turnover of the epithelium is slower in axenic animals, suggesting that the availability of circulating glutamine is not sufficient for optimal cell renewal [19].

Other more specific data support a role of butyrate, the presence of which could explain certain effects induced by the inoculation of microbial microflora [34].

Axenic animals were inoculated with *Clostridium paraputrificum*, a bacterial strain which selectively produces butyrate. In colonized animals, the expression of mitochondrial HMG-CoA synthase stabilized at a level identical to that observed in conventional animals (Figure 10).

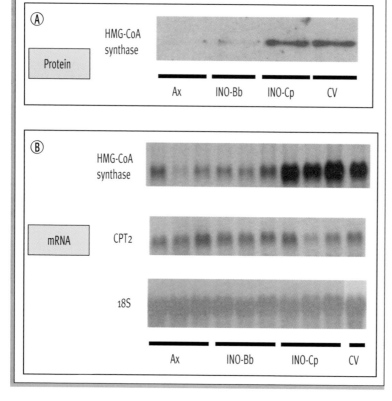

Figure 10.
Regulation of mitochondrial HMG-CoA synthase expression in the colonic mucosa: is butyrate involved? Axenic animals were inoculated with Clostridium paraputrificum (a bacterium that produces butyrate) or Bifidobacterium breve (which does not produce butyrate) and sacrificed three weeks later. HMG-CoA synthase expression was analysed by Western (A) and Northern (B) blotting. B : CPT2 and 18S are used as controls.
Ax: axenic rats;
CV: conventional rats;
INO-Cp: inoculated with Clostridium paraputrificum;
INO-Bb: inoculated with Bifidobacterium breve (taken from [34])

In contrast, when the animals were inoculated with *Bifidobacterium breve*, a strain which does not produce butyrate, the expression of mitochondrial HMG-CoA synthase remained identical to that observed in the untreated axenic animals (Figure 10). Butyrate could therefore modulate the expression of an enzyme involved in both its own metabolism and that of an enzyme involved in the metabolism of a nutrient of vascular origin. This dual butyrate activity, mimicking the effect of the inoculation of a complex microflora, points to the importance of bacterial metabolism in the functioning of the colonic epithelium.

Flora and modulation of gene expression

By studying gene expression profiles in the distal small intestines of axenic and conventional mice using DNA chip-based methods, a recent study extended our understanding of the role of the colonic microflora in the functioning of the intestinal epithelium [35]. The data obtained indicate that the bacterial microflora is able to modulate many aspects of the host's intestinal physiology. This research showed that the absence of microflora is accompanied by increases or decreases in the expression of about one hundred genes. These encode for proteins involved in:
- transport of nutrients (e.g., lipids, carbohydrates and iron) and the metabolism of enzymes involved in cellular energy production;
- epithelial barrier function;
- responses to hormones;
- composition of the extracellular matrix;
- signal transduction pathways.

The effects of different bacterial strains on the expression of target genes have been investigated and gene expression profiles differ according to the bacterial strain inoculated [35]. Thus, the intestine has specific responses to a given type of bacterium, drawing attention to the difficulty in analysing the role of a complex microflora in epithelial functioning and turnover.

Existence of a partnership—approaching a symbiotic relationship—between the bacterial microflora and the host's intestinal epithelium

The production of fucosylated glycoconjugates in enterocytes is a marker of intestinal maturation in the course of development. These glycoconjugates are also used by intestinal bacteria as a source of nutrients or as receptors for bacterial adhesins. They represent, therefore, a useful target for the study of interactions between the bacterial microflora and the host's intestinal epithelium. These experiments, carried out by the Gordon team at the University of Saint Louis (United States), reveal, by way of the example of glycoconjugate production, dynamic interactions between the two partners, microflora and epithelium. Ultimately, these interactions could allow certain bacteria to create an environment which is favourable to their own establishment [1, 36, 37].

In the distal part of the murine small intestine, fucosylated glycoconjugates (Fucα_1,2Galβ) appear in the crypts and villi in a sparse pattern between 17 and 21 days after birth. On day 21, expression of these glycoconjugates spreads to all ileal enterocytes and is sustained throughout at least the first year of life [38].

In the axenic mouse, the early stages of the production of glycoconjugate compounds are unaffected. However, as of day 21 and in contrast to what is seen in the conventional mouse, glycoconjugate production wanes to disappear completely [38]. When axenic animals are inoculated with the microflora from conventional mice, glycoconjugate production is induced and reaches the level seen in conventional animals. These induction events are associated with stimulation of the expression of α 1,2-fucosyltransferase, an enzyme involved in the synthesis of fucosylated, glycoconjugated compounds [38].

The role of *Bacteroides thetaiotaomicron,* a bacterium of the intestinal microflora in both mice and humans, in glycoconjugate production has also been investigated [38]. A strain was chosen that metabolizes diverse carbohydrates, including fucose which can come from both the host and dietary sources. When axenic animals were inoculated with this strain of *Bacteroides thetaiotaomicron*, the spatial and temporal profile of glycoconjugate production, and more particularly (Fucα_1,2Galβ), observed in the conventional animal was restored. In contrast, when animals were inoculated with a strain of *Bacteroides thetaiotaomicron* incapable of utilizing fucose, there was no induction of glycoconjugate production. These last findings suggest that there is a link between the capacity of bacteria to utilize fucose and their capacity to induce glycoconjugate production in the host.

The analysis of various mutants of *Bacteroides thetaiotaomicron* has shed light on the mechanisms underlying the action of this bacterium with respect to glycoconjugate production by the host [39]. This study revealed the existence of a protein, called FucR, which appears to coordinate both the enzymes of fucose metabolism in the bacterium and the "signal" molecule sent to the host to induce glycoconjugate production. The activity of FucR is itself regulated by fucose. In the absence of fucose, FucR represses the synthesis of the enzymes of fucose metabolism and stimulates synthesis of the "signal" molecule. In the presence of fucose, the activity of FucR is inhibited: expression of the enzymes of fucose metabolism is stimulated whereas that of the "signal" molecule is inhibited. Thus, according to the availability of fucose, initially derived from the host, FucR could orchestrate bacterial metabolism as well as glycoconjugate production by enterocytes.

All these data point to interactions between the bacteria of the microflora and intestinal epithelial cells. These interactions would involve—in response to environmental factors—the secretion of bacterial "signal" molecules capable of modulating the expression of target genes in the intestinal epithelium (Figure 11). The nature of these "signal" molecules, the existence of specific receptors at the epithelium, and the signal transduction pathways largely remain to be elucidated.

Thus, manipulation of the colonic microflora results in modification of metabolism in the colonic epithelium. Applying these findings with a view to preventing colonic pathology has been addressed over the last few years and this will be discussed hereafter.

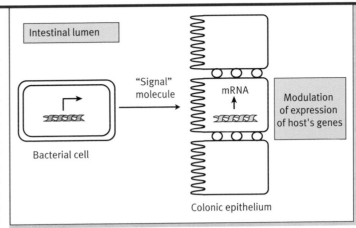

Figure 11.
Model of interactions between the bacterial microflora and the host's colonic epithelium. Interactions between the bacterial microflora and the host's colonic epithelium could involve the secretion of bacterial "signal" molecules capable of modulating host target gene expression. These interactions could constitute one of the molecular bases of the partnership which exists between the bacterial microflora and the colonic epithelium. The nature of the "signal" molecules, the existence of specific receptors on the epithelial tissue, signal transduction pathways and the nature of the target genes remain largely unelucidated

Can the intestinal microflora modulate the risk of colon cancer?

In France, colon cancer represents one of the most deadly diseases. The tumoural colonic epithelium is characterized by increased proliferative and metastatic capacities associated with diminished apoptotic phenomena. These changes reflect serial damage to multiple genes, either tumour suppressor or oncogene activator genes. This damage could be the consequence of high-level exposure to carcinogenic compounds. In practice, currently, only a small percentage of cases of colon cancer can be considered as true genetic diseases with precise familial and hereditary characteristics (familial adenomatous polyposis and other hereditary forms of cancer involving the colon). However, carcinogenesis is sometimes under the influence of a genetic predisposition which, taken alone, can prove insufficient to lead to complete progression of the tumoural process. The development of a malignancy, under the influence of the pro- and/or anticarcinogenic effects of numerous environmental factors, is a complex process which does not boil down to a few mutations or gene deletions. Neoplastic cells are in practice subject to the opposing actions of various factors, either stimulating the proliferation process or, in contrast, committing the cell to the apoptotic pathway. The balance between these various factors also constitutes a key parameter in tumour promotion and progression.

The data reviewed above indicate that the microflora and the production of bacterial metabolites (hydrogen sulphide, ammonia, polyamines, etc.) can play a role in the development of colonic tumours. The conversion of procarcinogens to carcinogens can involve exogenous agents derived from the diet and endogenous agents. Among these, secondary bile acids — generated by the colonic conversion of primary bile acids by bacterial 7 α-dehydroxylase — seem to induce hyperproliferation of the colonic epithelium and to promote the development of colonic tumours after chemical induction in animals [40]. The reduction of nitrobenzene, the products of the hydrolysis of glucuronide compounds, the conversion of nitrates to nitrites, derivatives of the bacterial catabolism of amino acids or the synthesis of potent mutagenic metabolites (e.g. fecapentenes) imply an active role of the microflora in tumour promotion [41]. On the other hand, the bacterial synthesis of protective factors (notably butyrate) from carbohydrate and/or protein substrates contributes to the protective role of the microflora towards cancer.

Bacterial colonization of the colon can constitute a risk factor for colon cancer

Rats exposed to various carcinogenic substances develop fewer neoplastic foci in the colon if they are maintained in axenic conditions [40], probably pointing to a role of the metabolic activity of the microflora in the generation of toxic metabolites. In addition, if the compositions of the faecal microfloras of different groups of subjects at different levels of risk for colon cancer are compared, high risks are associated with the presence of certain bacterial species (*Bacteroides vulgatus* and *Bacteroides stercoris*), and lower risks with the presence of *Lactobacillus acidiphilus, Lactobacillus SO6* and *Eubacterium aerofaciens* [42].

Finally, it is known that polyamine levels are higher in colon tumour tissue than that in healthy tissue, and this can be correlated with increased ornithine decarboxylase (ODC) activity in colonic cells. *In vitro*, the fact that the inhibition of ODC by DFMO leads to the arrest of tumour growth clearly illustrates the importance of polyamines in colon cancer. However, *in vivo*, the use of DFMO on its own has no effect and it is necessary, on the one hand to co-administer an antibiotic (to reduce bacterial polyamine synthesis) and, on the other to switch to a low-polyamine diet [43]. In this situation, the colonic microflora (or certain bacterial strains) mediates adverse effects at the colonic epithelium.

Beneficial modulation of the microbial microflora in the prevention of colon cancer: role of probiotics

The demonstration of a beneficial role of certain bacterial strains in the reduction of the risk of colon cancer [44] supports the taxonomic data discussed above. Thus, in animal models in which foci of abnormal crypts are induced by chemical means, it has been clearly shown that strains of lactic bacilli (*Lactobacillus acidophilus, Streptococcus thermophilus, Bifidobacterium breve*) mediate a protective effect. This is detected by a reduction in DNA damage or in the number of foci of abnormal crypts, i.e. neoplastic lesions from which an adenoma may develop. Can results obtained in animal models be extrapolated to human? Ingestion of *Lactobacillus* by healthy volunteers seems to reduce, in the short term, the mutagenic character of faeces, determined in situations in which large quantities of meat are consumed. However, the epidemiological data on the relationship between the consumption of fermented dairy products and the prevalence of colon cancer are inconsistent and need to be further consolidated.

In any case, the mechanisms whereby lactic bacteria could reduce the risk of colon cancer remain, to date, unknown. The possibilities proposed involve either a modulatory effect of physicochemical parameters in the colon (reduced pH which restricts bacterial growth, inactivation of mutagenic compounds) or modulation of the metabolic activities of the intestinal microflora and, more precisely, either those which release carcinogenic compounds in the colonic lumen (e.g. β-glucuronidase which can hydrolyse glucuronides) or, inversely, those which release anti-carcinogenic compounds. Finally, an immunomodulatory role of lactic bacteria which could lead to an anti-tumoural effect has also been proposed.

It is likely that the beneficial effect of consuming probiotics could be better characterized if the stage of tumour progression at which the probiotics are consumed is taken into account, as it has been possible with data collected in studies of dietary fibre.

Do certain pathogenic microbes have to be included in the list of bacteria with a protective effect against colon cancer?

In this context, mention should be made of recent data from Pitari *et al.* [45] addressing the action of the ST toxin—which is secreted by enterotoxigenic *Escherichia coli* (ETEC)—on the proliferation of colon tumour cells. This enterotoxin binds guanylyl cyclase C receptors expressed on the surface of microvilli and binding induces a marked increase in the intracellular concentration of cyclic guanosine monophosphate (cGMP). Up until now, the known physiological consequences mainly involved changes in the flow of ions and the appearance of diarrhoea; however, the induction of intracellular cGMP (that can also be mimicked using guanylyl cyclase C analogues) also leads to the arrest of the proliferation of intestinal cells which could, in countries in which the incidence of enteric infection is high, contribute to the low frequency there of colon cancer.

Key points

- Homeostasis of the colonic epithelium which is characterized by rapid turnover is regulated by complex cellular and molecular mechanisms. Abnormalities affecting these mechanisms lead to disorganisation of the epithelium and, sometimes, to pathology.

- Among the metabolites produced by the colonic microflora, butyrate is an essential compound in colonic homeostasis, constituting the preferred energy source of colonocytes and modulating the expression of numerous genes.

- The integrity of the colonic epithelium will largely depend on effects—sometimes opposing—of metabolites generated by the colonic microflora. Certain of these are able to cause genetic damage in cells in the proliferative compartment of the crypt.

- Interactions between colonic bacteria and intestinal cells have been demonstrated: these would involve the secretion by bacteria of "signal" molecules which modulate the expression of target genes in the intestinal epithelium.

- Better understanding of the underlying mechanisms in this field will make it possible to devise strategies—preventive and/or therapeutic—to reduce the risk of colon cancer.

References

1. Falk PG, Hooper LV, Midtvedt T, *et al*. Creating and maintaining the gastrointestinal ecosystem: what we know and need to know from gnotobiology. *Microbiol Mol Biol Rev* 1998 ; 62 : 1157-70.

2. Potten CS, Booth C, Pritchard DM. The intestinal epithelial stem cell: the mucosal governor. *Int J Exp Pathol* 1997 ; 78 : 219-43.

3. Marshman E, Booth C, Potten CS. The intestinal epithelial stem cell. *Bioessays* 2002 ; 24 : 91-8.

4. Cohn SM, Roth KA, Birkenmeier EH, *et al*. Temporal and spatial patterns of transgene expression in aging adult mice provide insights about the origins, organization, and differentiation of the intestinal epithelium. *Proc Natl Acad Sci USA* 1991 ; 88 : 1034-8.

5. Wong MH, Hermiston ML, Syder AJ, *et al*. Forced expression of the tumor suppressor adenomatosis polyposis coli protein induces disordered cell migration in the intestinal epithelium. *Proc Natl Acad Sci USA* 1996 ; 93 : 9588-93.

6. Merritt AJ, Potten CS, Watson AJ, *et al*. Differential expression of bcl-2 in intestinal epithelia. Correlation with attenuation of apoptosis in colonic crypts and the incidence of colonic neoplasia. *J Cell Sci* 1995 ; 108 : 2261-71.

7. Binder HJ, Sandle GI. Electrolyte transport in the mammalian colon. In : Johnson LR, ed. *Physiology of the gastrointestinal tract*, 3rd ed. New York : Raven Press, 1994 : 2133-71.

8. Yun CH, Tse CM, Nath SK, *et al*. Mammalian Na+/H+ exchanger gene family: structure and function studies. *Am J Physiol* 1995 ; 269 : G1-11.

9. Rajendran VM, Binder HJ. Characterization and molecular localization of anion transporters in colonic epithelial cells. *Ann NY Acad Sci* 2000 ; 915 : 15-29.

10. Hermiston ML, Simon TC, Crossman MW, *et al*. Model systems for studying cell fate specification and differentiation in the gut epithelium. In : Johnson LR, ed. *Physiology of the gastrointestinal tract*, 3rd ed. New York : Raven Press, 1994 : 521-69.

11. Bienz M, Clevers H. Linking colorectal cancer to Wnt signaling. *Cell* 2000 ; 103 : 311-20.

12. Korinek V, Barker N, Moerer P, *et al*. Depletion of epithelial stem-cell compartments in the small intestine of mice lacking Tcf-4. *Nat Genet* 1998 ; 19 : 379-83.

13. van de Wetering M, Sancho E, Verweij C, *et al*. The beta-catenin/TCF-4 complex imposes a crypt progenitor phenotype on colorectal cancer cells. *Cell* 2002 ; 111 : 241-50.

14. Lorentz O, Duluc I, Arcangelis AD, *et al*. Key role of the Cdx2 homeobox gene in extracellular matrix-mediated intestinal cell differentiation. *J Cell Biol* 1997 ; 139 : 1553-65.

15. Bonhomme C, Duluc I, Martin E, *et al*. The Cdx2 homeobox gene has a tumour suppressor function in the distal colon in addition to a homeotic role during gut development. *Gut* 2003 ; 52 : 1465-71.

16. Cuff MA, Lambert DW, Shirazi-Beechey SP. Substrate-induced regulation of the human colonic monocarboxylate transporter, MCT1. *J Physiol* 2002 ; 539 : 361-71.

17. Roediger WE. Utilization of nutrients by isolated epithelial cells of the rat colon. *Gastroenterology* 1982 ; 83 : 424-9.

18. Clausen MR, Mortensen PB. Kinetic studies on the metabolism of short-chain fatty acids and glucose by isolated rat colonocytes. *Gastroenterology* 1994 ; 106 : 423-32.

19. Cherbuy C, Darcy-Vrillon B, Morel MT, *et al*. Effect of germfree state on the capacities of isolated rat colonocytes to metabolize n-butyrate, glucose, and glutamine. *Gastroenterology* 1995 ; 109 : 1890-9.

20. Blottiere HM, Buecher B, Galmiche JP, *et al*. Molecular analysis of the effect of short-chain fatty acids on intestinal cell proliferation. *Proc Nutr Soc* 2003 ; 62 : 101-6.

21. Sakata T, von Engelhardt W. Stimulatory effect of short chain fatty acids on the epithelial cell proliferation in rat large intestine. *Comp Biochem Physiol A* 1983 ; 74 : 459-62.

22. Hass R, Busche R, Luciano L, *et al*. Lack of butyrate is associated with induction of Bax and subsequent apoptosis in the proximal colon of guinea pig. *Gastroenterology* 1997 ; 112 : 875-81.

23. Mandal M, Olson DJ, Sharma T, *et al*. Butyric acid induces apoptosis by up-regulating Bax expression *via* stimulation of the c-Jun N-terminal kinase/activation protein-1 pathway in human colon cancer cells. *Gastroenterology* 2001 ; 120 : 71-8.

24. Medina V, Edmonds B, Young GP, *et al*. Induction of caspase-3 protease activity and apoptosis by butyrate and trichostatin A (inhibitors of histone deacetylase): dependence on protein synthesis and synergy with a mitochondrial/cytochrome c-dependent pathway. *Cancer Res* 1997 ; 57 : 3697-707.

25. Sassone-Corsi P. The decline of induced transcription: a case of enzymatic symbiosis. *Nat Struct Biol* 2003 ; 10 : 151-2.

26. Ichikawa H, Sakata T. Stimulation of epithelial cell proliferation of isolated distal colon of rats by continuous colonic infusion of ammonia or short-chain fatty acids is nonadditive. *J Nutr* 1998 ; 128 : 843-7.

27. Darcy-Vrillon B, Cherbuy C, Morel MT, *et al*. Short chain fatty acid and glucose metabolism in isolated pig colonocytes : modulation by NH4+. *Mol Cell Biochem* 1996 ; 156 : 145-51.

28. Babidge W, Millard S, Roediger W. Sulfides impair short chain fatty acid beta-oxidation at acyl-CoA dehydrogenase level in colonocytes: implications for ulcerative colitis. *Mol Cell Biochem* 1998 ; 181 : 117-24.

29. Loser C, Eisel A, Harms D, *et al*. Dietary polyamines are essential luminal growth factors for small intestinal and colonic mucosal growth and development. *Gut* 1999 ; 44 : 12-6.

30. Hessels J, Kingma AW, Ferwerda H, *et al*. Microbial flora in the gastrointestinal tract abolishes cytostatic effects of alpha-difluoromethylornithine *in vivo*. *Int J Cancer* 1989 ; 43 : 1155-64.

31. Thomas T, Thomas TJ. Polyamines in cell growth and cell death: molecular mechanisms and therapeutic applications. *Cell Mol Life Sci* 2001 ; 58 : 244-58.

32. Alam M, Midtvedt T, Uribe A. Differential cell kinetics in the ileum and colon of germfree rats. *Scand J Gastroenterol* 1994 ; 29 : 445-51.

33. Sakata T. Effects of short-chain fatty acids on the proliferation of gut epithelial cells *in vivo*. In : Cummings JH, Rombeau JL, Sakata T, eds. *Physiological and clinical aspects of short-chain fatty acids*. Cambridge : Cambridge University Press, 1995 : 289-305.

34. Cherbuy C, Andrieux C, Ide C, *et al*. Expression of mitochondrial HMGCoA synthase and glutaminase in the colonic mucosa is modulated by bacterial species. *Eur J Biochem* 2004 ; 271 : 87-95.

35. Hooper LV, Wong MH, Thelin A, *et al*. Molecular analysis of commensal host-microbial relationships in the intestine. *Science* 2001 ; 291 : 881-4.

36. Gordon JI, Hooper LV, McNevin MS, *et al*. Epithelial cell growth and differentiation. III. Promoting diversity in the intestine: conversations between the microflora, epithelium, and diffuse GALT. *Am J Physiol* 1997 ; 273 : G565-70.

37. Hooper LV, Bry L, Falk PG, *et al*. Host-microbial symbiosis in the mammalian intestine: exploring an internal ecosystem. *Bioessays* 1998 ; 20 : 336-43.

38. Bry L, Falk PG, Midtvedt T, *et al*. A model of host-microbial interactions in an open mammalian ecosystem. *Science* 1996 ; 273 : 1380-3.

39. Hooper LV, Xu J, Falk PG, *et al*. A molecular sensor that allows a gut commensal to control its nutrient foundation in a competitive ecosystem. *Proc Natl Acad Sci USA* 1999 ; 96 : 9833-8.

40. Nancey S, Coffin B, Descos L, *et al*. Flore et cancer colique. *Gastroenterol Clin Biol* 2001 ; 25 : C79-C84.

41. Rowland IR, Mallett AK, Wise A. The effect of diet on the mammalian gut flora and its metabolic activities. *Crit Rev Toxicol* 1985 ; 16 : 31-103.

42. Guarner F, Malagelada JR. Gut flora in health and disease. *Lancet* 2003 ; 361 : 512-9.

43. Quemener V, Moulinoux JP, Havouis R, *et al*. Polyamine deprivation enhances antitumoral efficacy of chemotherapy. *Anticancer Res* 1992 ; 12 : 1447-53.

44. Rafter J. Probiotics and colon cancer. *Best Pract Res Clin Gastroenterol* 2003 ; 17 : 849-59.

45. Pitari GM, Zingman LV, Hodgson DM, *et al*. Bacterial enterotoxins are associated with resistance to colon cancer. *Proc Natl Acad Sci USA* 2003 ; 100 : 2695-9.

Influence of the Intestinal Microflora on Host Immunity: Normal Physiological Conditions

Marie-Christiane Moreau

Unité d'Écologie et de Physiologie du Système Digestif, INRA, Jouy-en-Josas, France.

The intestine remains a poorly understood organ. Its mucosa has a surface area of about 300 m^2 and acts as the interface between the outside world and our inside world, performing the vital function that is digestion and the absorption of nutrients at the same time as protecting us from invasion by pathogenic microorganisms. Thus, to maintain the homeostasis indispensable to its normal functioning, the intestine has developed other functions: it is both the body's primary immune organ as well as its "second brain" by virtue of the number of immune cells and neurones that it contains. Within the first days of life, the intestine also houses a considerable microflora, one hundred thousand billion bacteria, which mediates numerous beneficial effects in healthy individuals and allows them to live in a septic environment. Among the multiple effects of this microflora, its action on the immune system and, in particular on the intestinal immune system (IIS), is considerable. In physiological conditions, the relationship between the IIS and the microflora could be described as "symbiotic". The IIS does not mount inflammatory immune responses toward the microflora which, in turn, exerts many effects on the immune system at the intestinal level and also at the peripheral (or systemically) level, even if in the last case, the information is less complete.

Resident intestinal microflora: importance of the neonatal period

In children, it is estimated that the balance of the intestinal microflora is similar to that of adults by about two years of age. During this period, the relatively undiversified neonatal microflora (only about ten to twelve different microbial species) gradually becomes more complex, reaching a total of three to four hundred different species in the adult microflora. Diet plays a crucial role in this diversification process (*in* [1]). It is at around two years of age that a child's peripheral and intestinal immune systems are believed to be mature. Thus, from a physiological point of view, it is particularly important to consider the immune system microflora relationship during this first period of life.

At birth, the baby's bacterial environment is essentially derived from the mother's vaginal and faecal microfloras, but only a few bacteria colonize its digestive tract. The factors which dominate at the first selection are related to the baby (mucus), to delivery conditions (natural route, caesarean, environment) and to the mother's status (antibiotics). *Escherichia coli* and *Streptococcus* are among the first bacteria to colonize the digestive tract. Then, strict anaerobes (notably *Bacteroides, Clostridium* and *Bifidobacterium*) establish themselves during the first week of life after a second selection in the course of which the diet plays a fundamental role. It has been long known that the breast-fed baby is colonized with a strictly anaerobic microflora, essentially composed of bifidobacteria, whereas, in formula-fed babies, these are absent or present in a random fashion [2]. As indicated by the experimental and clinical studies discussed here, the microflora of the baby plays a considerable role in maturation of the immune system and perturbation of the fragile microbial equilibrium by diverse factors—delivery conditions, antibiotics, diet—can have important consequences, not only in the short term but also in the long term (Figure 1).

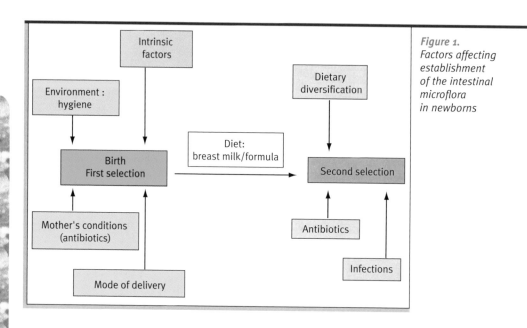

Figure 1.
Factors affecting establishment of the intestinal microflora in newborns

In healthy adult humans whose immune systems are fully developed and functional, the complex microflora, at least that of the left colon, is far less influenced in terms of composition by diet. Other factors can, however, perturb its equilibrium, the most obvious being antibiotics. Stress, unbalanced diet, changes in gastrointestinal transit and intestinal infections can also affect the composition of the faecal microflora. Considering the important role played by the intestinal microflora on the continual optimisation and regulation of the host's immune responses, modification of the bacterial microflora can then have consequences on these responses, making them sub-optimal or harmful. A well balanced intestinal microflora is thus an important factor indispensable to maintaining an optimal and adapted functioning immune system.

Brief review of immunity

Innate immunity

The host's first—and oldest—line of defence is mediated by the cells of innate immunity, i.e., monocytes/macrophages, dendritic cells (DC), natural killer (NK) cells and neutrophils. These are the body's sentinels. Thus, by virtue of the phagocytic activity of DCs and to an even greater extent of macrophages, foreign organisms are phagocytosed and destroyed.

Recent data show that macrophages and peripheral DCs are able to recognize bacterial components, abnormally present, through certain receptors expressed at the cell surface, including CD14 and approximately ten other receptors called the Toll-like receptors (TLR) (*in* [3]). The binding of bacterial components to these receptors leads to activation of the nuclear factor κB (NFκB) which induces the transcription of genes coding for proinflammatory chemokines such as IL-8, and cytokines such as TNFα, IL-1 and IL-6. The consequence of this synthesis is to attract neutrophils to the site of inflammation, and later B and T cells (Tcs), thereby launching an "acquired immune response". Additionally, the synthesis of other cytokines such as IL-12 is induced. It plays an important role on the modulation of the acquired immunity, especially on the Th1/Th2 balance (*see below*). Among all the TLRs, some are now well characterized. Thus, TLR2 recognizes the peptidoglycan of Gram-positive bacteria, TLR4 the lipopolysaccharide (LPS) of Gram-negative bacteria, TLR5 bacterial flagellae, and TLR9 unmethylated cytosine phosphoryl guanine DNA (CpG) which is only found in bacterial genomes. LPSs from different bacteria do not always have the same actions and one speaks of the "repertoire" of TLRs. In the intestine, enterocytes are also capable of recognizing bacterial components and activating the NFκB pathway but the activation is strongly controlled by several processes to avoid inflammatory reactions which can compromise the intestinal homeostasis [4].

NK cells are involved in anti-tumour immunity and can also, through the synthesis of gamma interferon (IFNγ), modulate the Th1/Th2 balance.

Thus, the innate immune system which is non-specific and not endowed with memory, is the first to intervene following antigenic aggression. It also plays an important role in acquired immunity through the presentation of antigens (Ags) to T cells (Tcs) and the synthesis of some cytokines.

Acquired immunity

Acquired responses concern Ag-specific humoral (antibody synthesis) and cell-mediated responses (cellular responses). After a first contact with an Ag, they take a long time to develop (seven to ten days) but they induce memory, allowing a very rapid response after a second contact with the same Ag. These responses require cooperation between antigen-presenting cells (APC), macrophages and DCs, and Tcs, *via* several interactions during which ligand receptor molecules are expressed by both the APCs and the Tcs. All these binding events lead to activation of Tcs of the CD8+ phenotype for cell-mediated responses, and CD4+ for both humoral and cell-mediated responses. These molecular and cellular interactions are multiple and participate in the modulation of immune responses. Thus, APCs play a key role in the acquired immune response through their capacity to present the Ag and synthesize diverse cytokines which are capable of modulating and directing immune responses.

Humoral response and Th1/Th2 balance

After activation by APCs, several subjects of CD4+ or helper Tcs (Th) modulate the synthesis of antibodies (Ab) by B cells (Bcs) *via* the production of cytokines (Figure 2).

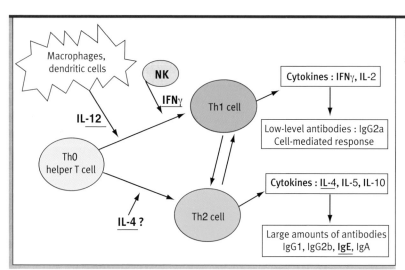

Figure 2.
Th1/Th2 balance:
role of cytokines

Several subsets of Th cells differ in the profile of cytokines they produce. Type 1 Th cells (Th1) mainly secrete IFNγ, a "pro-inflammatory" cytokine, and induce low-level Ab synthesis by Bcs (sub-class: IgG2a). They will be more recruited in the case of cell-mediated responses [5]. In contrast, the activation of type 2 Th cells (Th2) leads to the synthesis of the "anti-inflammatory" cytokines IL-4, IL-5, IL-10, IL-13 and to high-level production by Bcs of Ab belonging to the classes and sub-classes of IgG1, IgA, or IgE, the latter being involved in allergy. The activation of one population inhibits that of the other. Activation of the precursor Th0 cell to either Th1 or Th2 depends on environmental factors among which cells of innate immunity (macrophages, DCs and NK cells) play a considerable role through the synthesis of cytokines, including IL-12 and IFNγ, which act on the preferential direction towards a Th1 profile. The Th1/Th2 balance allows an immune response which is matched to each type of Ag: an inflammatory, cell-mediated Th1 response for intracellular infections, and a non-inflammatory, Th2 response with a marked IgG1 or IgA antibody synthesis in other cases. With respect to the IgE response, this must remain restrained at the risk of leading to undesirable allergic reactions. Among other factors, IL-

10 could be involved in this regulation [6]. The balance of cytokines therefore plays a considerable role in regulating and directing immune responses.

Roles of the intestinal microflora in host immunity

On the basis of data mainly derived from animal studies together with some recent clinical and epidemiological results from children, the action of the intestinal microflora can be characterized in three ways: "activation" of the immune system, "modulation" of immune responses, and "regulation" of responses allowing appropriate reactions to different antigenic stimuli in the short and long terms. The post-natal period seems to be crucial in the development of some of these regulatory mechanisms, notably those involved in atopic disease.

Most of the experimental data come from studies in germ-free or axenic (AX) animals. These animals (mice or rats) are reared into isolators in which the entire environment—air, food and equipment—is sterile. Comparisons of AX mice with conventionally (CV) mice or "humanized" mice (AX mice whose digestive tracts are colonized by a human faecal microflora) have shown the role played by the microflora on cellular development of the immune system and on its functionality. The AX mouse model is also useful because it allows *in vivo* analysis of the specific roles played by different bacteria composing the intestinal microflora on immune responses by colonizing the digestive tract with one or more known microbial species ("gnotobiotic" mouse models). Results show that, depending on the immune response studied, the immunomodulatory effect of the microflora is due to either the establishment of all the bacteria of the microflora from birth to the adult state or to the presence of some specific strain and species of bacteria, the effect being sometimes "strain-dependent". Effects of the microflora are seen in both the periphery and the intestine.

Role of the microflora on the peripheral immune system: innate immunity

Activating effect of the microflora on antigen-presenting cells

The mechanisms underlying activation of innate immunity by bacterial components probably play a key role in the permanent activation of the immune system in adults. They must participate in immune maturation in babies in whom the major cause of immaturity of the peripheral immune system would be APC immaturity [7]. Experimental results support this hypothesis. A few picograms of LPS are sufficient to activate APCs. In AX mice, colonization of the digestive tract by the microflora of a CV mouse induces the synthesis of the pro-inflammatory cytokines IL-1, IL-6 and TNFα by peritoneal macrophages (Table I). The same effect can be reproduced with the presence of only *Escherichia coli* in the digestive tract whereas a strain of *Bifidobacterium bifidum* from a baby has no effect [8]. Similarly, the presence of the microflora stimulates—through macrophages derived from splenic precursors—the synthesis of IL-12 which is known to play an important role in driving a response in the Th1 direction [9] (Figure 2). In children, this activation could play a key role in regulation of the Th1/Th2 balance (*see below*). In adults, the slight physiological inflammatory state existing at the level of the IIS could be explained by this sustained effect of the microflora. It is interesting to observe that two Gram-negative bacteria, *Escherichia coli* and *Bacteroides*, are part of the dominant microflora in children and adults respectively. In normal conditions, the colonization of the digestive tract of babies by *Escherichia coli* just after birth could therefore have a major impact on maturation of the peripheral immune system by generating a physiological inflammatory state indispensable to this activation.

Intestinal microflora	Cytokines			
	IL-1	IL-6	TNFα	
Conventional	18 200	6.33	72	
Axenic	8 300	2.62	< 50	
Bifidobacterium bifidum	8 000	2.46	< 50	
Escherichia coli	15 350	7.24	108	

Table I.
Influence of intestinal bacteria on the production of inflammatory cytokines by peritoneal macrophages. Results are expressed in Units/mL (taken from [10])

Consequences: regulation of the Th1/Th2 balance

Over the last fifty years, there has been a worrisome increase in the incidence of allergy in babies, especially in rich industrialized countries. The "classic" causes (genetics, pollution, smoking, etc.) cannot explain this increase (*in* [11]). A unbalanced Th1/Th2 response could be one of the causes of these atopic responses. Because of the importance of pro-inflammatory cytokines in directing immune responses towards a Th1 profile, it has been suggested that the bacterial environment could play a crucial role in regulating the Th1/Th2 balance in children. At birth, the baby is in a Th2 immunological context which is necessary to avoid rejection of the foetus during gestation; Th1 responses are largely repressed (*in* [11, 12]). After birth, the baby must quickly restore the balance between Th2 and Th1 and this process would occur during the post-natal period, in the first two years of life, especially the first year. Various epidemiological and clinical studies have shown that, in atopic children, the Th2 → Th1 switch does not occur and the child remains in an unbalanced Th2 context with a predisposition to develop IgE-based allergic responses [12]. Recent epidemiological studies point to an important role for the microbial environment during the first year of life in this regulatory process. Comparisons of children living in the same region but under different lifestyle conditions (urban or farming environments) show that children who live the first year of life in a traditional rural environment are less likely to develop allergic diseases than children living in town [13]. The existence of a rich microbial environment (contact with animals, ingestion of raw milk, etc.) seems to be important. The role of LPS has also been suggested as important but not sufficient. Currently, bacteriological studies on the faecal microflora in children are being undertaken in order to better understand possible interactions between the establishment and composition of the intestinal microflora and the development of atopy (*in* [14]). A change in the establishment of the microflora in the newborn is in practice observed in several European countries as characterized by a predominance of *Staphylococcus* and *Clostridium*, associated with a reduction in the number of *Escherichia coli* and bifidobacteria. The important role of the microbial equilibrium on directing Th2 responses towards Th1 ones was experimentally demonstrated by Sudo *et al*. [15]. In three-week-old mice, these authors showed how the modification of the bacterial equilibrium by ingestion of an antibiotic (kanamycin) distorts immune responses which remained Th2 in contrast to those in control animals in which both Th1 and Th2 responses developed. Finally, very recent clinical studies using some probiotics showed they were effective in the treatment or prevention of atopic dermatitis in babies, supporting the hypothesis that the intestinal bacterial equilibrium plays an important role in the appropriate regulation of immune responses [14, 16]. Indeed, a preventive effect was shown with a probiotic, *Lactobacillus rhamnosus* GG: in a group of 134 atopic mothers, half were given 10^{10} units of probiotic/day during one month before delivery and then six months after (mother or baby), and the other half was given a placebo. At the age of two, the prevalence of atopic dermatitis in the treated children was 23% compared with 46% in the placebo group [16]. The mechanism of action underlying this preventive effect of the probiotic is not yet understood.

Taking all these observations together, an important question arises: could not excessive hygiene and inappropriate usage of prophylactic antibiotics during delivery and the baby's life be causes leading to perturbation of the child intestinal bacterial equilibrium with irreversible, and disastrous consequences on the regulation of the Th1/Th2 balance? This is an important question! Probiotics could be also good palliative agents with respect to impaired equilibrium of the intestinal microflora. Now, it is important to understand the immunoregulatory mechanisms by which resident bacteria and probiotics act on the immune systems.

Roles of the microflora on the peripheral immune system: acquired immunity

Activating and regulatory effects of the microflora on the level of natural immunoglobulins and the B cell repertoire

Without any immunisation, so-called "natural" immunoglobulins (Ig) are found in the blood. Their level is relatively constant and stable in terms of the profile of isotypes and Ig sub-classes. It has been demonstrated that the intestinal microflora has an important action on the levels of natural IgG and IgA which are very low in AX mice. It has no effect on IgM levels (*in* [17]).

The presence of the intestinal microflora acts strongly—through natural Igs—on the Bc repertoire and therefore on the possibility for the individual to develop diversified humoral responses. In practice, analysis of the expression of certain VH genes, which code for synthesis of the so-called "variable" domains of Igs and therefore their antibody (Ab) site, has made it possible to evaluate the diversity of the repertoire of Igs secreted by Bcs [17, 18]. Strong use of one gene, the VH7183 gene is observed in the Bcs of the spleen of baby CV mice, pointing to a low diversity of secreted Abs. However, this usage drops sharply towards adulthood, indicating progressive diversification of the repertoire of peripheral Bcs and therefore of the "natural" Abs synthesized. This pattern is not seen in adult AX mice in which VH7183 remains strongly expressed, as in the newborn, indicating that the intestinal microflora would have a key role on the diversification of Ab synthesis. It was shown that it is the natural Abs mediate an effect on the expression of VH genes. Indeed, the injection of natural Igs from CV mice into AX mice reduces VH7183 expression to the level seen in adult CV mice. Consequently, by the way of the synthesis of natural Igs, especially IgG, the intestinal microflora would therefore be responsible for the diversification of the repertoire of peripheral Bcs which occurs over the course of life. These natural Abs would play their regulatory roles on the individual's Bc repertoire through interactions that are referred to as idiotypic (interactions between different Abs) [17, 18]. In humans, the regulatory role of these natural Igs is exploited in the treatment of some auto-immune diseases for which the intravenous injection of a pool of human IgG induces clinical improvement [19].

Microflora and susceptibility to certain diseases: example of an auto-immune disease

It is known that there is a relationship between some systemic bacterial infections and the appearance of auto-immune problems. However, the protective role of intestinal bacteria on susceptibility to these diseases is less well characterized. A very nice example was published a few years ago concerning experimental arthritis induced in rats by the injection of an aqueous suspension of streptococcal cell wall [20]. This auto-immune disease is characterized by an acute phase followed by a chronic phase. The latter is genetically determined and some lineages of rat are described as resistant (Fisher rats) whereas others are susceptible (Lewis rats). It was shown that, when Fisher rats are reared in AX conditions, resistance disappears. It appears again if the animals are colonized with a microflora from a CV animal. The protective effect of the microflora would be due to the existence of clones of Tcs which have become non reactive to certain bacterial Ags, including those of the streptococcal cell wall, in the presence of the bacterial microflora. In susceptible rats, this tolerance would either be absent or would be weak. In resistant rats, it is associated with the constant presence of the intestinal microflora. This example shows how genetic susceptibility to certain diseases could be tightly linked to an important environmental factor: the intestinal microflora. It also raises the question of the consequences that major modifications of the intestinal bacterial equilibrium could have on the appearance of auto-immune diseases following, for example, a course of antibiotic treatment.

Roles of the microflora on the intestinal immune system

Physiology of the intestinal immune system

Here we will only address the physiology of the IIS, since its anatomical description has been (and still is) the subject of many publications [21, 22].

Unlike the peripheral immune system, the IIS, in constant contact with the considerable antigenic mass of dietary and bacterial proteins, does not mount inappropriate inflammatory immune responses which would damage the integrity of the intestinal mucosa. Immune responses of the IIS are adapted to the intestinal environment and the presence of intestinal microflora plays a crucial role on its functions.

The functions of IIS are apparently contradictory [22]. The first function is to mount protective cell-mediated and humoral responses towards enteropathogenic viruses, bacteria or parasites. The intestinal humoral Ab response is characterized by the IgA isotype, which is secreted into the intestinal lumen associated with a glycoprotein, the secretory component which confers a resistance to proteolytic enzymes and a targeted action [21, 23]. Secretory IgA Abs (sIgA) form immune complexes with the Ag, thereby blocking mucosa adhesion of pathogenic bacteria, inhibiting viral proliferation inside enterocytes, and neutralising enterotoxins (immune exclusion). Cell-mediated responses mainly involve intra-epithelial lymphocytes, one primary function of which is to maintain the integrity of the intestinal epithelium by destroying infected or abnormal enterocytes [24].

In contrast, the second function of the IIS is to prevent the induction of immune responses against food and bacterial Ags which are permanently present in the digestive tract, by eliciting suppressive responses. One of these responses is called "oral intolerance" [22, 25]. It is defined by the state of both specific systemic peripheral and intestinal immune unresponsiveness induced after protein ingestion. It is a long-lasting process. This response plays a major role in intestinal homeostasis by preventing inflammatory mucosal reactions that are incompatible with the essential function of the intestine which is the digestion and absorption of nutrients. When it is defective, inflammatory problems appear, in particular food hypersensitivities manifesting at either the systemic level (atopic dermatitis) or in the intestine (diarrhoea, vomiting). Consequently, oral tolerance—which is known to exist in humans [26]—as well as Th1/Th2 balance, are important immuno-regulatory processes which prevent the mounting of inappropriate and therefore harmful immune responses, particularly against dietary proteins. The high percentage of hypersensitivities in babies (up to 15% during the first year) could be due to a failure in the establishment of these mechanisms (*reviewed in* [22, 25]).

Does the oral tolerance process apply to the resident bacteria of the microflora which we know to be as well tolerated as an individual's own tissues [27]? It could be believed so since some auto-immune diseases such as arthritis in the rat would be due to impaired tolerance to arthritogenic bacterial Ags [20]. However, the absence of inflammatory reactivity to intestinal bacteria could also be due to several other suppressive mechanisms developed by the IIS. For example, it was shown recently that the APCs of the IIS, in contrast to those in the periphery, do not express receptors for bacterial components (CD14 and TLRs) which could in part explain why they do not respond to the bacteria of the intestinal microflora [28].

Activating role of the microflora on the development of the intestinal immune system: example of IgA-producing plasma cells

Comparison of AX and CV mice shows that the presence of the intestinal microflora plays a crucial role in the development and activation of the IIS [1]. In the AX mouse, as in the baby, the IIS is underdeveloped: Peyer's patches are atrophied and the density of cells (Bcs, Tcs, IgA-producing plasma cells) in the *lamina propria* is low (Figure 3).

Colonization of AX mice with the microflora of an adult CV mouse induces activation of the IIS within three weeks: increased numbers of IgA-producing plasma cells and Tcs, expression of Class II molecules on the enterocytes at the tips of villi, and an increased number of intra-epithelial lymphocytes (*in* [1]). The effect of the microflora on the number and activation of the intestinal APCs is not still well known.

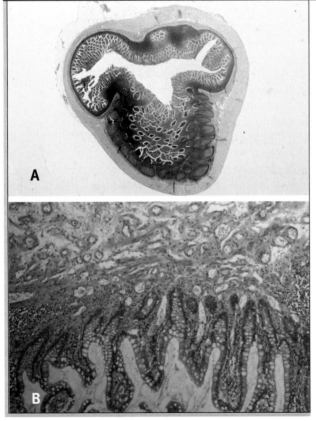

Figure 3.
A : cross-section of the ileum.
Peyer's patch (dark) seen in the lower part of the image, formed by clusters of lymphoid follicles in the region opposite the insertion zone of the mesentery (micrograph: C. Da Lage).
B : intestinal immune system:
Peyer's patch (micrograph: T. Piche, Nice)

Many plasma cells in the mucosa secrete IgAs which control the translocation of bacteria of the resident microflora. At birth, the CV mouse—like adult AX mouse—has a very low number of IgA-producing plasma cells which reach a number equivalent to that in the adult CV mouse at the age of about six weeks (i.e., three weeks after weaning). This situation is the same in children, in whom the number of intestinal IgA-producing plasma cells found in the adult is not reached until between the first and second year of life, in parallel to the sequential establishment of the intestinal microflora. The possible immaturity of the IIS, an inhibitory effect of breast milk Abs, or the sequential establishment of the gut microflora from birth to weaning could explain this long delay in activation of the IIS. To test the latter hypothesis, adult AX mice were colonized with the intestinal microflora of growing CV mice from one day to twenty-five days of age (gnotobiotic models). Results showed that the sequential colonization of the digestive tract by intestinal bacteria can be responsible for of the full maturation of the intestinal IgA-producing plasma cells [29] (Table II).

Table II. Role of the sequential establishment of the intestinal microflora in growing conventional mice (from birth to five days after weaning) on the maturation of IgA plasma cells measured in adult gnotobiotic mice (mean ± SEM) (taken from [28])	Intestinal microflora in gnotobiotic mice	Number of IgA-producing plasma cells/intestinal villus
	Microflora from a conventional adult mouse	41 ± 1
	Axenic mouse	4 ± 0.5
	Microflora from mice of between 1 and 4 days of age	15 ± 2
	Microflora from mice of between 7 and 23 days of age	23 ± 1
	Microflora from mice of 25 days of age	43 ± 1

Although some Gram-negative bacteria have been shown to play an adjuvant role in this IgA response [30], it is nevertheless necessary that the microflora be complex and diversified to obtain maximum stimulation ([29] and *in* [1]). Thus, in baby mice, the long six-week delay is explained by the time it takes to acquire an intestinal microflora close to that of the adult which occurs just after weaning (between three and four weeks). The additionnal three weeks are related to the time needed to develop a cellular IgA response. These data show the close relationship which exists between diet, diversification of the intestinal microflora and its effect on the IIS in the young. Perturbation of the establishment of the microflora and an early or late dietary divesification could have consequences on the quality of the microbial balance of the child's microflora and on development of the IIS. In adults, a relationship between unbalanced microflora and IgA deficiency has not been directly demonstrated, but it is known that the ingestion of probiotics can stimulate the secretion of total sIgA (*in* [31]).

Modulatory role of the microflora on the functions of the intestinal immune system: example of the specific IgA anti-rotavirus response

It has been known for a long time that rotavirus-induced diarrhoea, which affects all children in the world, is less frequent and less severe in breast-fed babies. Immune protection against rotaviruses is mainly due to specific intestinal IgA anti-rotavirus Abs and cell-mediated immune mechanisms. To distinguish the protective effect conferred by breast milk from that due to the intestinal microflora (which is particularly rich in *Bifidobacterium* in breast-fed children), experimental models of adult gnotobiotic mice colonized with either the faecal microflora of a breast-fed baby or the faecal microflora of a formula-fed baby were developed. They were then orally inoculated with a strain of rotavirus in order to compare the immunomodulatory effects of the baby microfloras on the levels of intestinal IgA anti-rotavirus Abs. Groups of gnotobiotic mice were similar in all points except the intestinal microfloras (Figure 4).

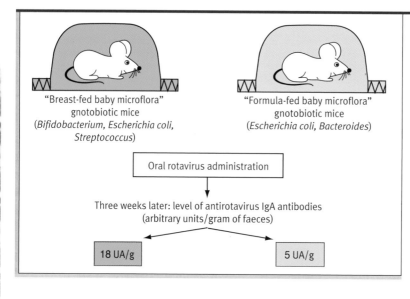

"Breast-fed baby microflora"
gnotobiotic mice
(*Bifidobacterium, Escherichia coli,*
Streptococcus)

"Formula-fed baby microflora"
gnotobiotic mice
(*Escherichia coli, Bacteroides*)

Oral rotavirus administration

Three weeks later: level of antirotavirus IgA antibodies
(arbitrary units/gram of faeces)

18 UA/g   5 UA/g

Figure 4.
Adjuvant effect of the faecal microflora of a microflora breast-fed baby on the intestinal IgA anti-rotavirus antibody response measured in faeces of adult gnotobiotic mice

Escherichia coli was present in both microfloras but a strain of *Bifidobacterium bifidum* was only found in the microflora from the breast-fed baby. After viral infection, kinetics of the faecal anti-rotavirus IgA response did not differ between the two groups of "breast-fed" and "formula-fed" gnotobiotic mice. However, the maximal level reached around 20 days after viral inoculation, was approximately 3-4 times higher in breast-fed than in formula-fed gnotobiotic mice [32].

In order to analyse the respective roles played by either *Bifidobacterium bifidum* or *Escherichia coli* in this Ab stimulation, other gnotobiotic mouse models were realized. Results clearly show that *Bifidobacterium bifidum* was responsible for a major adjuvant effect on the anti-rotavirus IgA response whereas, in contrast, *Escherichia coli* mediated a clear suppressive effect [32]. Thus, the presence of *Bifidobacterium* in the digestive tract of a breast-fed baby moderates the suppressive effect mediated by *Escherichia coli*. The results show the importance of the presence of *Bifidobacterium* in the microflora of babies to stimulate the important protective immune response towards rotaviruses. These results again reveal the considerable role played by the bacterial balance of the microflora on the modulation of a protective immune response. In adults, the species of *Bifidobacterium* present—very often different from those found in babies—do not seem to have the same immunostimulatory effect on the anti-rotavirus IgA response but rather have a suppressive effect (unpublished results). This "strain-dependent" immunomodulatory effect makes these studies and the interpretation of their results even more complex.

Regulatory role of the microflora in the intestinal immune system: oral tolerance

The intestinal microflora has a regulatory effect on the functions of the IIS, in particular mediating processes to suppress immune responses, such as oral tolerance which plays a key role in intestinal homeostasis. Oral tolerance is particularly important in the newborn in whom inappropriate immune responses to ingested dietary proteins encountered for the first time must be inhibited as soon as possible. The digestive microflora plays again an important role in the establishment of the suppressive responses as shown by results coming from gnotobiotic mice colonized with bacteria from the human faecal microflora.

The induction of oral tolerance can be reproduced experimentally by feeding a group of mice with a dietary protein, like ovalbumin (OVA), prior to a subsequent peripheral immunisation with the same protein seven days later. Comparison of the immune responses to OVA measured in the periphery in the OVA-fed group and a control buffer-fed group shows whether oral tolerance has become established. When it is the case, the cell-mediated and/or humoral response to OVA is significantly decreased or suppressed entirely in the OVA-fed animals compared with the control group. If oral tolerance is not established, the response to OVA immunisation is the same for both the OVA and the control groups. This experimental protocol has shown that the intestinal microflora is one of the important factors influencing oral tolerance establishment [1, 25].

Wannemuehler *et al.* [33] were the first to report that, unlike the case with the CV mouse, feeding AX mice with sheep erythrocytes did not result in oral tolerance. However, the tolerant state was re-established by prior ingestion of LPS. They concluded that Gram-negative bacteria may play a fundamental role in the mechanisms underlying oral tolerance. Then, using another Ag, namely OVA, it has been shown that it is possible to establish oral tolerance (as measured by the suppression of the circulating anti-OVA IgG response after OVA feeding) in adult AX mice but in contrast to what is found in CV mice and in "humanized" mice colonized with an adult human microflora, this suppression is very short-lived, i.e., about ten days as opposed to over five months in the CV mouse [34, 35]. Colonization of the digestive tract of

AX mice with only *Escherichia coli* or *Bacteroides* (two LPS-rich Gram-negative bacteria) prior to OVA feeding allows to restore suppression which is then as long-lived as that in CV mice. In contrast, a strain of *Bifidobacterium bifidum* had no effect (unpublished results). Recently, Sudo *et al.* [36], studying the role of the microflora in suppression of the anti-OVA IgE response, showed that, in their experimental conditions, AX mice fed with OVA did not induce suppression of the circulating anti-OVA IgE response in contrast to CV mice. Colonization of the digestive tract of AX mice with a strain of *Bifidobacterium infantis* restored the suppressive response but only when the bacteria had been established in the digestive tract since birth. Other studies have also shown that the intestinal microflora plays an important protective role against the abrogative effect of some enterotoxins (cholera toxin, *Escherichia coli* heat-labile enterotoxin) on the oral tolerance process, but in some cases, only if the microflora had been established since birth [1, 35].

All of these experiments strongly suggest the importance of the presence of some bacteria in the baby's microflora on the mechanisms underlying oral tolerance. They also reveal the crucial role played by the post-natal period in the establishment of these regulatory mechanisms. These observations [35, 36] support the epidemiological findings of Rieder *et al.* [13], which point to the importance of a rich bacterial environment surrounding the baby in its first months of life in the prevention of atopy.

The exact impact of the intestinal bacteria on the mechanisms of oral tolerance is as yet unknown since the mechanisms themselves have not been fully elucidated. Current studies are showing that intestinal APCs, in particular DCs, and specific regulatory Tcs (rTcl), could be involved. The mechanisms would mainly involve special Ag presentation by APCs leading to the non-activation of Tcs (clonal anergy) and/or the preferential secretion of cytokines, in particular IL-10, by intestinal DCs in response to the antigenic stimulus (bystander suppression). This cytokine would drive the Th response towards the production of IL-10 and TGF-β by Tcs of the Th3 type and by rTcs induced in this situation as recently described (*in* [22]). This anti-inflammatory and suppressive cytokine environment would then inhibit the activation of classic Tcs [1, 22, 25]. The importance of IL-10 secretion in the suppression of intestinal inflammatory responses is also confirmed by other experimental studies showing that one of the mechanisms of action of some probiotics in maintaining remission in patients with inflammatory bowel diseases could also be associated with this synthesis [37-39].

With respect to tolerance of the host's own intestinal microflora, the recent works of Neish *et al.* [40] and Dubuquoy *et al.* [41] have given interesting information on the role played by commensal or non-pathogenic intestinal bacteria in the regulation of the NFκB activation pathway which is involved in the synthesis of inflammatory cytokines. This regulation is submitted to many inhibiting or activating processes involving various effector molecules and/or receptors [4, 40]. In brief, at the level of APCs and especially the intestinal epithelial cells (enterocytes and colonocytes), Neish *et al.* [40] showed *in vitro* that the presence of a non-pathogenic strain of *Salmonella* blocked the NFκB activation pathway by inhibiting—through a phosphorylation mechanism—breakdown of the regulatory molecule IκBα [40]. In another *in vivo* study using AX mice, Dubuquoy *et al.* [41] showed that the presence of the intestinal microflora activated another regulatory pathway triggered by a receptor, the PPARγ (peroxisome proliferator-activated receptor) mainly expressed on the surface of colonocytes in humans, which blocks the NF-κB activation pathway.

All these data are providing more and more evidence that a cross-talk between intestinal bacteria and the IIS *via* epithelial cells plays a major role in regulation of the functioning of the IIS. In this case again, the observed efficacy of some probiotics, in particular VSL#3 which is a mixture of eight strains of lactic bacteria [42] or the yeast *Saccharomyces boulardii* [43], on the maintenance of remission in chronic pouchitis or ulcerative colitis, could be explained by re-establishment of the interrupted or perturbed cross-talk between the intestinal microflora and the epithelium.

Although all these experimental and clinical findings provide a solid basis to believe that the microflora has very important effects on the IIS, we are still a long way from understanding all the regulatory roles played by the bacteria on the particularities which differentiate the IIS from the peripheral immune system (Table III). Nevertheless, this point is important to understand because these particularities, especially the preferential induction of suppressive responses, are associated with correct functioning of the IIS and thus to keeping us in good health.

Table III. *Characteristics* *of the intestinal* *immune system.* *Roles of the gut* *microflora?*	• Special populations of DCs in the Peyer's patches (IL-10 synthesis) • Presence of regulatory Tcs (CD4+ and CD25+) • Non-expression of CD14 and CD89 by macrophages in the *lamina propria* • Large-scale Tc apoptosis in the *lamina propria* • Preferential stimulation of IgA antibodies: roles of TGFβ and IL-12

Conclusion

It is ever-increasingly accepted in the scientific and medical communities that the intestinal microflora plays a considerable role in the development and functioning of the IIS. Unfortunately, the too small number of researchers working in this field in past years has meant that it has not been possible to define a number of points which now need to be elucidated in order to obtain the fundamental understanding necessary to developing promising therapeutic applications, such as the use of probiotics. Three lines of research have to be developed. The first concerns the characterization of the intestinal microflora: what it is; its functional importance in children, adults and the elderly; its behaviour in response to everyday stress or after diseases affecting the digestive tract; the impact of bacterial metabolites on immunoregulation with, as corollary, an understanding of the metabolism of the microflora which is known to be highly diet-dependent in adults... The second concerns understanding of the IIS functions: how does it manage this amazing duality of mounting at the same time immune responses mediating both defence and tolerance? What are the links of the IIS with the peripheral compartment? How does the microflora mediate its effects in a constant fashion, what is the "good" microflora with respect to its preferential order of acquisition...? Understanding these points is indispensable to the third area of research concerning probiotics: in what conditions can probiotics act in the digestive tract? What are the immunomodulatory properties specific to each probiotic strain, because it is unlikely that any single strain would be able to act on all kind of immune responses? How important is their adhesion to the digestive tract? An enormous amount of work remains to be done, but it is important to hope that, given the promise of being able to "act" (notably using probiotics) on the intestinal microflora and therefore on its functions and therefore on our health, these three fields of research will develop in an interactive fashion and bring the awaited answers... and probably others that have not stopped surprising us!

Key points

- The intestinal immune system (IIS) fulfils two essential and opposed functions to maintain intestinal homeostasis: defence against pathogenic microorganisms (IgA antibodies and cell-mediated responses) and the establishment of suppressive responses to inhibit immune reactions against dietary proteins and bacterial components of the intestinal microflora which are permanently resident in the digestive tract.

- The sequential colonization of the baby's digestive tract (which is sterile at birth) by intestinal microflora plays a crucial role in maturation of the IIS, which is inactivated rather than immature. It probably also plays an important role in maturation of the systemic immune system, although this is less well characterized.

- The intestinal microflora has three fundamental roles on the intestinal and peripheral immune systems: a role in activation; a role in modulating specific responses (e.g. on the intestinal protective IgA anti-rotavirus response in babies); and finally, a regulatory role for the establishment of suppressive responses (e.g. tolerance induced by the oral route which prevents immune reactions to dietary proteins and components of our intestinal microflora).

- Depending on its action, the microflora will be involved in different ways:
  - it needs levels of diversity and complexity close to those of the adult microflora to mediate its full effect on IIS activation;
  - it only requires the presence, in the dominant microflora, of some bacteria which are able to mediate an adjuvant effect on defence responses such as the intestinal anti-rotavirus IgA response;
  - furthermore, it only requires the presence, in the dominant microflora, of bacteria (the same ones or others) able to induce the regulatory mechanisms with the condition, in some cases, that they are present from a very young age, illustrating the importance of the post-natal period in the acquisition of various regulatory mechanisms which will subsequently be operational throughout life.

- According to clinical studies, probiotics can have, in some cases, effects comparable to those of the bacteria which compose the intestinal microflora, thereby strengthening the idea that intestinal bacterial balance plays an important role in optimising and matching the host's immune responses according to the situations encountered. Probiotics represent new perspectives with respect to manipulating the intestinal microflora and its functions, and therefore our health.

References

1. Moreau MC, Gaboriau-Routhiau V. Influence of resident intestinal microflora on the development and functions of the Gut-Associated Lymphoid Tissue. *Microb Ecol Health Dis* 2001 ; 13 : 65-86.

2. Moreau MC, Thomasson M, Ducluzeau R, *et al*. Cinétique d'établissement de la microflore digestive chez le nouveau-né humain en fonction de la nature du lait. *Reprod Nutr Dévelop* 1986 ; 26 : 745-53.

3. Uderhill DM, Ozinsky A. Toll-like receptors: key mediators of microbe detection. *Curr Opin Immunol* 2002 ; 14 : 103-10.

4. Neish AS. The gut microflora and intestinal epithelial cells: a continuing dialogue. *Microb Infect* 2002 ; 4 : 309-17.

5. Romagnani S. The Th1/Th2 paradigm and allergic disorders. *Allergy* 1998 ; 53 : 12-5.

6. Pretolani M, Goldman M. IL-10: a potential therapy for allergic inflammation? *Immunol Today* 1997 ; 6 : 277-80.

7. Bondada S, Wu HJ, Robertson DA, *et al*. Accessory cell defect in unresponsiveness of neonates and aged to polysaccharides vaccines. *Vaccine* 2001 ; 19 : 557-65.

8. Nicaise P, Gleizes A, Forestier F, *et al*. The influence of *E. coli* implantation in axenic mice on cytokine production by peritoneal and bone marrow-derived macrophages. *Cytokine* 1995 ; 7 : 713-9.

9. Nicaise P, Gleizes A, Sandre C, *et al*. The intestinal microflora regulates cytokine production positively in spleen-derived macrophages but negatively in bone marrow-derived macrophages. *Eur Cytokine Netw* 1999 ; 10 : 365-72.

10. Nicaise P, Gleizes A, Forestier F, Quero AM, Labarre C. Influence of intestinal bacteria flora on cytokine (IL-1, IL-6 and TNF-α) production by mouse peritoneal macrophages. *Eur Cytokine Netw* 1993 ; 4 : 133-8.

11. Wold AE. The hygiene hypothesis revised: is the rising frequency of allergy due to changes in the intestinal flora? *Allergy* 1998 ; 46 : 20-5.

12. Renz H, vonMutius E, Illi S, *et al*. T (H) 1/T (H) 2 immune responses profiles differ between atopic children in eastern and western Germany. *J Allergy Clin Immunol* 2002 ; 109 : 338-42.

13. Riedler J, Braun-Fahrländer C, Eder W, *et al*. Exposure to farming in early life and development of asthma and allergy: a cross-sectional survey. *Lancet* 2001 ; 358 : 1129-33.

14. Isolauri E, Rautava S, Kalliomäki M, *et al*. Role of probiotics in food hypersensitivities. *Curr Opin Allergy Clin Immunol* 2002 ; 2 : 263-71.

15. Sudo N, Yu XN, Aiba Y, *et al*. An oral introduction of intestinal bacteria prevents the development of a long-term Th2-skewed immunological memory induced by neonatal antibiotic treatment in mice. *Clin Exp Allergy* 2002 ; 32 : 1112-6.

16. Kalliomaki M, Salminen S, Arvilommi H, *et al*. Probiotics in primary prevention of atopic disease: a randomised placebo-controlled trial. *Lancet* 2001 ; 357 : 1076-9.

17. Wostmann BS, Pleasants JR. The germ-free animal fed chemically defined diet: a unique tool. *Proc Soc Exp Biol Med* 1991 ; 198 : 539-46.

18. Freitas AA, Viale AC, Sunblad A, *et al*. Normal serum immunoglobulins participate in the selection of peripheral B-cell repertoires. *PNAS* 1991 ; 88 : 5640-4.

19. Kaveri SV, Lacroix-Desmazes S, Mouthon L, *et al*. Human natural antibodies: lessons from physiology and prospects for therapy. *Immunologist* 1998 ; 6 : 227-33.

20. Van der Broek MF, Van Bruggen MCJ, Koopman JP, *et al*. Gut flora induces and maintains resistance against streptococcal cell wall-induced arthritis in F344 rats. *Clin Exp Immunol* 1992 ; 88 : 313-7.

21. Cellier C, Cerf-Bensussan N, Brousse N, *et al*. Le système immunitaire intestinal. In : Rampal P, Beaugerie L, Marteau P, Corthier G, eds. *Colites infectieuses de l'adulte*. Paris : John Libbey Eurotext, 2000 : 27-38.

22. Mowat AM. Anatomical basis of tolerance and immunity to intestinal antigens. *Nature Rev Immunol* 2003 ; 3 : 331-41.

23. Phalipon A, Cardona A, Kraehenbuhl JP, *et al*. Secretory component: a new role in secretory IgA-mediated immune exclusion *in vivo*. *Immunity* 2002 ; 17 : 107-15.

24. Guy-Grand D, Vassali P. Gut intraepithelial lymphocyte development. *Curr Opin Immunol* 2002 ; 14 : 255-9.

25. Strobel S, Mowat A McI. Immune responses to dietary antigens : oral tolerance. *Immunol Today* 1998 ; 19 : 173-81.

26. Husby S, Mestecky J, Moldoveanu Z, *et al*. Oral tolerance in humans – T cell but not B cell tolerance after antigen feeding. *J Immunol* 1994 ; 152 : 4663-70.

27. Dutchmann R, Kaiser I, Hermann E, *et al*. Tolerance exists towards resident intestinal flora but is broken in active inflammatory bowel disease. *Clin Exp Immunol* 1995 ; 102 : 448-55.

28. Smith PD, Smythies LE, Mosteller-Barnum M, *et al*. Intestinal macrophages lack CD14 and CD89 and consequently are down-regulated for LPS- and IgA-mediated activities. *J Immunol* 2001 ; 167 : 2651-6.

29. Moreau MC, Raibaud P, Muller MC. Relation entre le développement du système immunitaire intestinal à IgA et l'établissement de la flore microbienne dans le tube digestif du souriceau holoxénique. *Ann Immunol (Inst. Pasteur)* 1982 ; 133D : 29-39.

30. Moreau MC, Ducluzeau R, Guy-Grand D, *et al*. Increase in the population of duodenal IgA plasmocytes in axenic mice monoassociated with different living or dead bacterial strains of intestinal origin. *Infect Immun* 1978 ; 21 : 532-9.

31. Moreau MC. Microflore intestinale, prébiotiques, probiotiques et immunomodulation. *NAFAS* 2001 ; 6 : 19-26.

32. Moreau MC. Effet immunomodulateur des bactéries intestinales : rôle des bifidobactéries. *J Péd Puér* 2001 ; 14 : 135-9.

33. Wannemuehler, MJ, Kiyono, H, Babb, JL, *et al*. Lipopolysaccharide (LPS) regulation of the immune response: LPS converts germfree mice to sensitivity to oral tolerance induction. *J Immunol* 1982 ; 129 : 959-65.

34. Moreau MC, Gaboriau-Routhiau V. The absence of gut flora, the doses of antigen ingested and aging affect the long-term peripheral tolerance induced by ovalbumin feeding in mice. *Res Immunol* 1996 ; 147 : 49-59.

35. Gaboriau-Routhiau V, Raibaud P, Dubuquoy C, *et al*. Colonization of gnotobiotic mice with human microflora at birth protects against *Escherichia coli* heat-labile enterotoxin-mediated abrogation of oral tolerance. *Pediatr Res* 2003 ; 54 : 739-46.

36. Sudo N, Sawamura SA, Tanaka K, *et al*. The requirement of intestinal bacterial flora for the development of an IgE production system fully susceptible to oral tolerance induction. *J Immunol* 1997 ; 159 : 1739-45.

37. Madsen K, Cornish A, Soper P, *et al*. Probiotic bacteria enhance murine and human intestinal epithelial barrier function. *Gastroenterology* 2001 ; 121 : 580-91.

38. Steidler L, Hans W, Schotte L, *et al*. Treatment of murine colitis by *Lactococcus lactis* secreting interleukin-10. *Science* 2000 ; 289 : 1352-5.

39. Tamboli CP, Caucheteux C, Cortot A, *et al*. Probiotics in inflammatory bowel disease: a critical review. *Best Pract Res Clin Gastroenterol* 2003 ; 17 : 805-20.

40. Neish AS, Gewirtz AT, Zeng T, *et al*. Prokaryotic regulation of epithelial responses by inhibition of I kB- aubiquitination. *Science* 2000 ; 289 : 1560-3.

41. Dubuquoy L, Jansson EA, Deeb S, *et al*. Impaired expression of peroxisome proliferator-activated receptor gin ulcerative colitis. *Gastroenterology* 2003, 124 : 1265-76.

42. Gionchetti P, Rizello F, Venturi A, *et al*. Oral bacteriotherapy as maintenance treatment in patients with chronic pouchitis; a double blind placebo controlled trial. *Gastroenterology* 2000 ; 119 : 305-9.

43. Guslandi M, Giollo P, Testoni PA. A pilot trial of *Saccharomyces boulardii* in ulcerative colitis. *Eur J Gastroenterol Hepatol* 2003 ; 15 : 697-8.

Influence of the Intestinal Microflora on Host Immunity in Inflammatory Bowel Disease

Pierre Desreumaux, Christel Rousseaux

Service des Maladies de l'Appareil Digestif et de la Nutrition, Équipe INSERM-Université 0114, CHU Lille, France.

Crohn's disease and ulcerative colitis are both inflammatory bowel diseases (IBD), characterized by flare-ups alternating with periods of remission. This special pattern leads to lesions of variable age that can be distinguished at the macroscopic level and by histological analysis as either acute or chronic lesions. IBD involves loss of regulation of the mucosal immune response which is then directed against components of the gut microflora, and it occurs in genetically predisposed subjects. Interactions between the gut microflora and the mucosal immune system therefore play an important role in the pathogenesis of these IBD.

Microflora and inflammatory bowel diseases

Observations suggesting that the microflora is involved in inflammatory bowel disease

Most of the animal models of colitis (spontaneously occurring or induced by chemical agents) depend on the presence of the bacterial microflora in the gut lumen [1, 2]. Only in those mouse models in which either the glial fibrillar acid glycoprotein (GFAP) or the Gαi2 protein have been knocked out are lesions developed (respectively in the jejunum and the colon) in the absence of any gut microflora [3, 4]. In the other models, there is no intestinal inflammation or it is extremely attenuated in axenic animals. In addition, one model of chronic granulomatous colitis which mimics Crohn's disease is based on the intraperitoneal administration of streptococcal cell wall material (PG-PS) in the distal colon of rats [2, 5]. Therefore, in animal models, the gut microflora is a crucial factor in the induction and maintenance of intestinal lesions.

Similar observations have been made in humans. The intestinal mucosa of an IBD patient is colonized by an abundant gut microflora, especially in ulcers and fistulae (Figure 1). Cartun *et al.* detected antigens of *Escherichia coli* and *Streptococcus* in 69% and 63% respectively of resected tissues from patients with Crohn's disease [6]. In a number of studies, high levels of antibodies directed against various bacteria of the saprophytic microflora

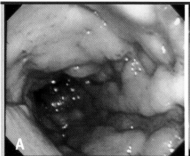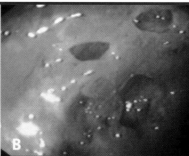

Figure 1.
Crohn's disease.
Endoscopic image
of severe colitis.
A : longitudinal ulcers,
forming a continuous
line.
B : pitted ulcers
(photographs by
A. Bitoun, Hôpital
Lariboisière, Paris.
Traité de Gastro-
entérologie, 2000,
J.C. Rambaud, ed.
Médecine-Sciences
Flammarion)

(notably *Bacteroides, Streptococcus faecalis* and *Escherichia coli*) have been measured in the blood of patients with Crohn's disease [7]. Most light has been shed on the pathogenic role of the gut microflora in Crohn's disease by work on the model of endoscopic recurrence following surgery. After surgical resection of the terminal ileum followed by ileocolonic anastomosis, endoscopic recurrence occurred within one year in 73% of cases. If the anastomosis was protected from faecal material by a surgical opening upstream, no lesions developed; however, recurrence soon occurred if digestive continuity was re-established leading to re-exposure of the anastomotic region to faecal material [8]. We recently showed that, in this situation, the neo-ileum—the focus of the recurrence—was colonized by a gut microflora similar to that in the colon which may play a role in reactivating the disease process [9]. Harper *et al.* showed that the instillation of ileal contents into the excluded colon led to clinical recurrence within one week in 60% of patients with Crohn's disease in remission. In contrast, no recurrence was observed if the ileal contents had been sterilized and ultrafiltered to remove particles of greater than 0.22 μm in size (i.e,. including bacteria) suggesting that the gut microflora has a primordial role in the phenomenon [10]. Finally, the efficacy of certain probiotics in the treatment and prevention of flare-ups of IBD together with their action against refractory pouchitis following total colectomy to correct ulcerative colitis (*see chapter entitled* "Probiotics and Digestive Problems") provide indirect evidence of the involvement of the gut microflora in such problems.

Changes in the endogenous microflora in inflammatory bowel disease

Most studies so far of the gut microflora of patients suffering from Crohn's disease have been based on faecal samples. Such studies have shown increased densities of anaerobic bacteria, notably of *Bacteroides vulgatus* and certain Gram-positive cocci (*Eubacterium, Peptostreptococcus* and *Coprococcus*) [11]. This pattern could be genetically determined since, in a prospective study, Van de Merwe *et al.* showed that one-third of the children (who were symptom-free) of patients with Crohn's disease had higher faecal densities of anaerobic bacteria than control subjects [12] although this observation has not yet been confirmed. Keighley *et al.* detected significant increases in the numbers of *Escherichia coli* and *Bacteroides fragilis* in the ileum and colon of patients with Crohn's disease [13].

Few studies have addressed the adherent microflora in IBD. In a series of patients with ulcerative colitis—twenty-five experiencing a first flare-up, twenty with recurrence, and forty-four in remission—Hartley *et al.* observed reduced numbers of *Bifidobacterium* and increased colonization by *Escherichia coli* in the involved segments during the flare-up [14]. In another study on the microflora associated with the ileal mucosa, enterobacteria were isolated more often from biopsies from patients with Crohn's disease than from control subjects [15]. Studying the microflora associated with the ileal mucosa in Crohn's disease focuses on the most common segment involved in this disease, eliminating interference with the abundant fermenting microflora in the colon. Our preliminary results suggest that non-sporulating, Gram-positive bacilli (*Eubacterium* and *Bifidobacterium*) are isolated less frequently whereas enterobacteria—especially *Escherichia coli*—are more common [16].

Another possible approach to the study of the microflora focuses on metabolic functions. Several studies have revealed reduced exoglycosidase activity (β-galactosidase, N-acetyl-β-glucosaminidase and α-mannosidase) in the faeces of patients with active Crohn's disease, a reduction which correlates with decreased numbers of *Bifidobacterium* in the faecal microflora [17]. The levels of mucin-degrading enzymes are elevated in ulcerative colitis but remain the same in Crohn's disease. Short-chain fatty acids (SCFA) (acetic, propionic and butyric acids) are the main products of colonic bacterial fermentation. Butyrate provides 70% of the energy requirement of colonocytes. In flare-ups of ulcerative colitis, the faecal SCFA concentration is reduced and the lactate concentration is increased. According to Roediger, ulcerative colitis results from energy deficiency in the colonic epithelium, according to which hypothesis colonocytes from patients with ulcerative colitis would metabolize SCFAs less efficiently than colonocytes from normal subjects [18]. This metabolic change could be induced by excess sulphides produced by large numbers of sulphate-reducing bacteria: in patients with ulcerative colitis, this type of bacterium would represent up to 97% of all the bacteria in the faeces compared with 50-70 % in control subjects. This theory is being tested in therapeutic trials of SCFA enemas to treat ulcerative colitis, although the results hitherto are disappointing.

Specific roles of components of the gut microflora in inflammatory bowel disease

Obligate anaerobes

A number of observations point to anaerobic bacteria having a specific role in IBD. Trials based on the selective implantation of microfloras in HLA-B27 transgenic mice have shown that the presence of anaerobic bacteria (notably *Bacteroides*) is critical for the onset of inflammation [19]. The faecal density of *Bacteroides vulgatus* is increased in flare-ups of Crohn's disease, and the therapeutic efficacy of metronidazole correlates with reductions in the density of this species [20]. Certain strains of *Bacteroides vulgatus* have been shown to have special adhesion properties but none of these have yet been isolated from patients with IBD. Other experimental evidence also suggests that certain strains of some clostridial species like *Clostridium ramosum* might have special pro-inflammatory activity [21].

Facultative anaerobes

The possibility that *Escherichia coli* is specifically involved in IBD is currently under investigation. *Escherichia coli* is one of the bacteria which is reproducibly found at high levels in patients' luminal and adherent microfloras [22], and higher levels of antibodies against *Escherichia coli* are found in patients with Crohn's disease than in normal subjects [7]. *Escherichia coli*-specific antibodies have been detected in the mucosa of Crohn's disease, associated with macrophages, ulcerous giant cells in the bottom of ulcerations, granulomas and the *lamina propria* [6]. Several *in vitro* studies have shown that *Escherichia coli* strains isolated from the faeces of patients suffering from IBD had similar adhesion properties to those of enteropathogenic strains [23, 24]. More than 80% of *Escherichia coli* isolates from the ileal mucosa of patients with Crohn's disease bound Caco-2 cells compared with only 33% of reference *Escherichia coli* strains: entero-invasive (EIEC), enteropathogenic (EPEC), enterotoxinogenic (ETEC), entero-aggregating (EaggEC), enterohaemorrhagic (EHEC) or diffusely adhering (DAEC). None of these strains were carrying any of the virulence genes associated with enteropathogenic strains of *Escherichia coli*, and one-quarter of them were synthesizing an α-haemolysin which was cytotoxic for cultured cells [25]. Thus, at the same time as strains of *Escherichia coli* expressing certain pathogenicity factors are acquired, the development of Crohn's disease could also be linked to enhanced susceptibility of the patient's mucosa to colonization.

Immunity and inflammatory bowel disease

In IBD, the mucosal immune system is destabilized by a cascade of mechanisms. The first is abnormal stimulation of cells resident in the intestinal mucosa, leading to the activation of signal transduction pathways, including the nuclear factor kappa B (NFκB) and mitogen-activated protein kinase (MAPK or stress kinase) pathways. Activation leads to the production of inflammatory mediators (cytokines and chemokines) which will then recruit new inflammatory cells from the blood into intestinal wall tissue as a result of the up-regulation of adhesion molecules (Figure 2).

These two mechanisms lead to the infiltration of activated, pro-inflammatory cells into the gut wall. A final pathogenic mechanism, namely inhibition of apoptosis (physiological cell death) results in enhanced survival of these pro-inflammatory cells in the intestinal mucosa, thereby sustaining the inflammatory process.

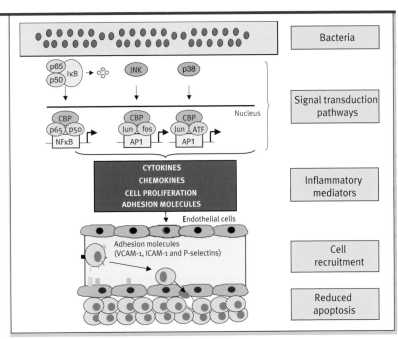

Figure 2.
Cascades in intestinal inflammation. Intestinal inflammation is mediated by the activation of resident cells by luminal bacteria (red circles). Activation leads to breakdown of inhibitory kappa B protein (IκB) and translocation of nuclear factor kappa B (NFκB) (which is composed of two sub-units, one of 50 kD [p50] and another of 65 kD [p65]). It also induces activation of mitogen-activated protein kinases (MAPK) leading to entry of p38 and the c-jun-NH2-terminal kinase (JNK) into the nucleus where certain co-activators are mobilised: the cyclic AMP response element binding protein (CREB) - binding protein (CBP) or the dimeric transcription factors jun-fos or jun-activating transcription factor (ATF) which bind a DNA region called the Activating protein (AP)-1 involved in the regulation of inflammation and cell proliferation. These cellular signal transduction pathways lead to the transcription (→) of genes encoding inflammatory mediators (cytokines and chemokines), growth factors, and adhesion molecules capable of inducing the recruitment of cells from the blood into the intestinal wall. Impaired clearance of intestinal inflammatory cells resulting from the inhibition of apoptotic mechanisms are also involved in digestive tract inflammation.

Activation of signal transduction pathways

The two main signal transduction pathways involved in inflammatory phenomena are the NFκB/IκB (inhibitory protein kappa B) and MAPK pathways. The NFκB/IκB heterodimer is found in the cytoplasm of all human cells. After activation of a cell, a cascade of phosphorylation reactions leads to breakdown of the IκB inhibitory protein resulting in translocation of NFκB (which is composed of two sub-units, one of 50 kD [p50] and another of 65 kD [p65]) from the cytoplasm into the nucleus where it interacts with certain nuclear transcription cofactors (such as the cyclic AMP response element binding protein [CREB] - binding protein [CBP]), in an inflammatory response triggered by two inflammatory cytokines (TNFα and IL-1β). The MAPK pathway involves about fifty cytoplasmic transcription factors organised in three modules: the MAP kinase kinase kinases (MAPKKK), the MAP kinase kinases (MAPKK) and the MAP kinases (MAPK). Activation of these three modules by stress factors gives rise to three main factors, namely p38, c-jun-NH2-terminal kinase (JNK) and extracellular-signal regulated kinase (ERK) which are then allowed to move into the cell nucleus. In the nucleus, p38 and JNK mobilise co-activators such as CBP or the dimeric transcription factors jun-fos or jun-activating transcription factor (ATF) which bind a DNA region called the activating protein (AP)-1 which is involved in the regulation of inflammation and cell proliferation (Figure 2).

Several studies in IBD patients have revealed increased activation of the NFκB/IκB and MAPK pathways in the intestinal mucosa. Most of the information about the pathological role of such local activation has come from experimental models of colitis in which inhibition of either the NFκB pathway (e.g. by an antisense oligonucleotide to the p65 of NFκB or an enzyme inhibitor [OXIS]) or the MAPK pathway (anti-p35) has proved effective in reversing the disease process. A number of therapeutic trials are currently underway in patients with Crohn's disease and ulcerative colitis [26].

Cytokine and chemokine production

Classification

Cytokines are soluble, low molecular weight proteins involved in communication between cells. They can be produced by various cell types. Small quantities are produced locally and they have a short half-life, all of which makes them difficult to assay, so methods based on gene amplification (e.g. the PCR) are particularly valuable when it comes to analysing these molecules. In normal conditions, cytokines are produced in the intestinal mucosa and quantitative methods are needed if their pathophysiological roles are to be elucidated. Since the discovery of the first cytokine in 1957, various classification systems based on structure and function have been proposed. Despite the existence of numerous regulatory loops and extreme functional pleiotropy, three major groups have been characterized: the inflammatory and anti-inflammatory cytokines; the immunoregulatory cytokines; and the chemokines. The balance between inflammatory cytokines (IL-1, IL-6, IL-8, TNFα) and anti-inflammatory cytokines (IL-1 receptor antagonist [IL-1RA], IL-10 and TGFβ) locally dictates the intensity and duration of the inflammatory reaction. It can also affect systemic parameters, e.g. reducing albumin synthesis and increasing the production of inflammatory proteins. The immunoregulatory cytokines are involved in susceptibility and resistance to infectious agents, allergic mechanisms and the regulation of inflammatory cytokines. They are divided into two different types referred to, in humans, as type 1 or type 2 by analogy with the classification system developed by Mossman *et al.* for clones of CD4+ T lymphocytes in mice (Th1 and Th2 profiles). The type 1 immunoregulatory cytokines are IL-2 and IFNγ which are involved in activating the cells of the immune system and the resistance to bacterial infection, delayed hypersensitivity reactions, and the synthesis of IgG2a. Type 2 cytokines (IL-4, IL-5 and IL-13) stimulate IgE synthesis, the activation and recruitment of eosinophils, resistance to parasitic infections, allergic mechanisms and susceptibility to bacterial infections. The chemokines represent a sub-group of about fifty mediators characterized by chemo-attractive activity [27]. Distinction is made between two distinct families on the basis of structural considerations: the CXC chemokines, notably IL-8 and growth-related oncogenes (GRO) α, β and γ, which are involved in the recruitment and activation of neutrophils; and the CC chemokines which include monocyte chemotactic proteins (MCP)-4 and 5, RANTES and eotaxin which, together with IL-5, recruits and activates eosinophils in the tissues.

Cytokines act on target cells when they bind to specific receptors, thereby activating a cascade of intracellular events, notably triggering the NFκB/IκB and MAPK pathways. There are autocrine and/or paracrine loops between these signal transduction pathways which affect the production of inflammatory cytokines; how these are regulated remains poorly understood.

Cytokines and animal models of colitis

Fifty-odd animal models of inflammatory colitis have been described, falling into three broad groups [28]. The first group covers spontaneous colitis models occurring in genetically modified animals. In these animals, a gene may have been knocked out or one may be abnormally expressed (transgenic animals or tissular gene transfer). In both other groups, colitis is induced, by the administration of either activated cells (e.g. of T lymphocytes into SCID mice), chemical agents (indomethacin, trinitrobenzene sulphonic acid [TNBS], dextran sulphate sodium [DSS] or acetic acid), or bacterial products (peptidoglycan-polysaccharide [PG-PS]). In these animal models, most of the chronic lesions are found in the colon.

In all of these models, the intestinal lesions are associated with increased production of inflammatory cytokines. When it comes to the immunoregulatory cytokines, the lesions of chronic colitis are associated with an increase in the synthesis of type 1 cytokines (IL-2 or IFNγ) [29]. IFNγ plays an important role in triggering and maintaining lesions in mice in which the gene coding for either IL-10 or the Gαi2 transduction-inhibiting protein has been knocked out, as well as when activated T cells (CD45RB[high]) are transferred into SCID mice. Several more recent studies have revealed the importance of type 2 cytokines in the triggering of colonic lesions. In models of spontaneous colitis (mice in which the gene for T cell receptor chain a has been knocked out) or in which colitis has been induced using a chemical agent (TNBS), cytokine profiles change with the age of the intestinal lesions: acute lesions are associated with elevated IL-4 synthesis and local IgE production (type 2); before the lesions become chronic, the profile of immunoregulatory cytokines being produced switches from type 2 towards type 1. Finally, inflammatory ileal and colonic lesions resembling IBD have been reported in mice that are transgenic for IL-4 and IL-5 (two type 2 cytokines).

Cytokines/chemokines and inflammatory bowel diseases

The levels of cytokines detected in the blood do not reflect immunologic changes in the gut. This review will only discuss local studies focusing on the intestinal mucosa of patients with IBD.

The inflammatory cytokines TNFα, IL-6 and IL-1β are involved in the chronic, inflammatory lesions in patients with Crohn's disease and ulcerative colitis. In Crohn's disease, TNFα is expressed in lesions in the mucosa, the sub-mucosa and the serosa. The macrophage is the main secreting cell in the *lamina propria*. An immunohistochemical signal is also detected in other structures, including granulomas, the germinative centres of lymphoid follicles and the mesenteric adipose tissue of patients with Crohn's disease [30]. The role of this abnormal TNFα synthesis by mesenteric adipocytes and macrophages is not understood but it could partly account for the preferential localization of intestinal mucosal lesions in Crohn's disease along the mesenteric border, and the frequency of adhesions in the intestinal loops. Quantitatively, it seems that more TNFα might be produced in the damaged mucosae of patients with chronic Crohn's disease than in ulcerative colitis. Similar results have been obtained for IL-6 and IL-1β. Although contradictory results have been published, there does not seem to be any primary abnormality in the synthesis of inflammatory cytokines or TGFβ in the healthy mucosal tissue of patients with Crohn's disease or ulcerative colitis. The presence of IL-1RA has also been investigated in the damaged mucosa of patients with IBD. Although controversial, there may be a relative reduction in the level of IL-1RA with a diminished IL-1RA/IL-1 ratio compared with that seen in other inflammatory conditions. In conclusion, the intestinal lesions of Crohn's disease and ulcerative colitis are associated with increased synthesis of inflammatory cytokines and, probably, relative deficiency in the production of anti-inflammatory cytokines. This abnormal balance between inflammatory and anti-inflammatory cytokines seems to be secondary to the inflammation and is not observed in the healthy mucosal tissue of patients with IBD.

As in the animal models, immunoregulatory cytokine profiles vary in the course of Crohn's disease [31]. Acute ileal lesions that develop three months after surgery are associated with type 2 cytokine production, notably IL-4, and an increase in the expression of productive IgE mRNA is observed. These cytokines are mainly synthesized by T lymphocytes, mast cells and eosinophils. In the same patients, chronic lesions are associated with a type 1 cytokine profile which could be induced by IL-12 and IL-18 produced by macrophages in the *lamina propria*. These findings suggest that various immunologic mechanisms lead to the triggering and maintenance of lesions, so different therapeutic protocols could be required to prevent post-surgical recurrence or to treat chronic lesions.

IL-8 is the chemokine which has been the most extensively studied in IBD. Several studies have shown increased IL-8 production (at both the mRNA and protein levels) in the inflamed colonic mucosa of patients with Crohn's disease and ulcerative colitis. Macrophages and neutrophils are the main cells responsible. Increased production is secondary to the inflammation since comparable levels of IL-8 are seen in the healthy mucosae of patients with IBD and controls. The synthesis of other chemokines involved in the recruitment and activation of neutrophils and macrophages in the intestinal mucosa (such as GRO, MCP-1, macrophage inflammatory protein (MIP)-1 α and β) is also elevated in IBD. The synthesis of C-C chemokines involved in the recruitment and activation of eosinophils in the intestinal mucosa has not been extensively investigated although three studies have shown increased RANTES production in Crohn's disease and increases in eotaxin levels, more marked in ulcerative colitis than in Crohn's disease. These findings explain the pleiotropic nature of the cells which make up the inflammatory infiltrate in patients with IBD. Further work will be necessary to determine the cascade of events underlying the inflammatory reaction in the course of the disease.

Increased expression of adhesion molecules

In Crohn's disease and ulcerative colitis (Figure 3), the intestinal lesions are characterized by infiltration of the mucosa by peripheral leukocytes.

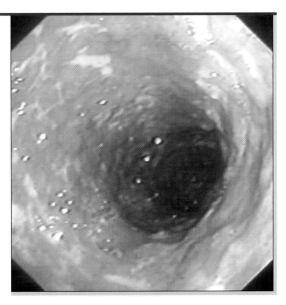

Figure 3.
Moderately severe ulcerative colitis:
erythema and superficial ulceration.
(photograph: A. Bitoun,
Hôpital Lariboisière, Paris.
Traité de Gastro-entérologie, 2000,
J.C. Rambaud, ed.
Médecine-Sciences Flammarion)

These leukocytes from the blood—mainly neutrophils and lymphocytes—bind to gut endothelial cells *via* various different cell surface receptors referred to as adhesion molecules (Figure 2). Expression of these adhesion molecules is partly regulated by cytokines. Distinction is made between two main families of adhesion molecule: molecules which are related to immunoglobulins and the selectins [32]. Binding of the lymphocyte function antigen (LFA)-1 by an intercellular adhesion molecule (ICAM-1 or ICAM-2) leads to recruitment of peripheral leukocytes into intestinal tissues. Other interactions between very late antigen (VLA)-4 or α4β7 and the vascular cell adhesion molecule (VCAM)-1 play a more selective role, attracting lymphocytes into the gut wall, whereas the macrophage-1(Mac-1)/ICAM-1 interaction leads to an infiltrate which is rich in neutrophils. The discovery of these adhesion molecules and their ligands has provided enormous insight into the mechanisms whereby cells are recruited from the blood into gut wall tissue, and has made a great contribution to the development of compounds to block formation of the cellular infiltrate. The therapeutic potential of certain compounds, notably ones targeting α4β7, is currently being evaluated in patients with Crohn's disease.

Inhibition of mechanisms of apoptosis

Apoptosis is the process of programmed cell death which, unlike necrosis, is an active, energy-dependent process. It manifests morphologically as a loss of cell volume and nuclear condensation with DNA fragmentation. Apoptosis is a physiological mechanism which rapidly eliminates ageing cells and protects the surrounding tissues, notably against inflammation induced by the release of cytoplasmic proteolytic enzymes.

In Crohn's disease, the rate of apoptosis is reduced in certain T lymphocytes (TL) in the *lamina propria* which are responsible for inflammatory reactions [33]. The reasons for this reduction are probably multiple but IL-6—which is mainly produced by macrophages and TLs—is known to be involved. The IL-6 produced binds to its receptor which is a heterodimer formed between an IL-6-binding peptide (IL-6R) and another peptide which transduces the signal (gp130). The IL-6R detaches from the cell membrane as a soluble complex with the IL-6 molecule; this complex binds gp130 expressed by a TL to activate anti-apoptotic factors, such as signal transducer and activator of transcription (STAT)-3 and the genes *bcl-2* and *bcl-xl* [33].

Mechanisms underlying gut microflora-induced inflammation in inflammatory bowel diseases

The gut microflora and the mucosal immune system interact with one another and the gut microflora is known to be able to induce intestinal inflammation by many different mechanisms. In the reverse case, it is also possible that an inappropriate immune response against the resident microflora can render the digestive tract susceptible to non-pathogenic bacteria.

Action of the gut microflora on the immune system

Pro-inflammatory role of bacterial components

Lipopolysaccharides (LPS) are the main constituents of the cell wall of Gram-negative bacteria. These endotoxins are powerful activators of macrophages, polymorphonuclear cells, endothelial cells, and T and B lymphocytes. LPS activation of monocytes/macrophages is partly dependent on the presence of the CD14 receptor and Toll-like receptor (TLR) 4 (Figure 4).

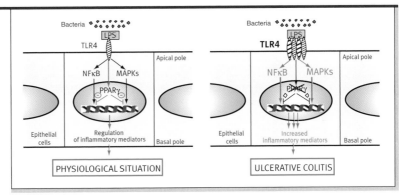

Figure 4. Role of the peroxisome proliferator-activated receptor (PPARγ) in inflammation. In physiological conditions, epithelial cells express the TLR4 receptor which, once bound by LPS, induce activation of the NFκB and MAPK pathways. However, this activation of signal transduction pathways is regulated by the induction of PPARγ by the binding of TLR4 by luminal bacteria, thereby maintaining intestinal homeostasis. In ulcerative colitis, TLR4 is over-expressed and it fails to induce the expression of PPARγ. Thus, regulation of the NFκB and MAPK pathways is perturbed leading to the production of inflammatory mediators

In normal physiological conditions, the macrophages of the *lamina propria* express little CD14 and this low level of expression might explain the relatively weak, local activating effect of bacterial LPS. In IBD, primary elevation of CD14 expression on macrophages extracted from the healthy and the damaged colonic *lamina propria* could partly explain the role of the gut microflora in initiating the chronicity of lesions [34]. In the same way, increased expression of TLR4 by macrophages and cells of the intestinal epithelium in patients with Crohn's disease could result in susceptibility to bacterially induced inflammation [35-37]. Recently, an abnormal balance between TLR4 expression and expression of the peroxisome proliferator-activated gamma receptor (PPARγ) was detected in ulcerative colitis [38]. PPARγ is a nuclear receptor with anti-inflammatory activity [39] which, in physiological conditions, is expressed by colonic epithelial cells [40] and whose expression is regulated by TLR4 (at least in part). In ulcerative colitis, the over-expression of LPS-activated TLR4 and the deficit in PPARγ expression by epithelial cells would result in absence of the regulation of the NFκB and MAPK pathways, which would be the reason for the chronicity of the inflammatory reaction (Figure 4). Another protein derived from the cell walls of Gram-negative and Gram-positive bacteria could also play an important role in the pathogenesis of Crohn's disease, namely peptidoglycan and more specifically the muramyl dipeptide, which can activate the cytoplasmic CARD15 receptor leading to the secretion of inflammatory mediators (see below).

Formyl-methionyl-leucyl-phenylalanine (FMLP) is an oligopeptide secreted by certain intestinal bacteria, including *Escherichia coli*. This and related peptides are potent chemotactic agents for neutrophils [41] and have been shown to induce acute colitis following intraluminal instillation into laboratory animals [42]. Anton *et al.* demonstrated that circulating neutrophils from patients with Crohn's disease express more surface FMLP receptors than cells from either patients suffering from ulcerative colitis or control subjects [43]. Moreover, the activity of FMLP-degrading enzymes (FMLP-ase) is lower in the ileum of patients with Crohn's disease compared with patients with ulcerative colitis or healthy controls [44]. All these factors together with the increased permeability of the mucosa to bacterial components (see below) could contribute to increased neutrophil chemotaxis which could trigger inflammation.

Other bacterial cell wall components (PG-PS) can be used to induce experimental colitis following injection into the colonic wall [2, 5].

Microflora and intestinal permeability

Certain bacteria, such as *Klebsiella spp*. and streptococci, increase intestinal permeability as measured in rats by means of a dextran-mannitol test [45]. Increased permeability could lead to the presence of more bacterial or dietary antigens in intestinal wall tissue and abnormal stimulation of the mucosal immune system.

Recruitment of inflammatory cells

Bacteria can influence the homing of peripheral inflammatory cells towards the digestive tract. In axenic mice, fewer polymorphonuclear cells are found in the *lamina propria* than in conventional mice. In immunodeficient SCID mice, the peripheral injection of immunocompetent CD45 RB[high] T lymphocytes triggers colitis. These parenterally administered peripheral cells only home to the digestive tract in the presence of gut microflora; they disappear in axenic mice [46]. The bacterial mechanisms leading to homing to the digestive tract could involve adhesion molecules. In rats, the presence of a colonic microflora induces mucosal expression of ICAM-1, the ligand of the $\beta2$ integrins LFA-1 and Mac-1 which are mainly expressed on polymorphonuclear cells [47].

Abnormal host immune responses against the microflora

Break of tolerance

Commensal bacteria can stimulate T lymphocytes of the intestinal mucosa and could cause lesions in IBD. Mononuclear cells extracted from the intestinal mucosa of a healthy human subject are normally tolerant of the homologous microflora but will proliferate and become activated in response to a heterologous microflora. In Crohn's disease, mononuclear cells extracted from damaged areas of the colon–but not those from healthy areas–are activated by even the homologous microflora. Such activation could reflect a break of tolerance to the subject's own microflora secondary to the development of lesions [48]. Similar results were obtained in mice with TNBS-induced colitis [49] in which the break of tolerance induced by the injection of TNBS was mediated by IL-12 and inhibited by IL-10. This phenomenon could therefore play an important role in the maintenance of inflammatory lesions.

Cytokine modulation of bacterial susceptibility and resistance

The triggering of inflammation by commensal bacteria could also be due to an inappropriate intestinal immune response on the part of the host. Certain cytokine profiles determine whether the body will be susceptible or resistant to a bacterium. Type 1 immunoregulatory cytokines (IL-2 and IFNγ) and inflammatory cytokines (IL-1, IL-6 and TNFα) partly determine host resistance to various bacteria and viruses. Most bacteria—especially intracellular bacteria like mycobacteria and *Listeria*—induce a type 1 immune response which eliminates the infectious agent at the same time as preventing a chronic inflammatory response. Animals in which the gene for IFNγ [50], IL-6 [51] or TNFα [52] has been knocked out are all susceptible to these pathogenic bacteria as well as *Candida albicans*. In contrast, type 2 immune responses (characterized by the production of IL-4) are associated with chronic infections, not only with pathogenic bacteria but also with bacteria of the saprophytic gut microflora. *In vitro*, IL-4 is a required supplement for culture of the bacterium which causes Whipple's disease [53]. In pigs, the intestinal expression of type 2 cytokines which is induced by the non-pathogenic whipworm (*Trichuris suis*) makes the animal's commensal microflora "pathogenic" and triggers necrotic proliferative colitis [54]. The known existence of a type 2 intestinal immune response in acute Crohn's disease lesions could make the digestive tract abnormally susceptible to its gut microflora [31].

Abnormal recognition of bacterial components by the innate immune system

One year ago, three European and American research teams identified the first gene for susceptibility to Crohn's disease, Nod2, which has since been renamed CARD15 by an international harmonisation committee [55-57]. Three main mutations and thirty-odd minor mutations of CARD15 have been detected in patients with Crohn's disease. About 50% of patients carry one of these mutations on one of their chromosomes (heterozygotes) and 15% have either the same mutation (homozygotes) or two different mutations (composite heterozygotes) on both their chromosomes. On the basis of these frequencies, the risk of developing Crohn's disease can be estimated at one-and-a-half to three times greater in simple heterozygotes than in subjects without any mutation, and about forty times greater in homozygotes or composite heterozygotes, making the genotype at this locus the most important risk factor yet identified. The first phenotypic studies carried out on the three main mutations make it possible to define a sub-population of patients who develop the disease at a younger age, which in this group is more often localized in the ileum and more likely to cause stenosis (Figure 5) [58-62].

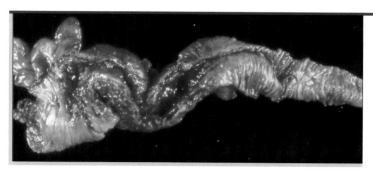

Figure 5.
Crohn's disease.
Resected ileum/caecum.
Lesions involving the terminal ileum and the ileocaecal valve; parietal thickening causing stenosis
(photograph:
A. Lavergne-Slove,
Hôpital Lariboisière, Paris.
Traité de Gastro-entérologie,
2000, J.C. Rambaud, ed.
Médecine-Sciences
Flammarion)

CARD15 is a cytoplasmic receptor expressed by monocytes/ macrophages, dendritic cells, Paneth cells, epithelial cells and T lymphocytes. Although CARD15 is spontaneously expressed in monocytes/macrophages and dendritic cells (cells which specialize in the presentation of antigens to lymphocytes), its expression in T lymphocytes and, to an even greater extent in colonic epithelial cells, is induced by TNFα, the central mediator of inflammation. Thus, CARD15 is expressed in cells which play a key role in immune responses and which are responsible for the surveillance for infectious phenomena in the gut. In functional terms, although the receptor's role remains poorly understood, it seems to be involved in the response to bacterial infection. CARD15 is a member of a recently described family, including Nod1/CARD4, ICE protease activating factor (Ipaf)-1/CARD12 and Apoptotic protease activating factor (Apaf)-1, which has structural homology with plant molecules which are involved in resistance to pathogenic bacteria [63]. CARD15 contains two N-terminal domains which mediate recruitment and activation of caspases (CARD, caspase-recruitment domain) linked to a nucleotide-binding domain (NBD) and a C-terminal domain based on leucine-rich repeat (LRR) sequences (Figure 6). The functional roles of the LRRs have not as yet been entirely elucidated but the proposed hypothesis is that they are involved in recognizing bacterial components such as peptidoglycan [55]. Recognition of a bacterial compound would trigger a cascade of events in the cell's cytoplasm, notably mobilisation of a transcription factor called RICK which, through a CARD-CARD interaction, leads to phosphorylation events and the activation of NFκB (Figure 6). Two studies conducted in mice suggest that RICK-less animals are more susceptible to bacterial infection, especially with intracellular species such as *Listeria monocytogenes* [64, 65]. Thus RICK, the partner of CARD15, is involved in the control of infectious phenomena, in particular by regulating the production of cytokines which are essential to an effective immune response (IFNγ, IL-12 and IL-18). These results expand our understanding of the pathogenesis of Crohn's disease. The absence of functional CARD15 in epithelial cells and key immune cells could explain the role played by luminal bacteria in the triggering and maintenance of intestinal lesions. In addition, the existence of a regulatory loop between TNFα and CARD15 in the epithelial cell suggests that the opportunist infections which take hold after anti-TNFα treatment could be secondary to inhibition of the expression of CARD15, the key receptor in controlling bacterial infections originating in the mucosa.

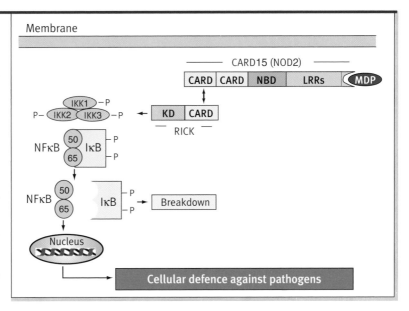

Figure 6. NOD2/CARD15 and the innate immune response. CARD15 is a cytoplasmic receptor formed by two N-terminal domains (CARD, caspase-recruitment domain) linked to a nucleotide-binding domain (NBD) and a C-terminal domain based on leucine-rich repeat (LRR) sequences. The C-terminal LRR region is involved in the recognition of muramyl dipeptide (MDP) which is derived from peptidoglycans in the membranes of Gram-positive and Gram-negative bacteria. CARD15-mediated recognition of bacterial components would trigger a cascade of events in the cell's cytoplasm, notably mobilisation of a transcription factor called RICK which, through a CARD-CARD interaction, leads to phosphorylation of the IκB kinase complex (IKK1-2-3), breakdown of the inhibitory IκB protein and release of the NFκB complex formed by the p50/p65 heterodimer. Thus, CARD15 would be involved in the innate, non-specific immune response against bacteria through activation of the NFκB pathway leading to production of inflammatory mediators capable of controlling the pathogenic potential of bacteria

Conclusion

Many studies have revealed the extensive interactions between bacteria and the gut mucosal immune system in the pathogenesis of IBD. This idea has been consolidated by discovery of the Crohn's disease-associated gene CARD15 which is involved in the inflammatory response induced by bacterial peptidoglycan. However, the exact mechanisms underlying perturbation of the interaction between infectious microorganisms and the host remain hypothetical. Would the guilty party be a pathogenic bacterium persisting in the mucosa leading to abnormal activation of immune cells; or, in contrast, could abnormal immune responses against the host's own gut microflora be involved? The availability of molecular tools for the study of gut microflora microorganisms that cannot be cultured using conventional bacteriological techniques; comparison of the expression profiles of the faecal and adherent microfloras in specimens and the mucosae (both healthy and inflamed) of healthy subjects and patients; descriptive and functional analyses of genes associated with the immune system which are regulated by infectious agents, and of receptors for bacteria, viruses and DNA in patients with IBD; and finally, the phenotyping of genetically modified mice—in particular *vis-à-vis* CARD15—should soon yield information about interactions between the microflora and the intestine, and therefore about the pathogenesis of IBD.

Key points

- There are many indications that the endogenous or saprophytic colonic microflora plays a role in inflammatory bowel diseases (IBD). In particular, the microflora is indispensable to the development of most forms of experimental colitis. In humans, upstream diversion of faecal material protects against ileal recurrence following ablation of the ileum and right colon to treat Crohn's disease.

- Data on possible deleterious changes in the endogenous ileo-colonic microflora in the course of IBD are as yet scarce although strictly anaerobic bacteria and entero-adherent strains of *Escherichia coli* are known to play a role.

- Levels of the inflammatory cytokines TNFα, IL-6 and IL-1β are high in the persistent lesions of IBD. Early post-operative ileal lesions are associated with the synthesis of a type 2 cytokine profile, notably IL-4.

- Levels of the chemokine IL-8 are high in the damaged mucosa of IBD. In parallel, increased expression of adhesion molecules leads to the recruitment of leukocytes from the blood at the same time as the apoptosis of certain T lymphocytes is inhibited.

- In the course of IBD, bacterial lipopolysaccharide-induced over-expression of CD14 and TRL-4, and under-expression of PPARγ perturb the NFκB and MAPK signal transduction pathways, causing chronic inflammation. Break of the tolerance to the homologous, endogenous microflora (which may be mediated by IL-12 and inhibited by IL-10) has been observed in Crohn's disease.

- CARD15—a molecule which plays a key role in immune responses and in the intestinal surveillance of infectious phenomena—is mutated and non-functional in a sub-group of patients suffering from Crohn's disease, another observation indicating that intraluminal bacteria may play an important role in this condition.

References

1. Elson CO, Sartor RB, Tennyson GS, Riddell RH. Experimental models of inflammatory bowel disease. *Gastroenterology* 1995 ; 109 : 1344-67.

2. Sartor RB. Insights into the pathogenesis of inflammatory bowel diseases provided by new rodent models of spontaneous colitis. *Inflamm Bowel Dis* 1995 ; 1 : 64-75.

3. Bush TG, Savidge TC, Freeman TC, *et al*. Fulminant jejuno-ileitis following ablation of enteric glia in adult transgenic mice. *Cell* 1998 ; 93 : 189-201.

4. Rudolph U, Finegold MJ, Rich SS, *et al*. Ulcerative colitis and adenocarcinoma of the colon in G alpha i2-deficient mice. *Nat Genet* 1995 ; 10 : 143-50.

5. Sartor RB. Microbial agents in the pathogenesis, differential diagnosis, and complications of inflammatory bowel disease. In : Blaser MJ, Smith PD, Ravdin JI, Greenberg HB, Guerrant RL, eds. *Infections of the gastrointestinal tract*. New York : Raven Press, 1995 : 435-58.

6. Cartun RW, Van Kruiningen HJ, Pedersen CA, Berman MM. An immunocytochemical search for infectious agents in Crohn's disease. *Mod Pathol* 1993 ; 6 : 212-9.

7. Tabaqchali S, O'Donoghue DP, Bettelheim KA. *Escherichia coli* antibodies in patients with inflammatory bowel disease. *Gut* 1978 ; 19 : 108-13.

8. Rutgeerts P, Geboes K, Peeters M, *et al*. Effect of faecal stream diversion on recurrence of Crohn's disease in the neoterminal ileum. *Lancet* 1991 ; 338 : 771-4.

9. Lederman E, Neut C, Desreumaux P, *et al*. Bacterial overgrowth in the neoterminal ileum after ileocolonic resection for Crohn's disease. *Gastroenterology* 1997 ; 112 : A1023.

10. Harper PH, Lee EC, Kettlewell MG, Bennett MK, Jewell DP. Role of the faecal stream in the maintenance of Crohn's colitis. *Gut* 1985 ; 26 : 279-84.

11. Ruseler-van Embden JG, Both-Patoir HC. Anaerobic gram-negative faecal flora in patients with Crohn's disease and healthy subjects. Antonie van Leeuwenhoek 1983 ; 49 : 125-32.

12. Van de Merwe JP, Schroder AM, Wensinck F, Hazenberg MP. The obligate anaerobic faecal flora of patients with Crohn's disease and their first-degree relatives. *Scand J Gastroenterol* 1988 ; 23 : 1125-31.

13. Keighley MR, Arabi Y, Dimock F, Burdon DW, Allan RN, Alexander-Williams J. Influence of inflammatory bowel disease on intestinal microflora. *Gut* 1978 ; 19 : 1099-104.

14. Hartley MG, Hudson MJ, Swarbrick ET, *et al*. The rectal mucosa-associated microflora in patients with ulcerative colitis. *J Med Microbiol* 1992 ; 36 : 96-103.

15. Peach S, Lock MR, Katz D, Todd IP, Tabaqchali S. Mucosal-associated bacterial flora of the intestine in patients with Crohn's disease and in a control group. *Gut* 1978 ; 19 : 1034-42.

16. Neut C, Bulois P, Desreumaux P, *et al*. Changes in the bacterial flora of the neoterminal ileum after ileocolonic resection for Crohn's disease. *Am J Gastroenterol* 2002 ; 97 : 939-46.

17. Favier C, Neut C, Mizon C, Cortot A, Colombel JF, Mizon J. Fecal β-D-galactosidase production and Bifidobacteria are decreased in Crohn's disease. *Dig Dis Sci* 1997 ; 42 : 817-22.

18. Roediger WEW. Role of anaerobic bacteria in the metabolic welfare of the colonic mucosa in man. *Gut* 1980 ; 21 : 793-8.

19. Rath HC, Herfarth HH, Ikeda JS, *et al*. Normal luminal bacteria, especially *Bacteroides* species, mediate chronic colitis, gastritis, and arthritis in HLA-B27/human β2 microglobulin transgenic rats. *J Clin Invest* 1996 ; 98 : 945-53.

20. Krook A, Lindstrom B, Kjellander J, Jarnerot G, Bodin L. Relation between concentrations of metronidazole and *Bacteroides* spp in faeces of patients with Crohn's disease and healthy individuals. *J Clin Pathol* 1981 ;34 : 645-50.

21. Senda S, Fujiyama Y, Ushijima T, *et al*. *Clostridium ramosum*, an IgA protease-producing species and its ecology in the human intestinal tract. *Microbiol Immunol* 1985 ; 29 : 1019-28.

22. Burke DA, Axon AT. Adhesive *Escherichia coli* in inflammatory bowel disease and infective diarrhoea. *Br Med J* 1988 ; 297 : 102-4.

23. Giaffer MH, Holdsworth CD, Duerden BI. Virulence properties of *Eschericia coli* strains isolated from patients with inflammatory bowel disease. *Gut* 1992 ; 33 : 646-50.

24. Lobo AJ, Sagar PM, Rothwell J, *et al*. Carriage of adhesive *Escherichia coli* after restorative proctocolectomy and pouch anal anastomosis: relation with functional outcome and inflammation. *Gut* 1993 ; 34 : 1379-83.

25. Boudeau J, Glasser AL, Masseret E, Joly B, Darfeuille-Michaud A. Invasive ability of an *Escherichia coli* strain isolated from the ileal mucosa of a patient with Crohn's disease. *Infect Immun* 1999 ; 67 : 4490-510.

26. Van Montfrans C, Peppelenbosch M, te Velde AA, van Deventer S. Inflammatory signal transduction in Crohn's disease and novel therapeutic approach. *Biochem Pharmacol* 2002 ; 64 : 789-95.

27. Desreumaux P. Cytokines, chimiokines et signaux de transduction. *Lett Hépato-Gastroentérol* 1998 ; 6 : 295-7.

28. Strober W, Fuss IJ, Blumberg RS. The immunology of mucosal models of inflammation. *Annu Rev Immunol* 2002 ; 20 : 495-549.

29. Desreumaux P, Nutten S, Cortot A, Colombel JF. Cytokines, chimiokines et anticytokines dans les maladies inflammatoires chroniques de l'intestin. *HepatoGastro* 1999 ; 6 : 6-15.

30. Dubuquoy L, Dharancy S, Nutten S, Auwerx J, Desreumaux P. PPARγ/RXR in inflammatory digestive diseases: a new therapeutic target in hepatogastroenterology. *Lancet* 2002 ; 360: 1410-8.

31. Desreumaux P, Brandt E, Gambiez L, *et al*. Distinct cytokine patterns in early and chronic ileal lesions of Crohn's disease. *Gastroenterology* 1997 ; 113 : 118-26.

32. Cellier C, Cervoni JP, Barbier JP, Brousse N. Adhérences cellulaires et maladies inflammatoires chroniques intestinales. *Gastroenterol Clin Biol* 1997 ; 21 : 832-42.

33. Atreya R, Mudter J, Finotto S, *et al*. Blockage of IL-6 trans signaling suppresses T-cell resistance against apoptosis in chronic intestinal inflammation: evidence in Crohn disease and experimental colitis *in vivo*. *Nat Med* 2000 ; 6 : 583-8.

34. Grimm MC, Pavli P, Van de Pol E, Doe WF. Evidence for a CD14+ population of monocytes in inflammatory bowel disease mucosa: implications for pathogenesis. *Clin Exp Immunol* 1995 ; 100 : 291-7.

35. Means TK, Golenbock DT, Fenton MJ. The biology of Toll-like receptors. *Cytokine Growth Factor Rev* 2000 ; 11 : 219-32.

36. Cario E, Podolsky DK. Alteration in intestinal epithelial cell expression of Toll-like receptors in inflammatory bowel disease. *Gastroenterology* 2000 ; 118 : 3684.

37. Bogunovic M, Reka S, Evans KN, Mayer LF, Sperber K, Plevy SE. Functional Toll-like receptors (TLR) are expressed on intestinal epithelial cells. *Gastroenterology* 2000 ; 118 : 4269.

38. Dubuquoy L, Jansson EA, Deeb S, *et al*. Impaired expression of peroxisome proliferator-activated receptor gamma in ulcerative colitis. *Gastroenterology* 2003 ; 124 : 1265-76.

39. Desreumaux P, Dubuquoy L, Nutten S, *et al*. Attenuation of colon inflammation through activators of the retinoid X receptor (RXR)/peroxisome proliferator-activated receptor gamma (PPARgamma) heterodimer. A basis for new therapeutic strategies. *J Exp Med* 2001 ; 193 : 827-38.

40. Dubuquoy L, Dharancy S, Nutten S, Pettersson S, Auwerx J, Desreumaux P. Role of peroxisome proliferator-activated receptor gamma and retinoid X receptor heterodimer in hepatogastroenterological diseases. *Lancet* 2002 ; 360 : 1410-8.

41. Marasco WA, Phan SH, Krutzsch H, *et al*. Purification and identification of formyl-methionyl-leucyl-phenylalanine as the major peptide neutrophil chemotactic factor produced by *Escherichia coli*. *J Biol Chem* 1984 ; 259 : 5430-9.

42. Hobson CH, Butt TJ, Ferry DM, Hunter J, Chadwick VS, Broom MF. Enterohepatic circulation of bacterial chemotactic peptide in rats with experimental colitis. *Gastroenterology* 1988 ; 94 : 1006-13.

43. Anton PA, Targan SR, Shanahan F. Increased neutrophil receptors for and response to the proinflammatory bacterial peptide formyl-methionyl-leucyl-phenylalanine in Crohn's disease. *Gastroenterology* 1989 ; 97: 20-8.

44. Chadwick VS, Schlup MM, Cooper BT, Broom MF. Enzymes degrading bacterial chemotactic F-met peptides in human ileal and colonic mucosa. *J Gastroenterol Hepatol* 1990 ; 5 : 375-81.

45. Garcia-Lafuente A, Antolin M, Crespo E, Guarner F, Malagelada JR. Intestinal permeability is modulated by the composition of the commensal flora. *Gastroenterology* 1997 ; 112 : 979.

46. Morrissey PJ, Charrier K. Induction of wasting disease in SCID mice by the transfer of normal CD4+/CD45RB[hi]T cells and the regulation of this autoreactivity by CD4+/CD45RB[lo]T cells. *Res Immunol* 1994 ; 145 : 357-62.

47. Komatsu S, Panes J, Mori N, Grisham MB, Russel JM, Granger DN. Effects of intestinal stasis on ICAM-1 expression: role of enteric bacteria. *Gastroenterology* 1997 ; 112 : 1018.

48. Duchmann R, Kaiser I, Hermann E, Mayet W, Ewe K, Meyer zum Büschenfelde KH. Tolerance exists towards resident intestinal flora but is broken in active inflammatory bowel disease. C*lin Exp Immunol* 1995 ; 102 : 448-55.

49. Duchmann R, Schmitt E, Knolle P, Meyer zum Büschenfelde KH, Neurath M. Tolerance towards resident intestinal flora in mice is abrogated in experimental colitis and restored by treatment with interleukin-10 or antibodies to interleukin-12. *Eur J Immunol* 1996. ; 26 : 934-8.

50. Harty JT, Bevan MJ. Specific immunity to *Listeria monocytogenes* in the absence of IFN gamma. *Immunity* 1995 ; 3 : 109-17.

51. Ladel CH, Blum C, Dreher A, Reifenberg K, Kopf M, Kaufmann SH. Lethal tuberculosis in interleukin-6-deficient mutant mice. *Infect Immun* 1997 ; 65 : 4843-9.

52. Marino MW, Dunn A, Grail D, *et al*. Characterization of tumor necrosis factor-deficient mice. *Proc Natl Acad Sci USA* 1997 ; 94 : 8093-8.

53. Schoedon G, Goldenberger D, Forrer R, *et al*. Deactivation of macrophages with interleukin-4 is the key to the isolation of *Tropheryma whippelii*. *J Infect Dis* 1997 ; 176 : 672-7.

54. Mansfield LS, Urban JF. The pathogenesis of necrotic proliferative colitis in swine is linked to whipworm induced suppression of mucosal immunity to resident bacteria. *Vet Immunol Immunopathol* 1996 ; 50 : 1-17.

55. Hugot JP, Chamaillard M, Zouali H, *et al*. Association of NOD2 leucine-rich repeat variants with susceptibility to Crohn's disease. *Nature* 2001 ; 411 : 599-603.

56. Ogura Y, Bonen DK, Inohara N, *et al*. A frameshift mutation in NOD2 associated with susceptibility to Crohn's disease. *Nature* 2001 ; 411 : 603-6.

57. Hampe J, Cuthbert A, Croucher PJ, *et al*. Association between insertion mutation in NOD2 gene and Crohn's disease in German and British populations. *Lancet* 2001 ; 357 : 1925-8.

58. Lesage S, Zouali H, Cezard JP, *et al*. CARD15/NOD2 mutational analysis and genotype-phenotype correlation in 612 patients with inflammatory bowel disease. *Am J Hum Genet* 2002 ; 70 : 845-57.

59. Cuthbert AP, Fisher SA, Mirza MM, *et al*. The contribution of NOD2 gene mutations to the risk and site of disease in inflammatory bowel disease. *Gastroenterology* 2002 ; 122 : 867-74.

60. Vermeire S, Wild G, Kocher K, et al. CARD15 genetic variation in a Quebec population: prevalence, genotype-phenotype relationship, and haplotype structure. *Am J Hum Genet* 2002 ; 71 : 74-83.

61. Radlmayr M, Torok HP, Martin K, Folwaczny C. The c-insertion mutation of the NOD2 gene is associated with fistulizing and fibrostenotic phenotypes in Crohn's disease. *Gastroenterology* 2002 ; 122 : 2091-2.

62. Abreu MT, Taylor KD, Lin YC, *et al*. Mutations in NOD2 are associated with fibrostenosing disease in patients with Crohn's disease. *Gastroenterology* 2002 ; 123 : 679-88.

63. Girardin SE, Sansonetti PJ, Philpott DJ. Intracellular vs extracellular recognition of pathogens-common concepts in mammals and flies. *Trends Microbiol* 2002 ; 10 : 193-9.

64. Cin AI, Dempsey PW, Bruhn K, Miller JF, Xu Y, Cheng G. Involvement of receptor-interacting protein 2 in innate and adaptive immune response. *Nature* 2002 ; 416 : 190-3.

65. Kobayashi K, Inohara N, Hernandez LD, *et al*. RICK/Rip2/CARDIAK mediates signalling for receptors of the innate and adaptive immune systems. *Nature* 2002 ; 416 : 194-8.

Commensal Colonic Microflora and Infectious Diarrhoea

Philippe Seksik

Département
de Gastro-entérologie,
Hôpital Européen
Georges Pompidou,
Paris, France.

I n acute infectious diarrhoea, a pathogen may be detected in a bacteriological stool analysis without it being possible to appreciate perturbations of the colonic microflora. Although the microorganisms that can cause diarrhoea are now more fully characterized, modifications of the commensal microflora remain poorly understood. The recognition of pathogenic bacteria has allowed rational development of antibiotic treatments. Thus, by analogy, a better understanding of modifications of the colonic microflora as a whole could theoretically lead to the use of prebiotics or probiotics to re-establish balance in this ecosystem. The study of modifications of the commensal colonic microflora in infectious diarrhoea is therefore the subject of this chapter.

Commensal colonic microflora

Introduction

The digestive tract is colonized by a large number of bacteria, corresponding to ten times the number of cells in the human body. This ecosystem is characterized by great biodiversity. Thus, nearly five hundred species would be present and the new techniques of molecular biology are revealing many species not hitherto isolated by culture-based methods [1]. Since physicochemical conditions vary considerably along the length of the digestive tract, there are major qualitative and quantitative variations in the digestive microflora at different sites. The colon is the most highly populated segment, housing about 10^{11} bacteria per gram of contents [2]. Some consider that the faecal microflora is representative of the colonic microflora as a whole but it probably only represents the luminal microflora of the distal colon (the left and sigmoid colons, and the rectum). In fact, populations are smaller by a factor of about two logarithmic units in the proximal colon than in the distal colon (or the rectum), and facultative anaerobic microorganisms (which are codominant with obligate anaerobes in the right colon) do not evolve in population as far as the rectum while obligate anaerobes dominate in the left colon and faecal matter [3].

Within the commensal microflora, distinction is made between a dominant microflora consisting of obligate anaerobes (more than 10^8 bacteria per gram of faeces) and a sub-dominant microflora which consists of facultative anaerobes (one hundred to one thousand times less abundant). To these autochtonous bacteria, an allochthonous microflora has to be added derived from food and in transit through the digestive tract.

In adults, phenotypic bacterial taxonomy makes it possible to establish a profile of the faecal microflora which is relatively stable at the level of the major microbial groups. The dominant microorganisms of the human faecal microflora are, for the Gram-negative, bacilli of the genus *Bacteroides*, for the Gram-positive, non-spore-forming bacilli of the genera *Eubacterium* and *Bifidobacterium*, cocci of the genera *Peptostreptococcus* and *Ruminococcus* and, finally, spore-forming bacilli of the genus *Clostridium*. The genera *Lactobacillus* and *Streptococcus* and the enterobacteria are frequently represented by sub-dominant species [4]. The step involving isolation in strictly anaerobic conditions has been a restrictive factor limiting this approach.

Limitations of the culture-based methods manifest both in the inability to culture the entirety of the microflora that can be seen in the microscope, and by the sophistication of the equipment necessary for the isolation and storage of all the dominant bacteria that can be cultured. The development of molecular tools has recently made it possible to bypass the constraints of culture [5]. The most developed methods today are based on the recognition of 16S ribosomal RNA molecules by oligonucleotide probes which are specific for domains, groups, sub-groups and species, making it possible to characterize, on the one hand the global composition of the human digestive microflora, and on the other hand the biodiversity of species.

Stability of the commensal colonic microflora

Old studies showed the specificity of each microflora at the individual level, and the stability over time of this microbial ecosystem. Using culture-based methods, Gorbach *et al*. studied the faecal microflora of seventy subjects of between twenty and one hundred years of age [6]. Quantitative and qualitative analyses revealed significant differences between individuals within a given age range, compared with, in any given individual, remarkable stability of the faecal microflora over time (period of seven weeks to seven months). These first results were recently confirmed as a result of the advent of molecular techniques. The biodiversity of the dominant microflora, specific from one individual to another, is perfectly stable over time in a given individual. If fragments of ribosomal DNA extracted from the faecal microflora of a healthy subject are made to migrate through an electrophoretic gel, a profile is obtained which is similarly specific to the individual and stable over time (Figure 1) [7]. Trials of the implantation of microorganisms into adults remain experimental. Modifications of the microbial equilibrium by dietary factors remain poorly understood or confined to the right colon. Other exogenous factors could disrupt this equilibrium, such as antibiotic treatment or an episode of infectious diarrhoea. In order to ensure the stability of such a complex ecosystem, a protective mechanism is mediated by the commensal microflora; this is referred to as the barrier effect.

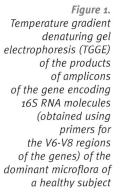
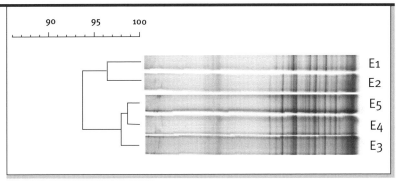

Figure 1.
Temperature gradient
denaturing gel
electrophoresis (TGGE)
of the products
of amplicons
of the gene encoding
16S RNA molecules
(obtained using
primers for
the V6-V8 regions
of the genes) of the
dominant microflora of
a healthy subject
collected at several different time points spread over a period of two years. E1 : sample collected in 1997;
E2-E5 : samples collected in 1999 on d1, d23, d58 and d78 respectively.
The dendrogram shows an optimal statistical representation of similarities between the TTGE profiles

Barrier effect

Although the mechanisms underlying the barrier effect remain poorly understood, they are subject to the same principle: the bacterium mediating the barrier effect must be in the dominant microflora. The balance of the gut microflora results from microbial interactions within the commensal microflora in the form of competition (for nutrient substrates or adhesion sites) and modification of the ecosystem by products of bacterial metabolism (pH, bacteriocins, organic acids, etc.) [8, 9]. Distinction is made between two different types of barrier: intraspecific and interspecific.

A number of animal experiments have shed light on intraspecific barriers. In practice, in mouse and gnotoxenic piglets, strains of *Escherichia coli* without any virulence factor can mediate a barrier effect against strains of *Escherichia coli* carrying plasmids encoding virulence factors. In humans, this work has had medical repercussions and the inoculation of a plasmid-free *Escherichia coli* strain into young children has been shown to reduce the carriage of antibiotic-resistant *Escherichia coli* [10]. Similarly, in gnotoxenic mice and later in humans, it has been possible to show that non-toxinogenic strains of *Clostridium difficile* can prevent the proliferation of toxinogenic strains [11-14]. Interspecific barriers are more difficult to investigate. In humans, *Bacteroides thetaiotamocron* and *Fusobacterium necrogenes* have been identified as being responsible for a barrier effect against *Clostridium perfringens* [15].

Modifications of the commensal colonic microflora in infectious diarrhoea

Infectious diarrhoea

Acute diarrhoea is defined by the WHO as the production of at least three soft-to-liquid stools every twenty-four hours for less than two weeks.

Infection represents the most common cause of acute diarrhoea. In France, the results of a survey of the weekly incidence of acute diarrhoea by the Sentinelle network show that there is a peak in winter of about five-hundred thousand cases with a recrudescence in summer. This bipolar pattern—together with indirect evidence—points to the cause of acute diarrhoea being infectious: viral in winter and bacterial in summer. Systematic microbiologic studies were conducted in three European cohorts with acute colitis [16-18]. Bacterial, viral and parasitic agents were sought, including analyses of stools and colon biopsies inoculated onto specific culture media, histological analysis of biopsies, and a parasitological examination of stool samples. Analysis of the results from these three cohorts shows that documented cases of infectious colitis represent half of all the cases of acute colitis investigated. These cases of infectious colitis were dominated by the following bacterial agents: *Campylobacter, Clostridium difficile, Salmonella* (Figures 2 & 3), *Shigella, Yersinia, Klebsiella oxytoca* and *Escherichia coli* (Figure 4).

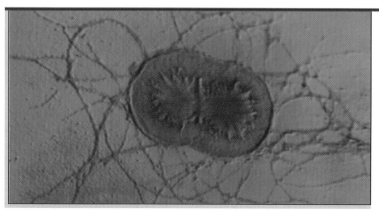

Figure 2.
Salmonella: scanning
electron micrograph
(photograph: T. Piche, Nice)

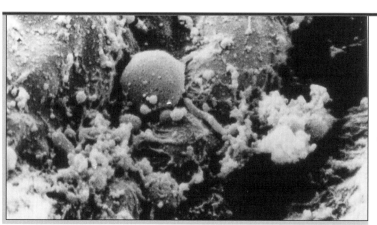

Figure 3.
SEM: mucosa
of the sigmoid colon
infected with Salmonella
enteritidis (Type B).
Bacterium in direct contact
with the basement
membrane which
probably corresponds
to a salmonella cell
(photograph: G. Brandi,
Bologne)

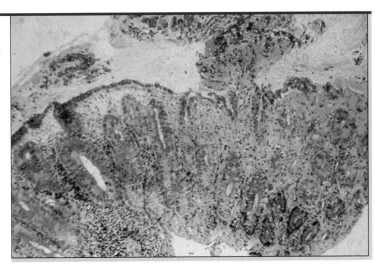

Figure 4.
Colon biopsy from a patient
infected with Escherichia coli
0157:H7. Pseudomembrane
covering the mucosa
(photograph:
C. Surawicz, Seattle)

These data provide information on the presence of a pathogenic microorganism in the faeces or associated with the colonic mucosa in bacterial diarrhoea. Pathogenic bacteria are isolated from specimens gathered immediately after the bowel movement and stored at +4 °C for no longer than twelve hours. Microscopic examination after Gram staining shows drastic changes in the balance of the commensal microflora but does not give any precise information about the nature of said changes. As a result, changes in the commensal colonic microflora in infectious diarrhoea can only be analysed in a systematic fashion, either by conventional microbiologic methods or by the techniques of molecular biology.

Modifications of the commensal colonic microflora

Few studies have focused on modifications of the commensal microflora in infectious diarrhoea [19]. Simplistically, it could be imagined that a pathogenic bacterium qualitatively and quantitatively replaces the normal colonic microflora during an episode of infectious diarrhoea. In fact, it has been observed in patients with cholera that the faecal density of *Vibrio cholerae* can reach 3.10^7 CFU/mL, whereas the density of *Bacteroides* drops to 10^5 CFU/mL. After cure, it has been observed that the normal microflora is rapidly restored [20].

Gorbach *et al.* studied the faecal microfloras of seventeen adults during an episode of acute diarrhoea and then during the recovery period [21]. During the diarrhoea, eight subjects presented a microflora in which *Escherichia coli* was dominant whereas the others presented varied microfloras combining *Klebsiella spp.*, *Pseudomonas spp.*, *Enterobacter cloacae* and *Alcaligenes faecalis*. In the first group, the density of *Escherichia coli* at the time of the diarrhoea was one to three logarithmic units higher than that of other aerobic and anaerobic bacteria. This would be due to a combination of effects: an increase in aerobic bacteria and a decrease in anaerobic ones. During recovery, the level of coliforms dropped, several species appeared, and the levels of *Bacteroides*, *Lactobacillus* and *Clostridium* significantly rose. In the second group, the levels of *Escherichia coli* in the faeces were not increased although the levels of *Bacteroides*, *Clostridium* and microaerophilic bacteria were lower than those observed during the recovery period. To summarize these results, it could be said that there is a global increase in aerobic bacteria paralleled by a decrease in anaerobic bacteria in infectious diarrhoea. These results have been confirmed by several teams.

Fujita *et al.* studied the faecal microflora in fourteen Kenyan children suffering from acute diarrhoea caused by different pathogens, namely *Shigella*, *Campylobacter*, enterotoxigenic *Escherichia coli* and rotavirus (in three cases, the etiology was not defined) [22]. The faecal microflora was studied at the time of the diarrhoea and during recovery. During the diarrhoea, not counting the pathogenic bacteria, the levels of aerobic bacteria were the same in the two observation periods. The levels of the anaerobic bacteria *Bacteroides* and *Bifidobacterium* were significantly lower in the course of the episode of diarrhoea than during the recovery period. A similar tendency was observed for *Lactobacillus* and *Eubacterium* species. The physicochemical properties of the stool specimens were also investigated: during the diarrhoea, the pH was higher and volatile fatty acids were lower in comparison with the recovery phase. These results were observed no matter which pathogenic agent was causing the diarrhoea.

Albert *et al.* studied the composition of the faecal microflora in forty-nine children with acute infectious diarrhoea as well as in twenty-nine healthy children [23]. In this study, in the children with acute diarrhoea, anaerobic bacteria were reduced in such a way that the ratio of anaerobes to aerobes was reversed compared with healthy subjects. No qualitative difference was detected between the compositions of the faecal microfloras of children with bacterial diarrhoea and those of children with viral diarrhoea. Similarly, in a global fashion, modifications of the commensal colonic microflora were identical whether the pathogenic agent had been identified or not.

At the end of the analysis of these studies, a few general remarks could be made. Our understanding of the colonic microflora in the course of episodes of infectious diarrhoea comes from old studies which focused on the faecal microflora of adults and/or children in developing countries. In the course of these studies, bacteria were mainly counted using the methods of conventional bacteriology. Globally the modifications seem to be similar whatever the etiologic agent: an increase in aerobes coupled with a decrease in obligate anaerobes.

These observations point to pathogenetic hypotheses. Modifications of the commensal microflora could reflect perturbation of the colonic ecosystem resulting from degraded physicochemical properties: changes in substrates (blood), and variation of the pH and/or the redox potential. The high levels of aerobic bacteria can be linked, by analogy, with the composition of the microflora of the right colon [23]. On the basis of these observations, it could be imagined that, in the course of episodes of infectious diarrhoea, because of the influx of water and electrolytes or as a result of motility problems, part of the usual microflora in the right colon arrives in the left colon and in the stools. However, in interpreting these results, it should be remembered that not all the microorganisms of the microflora can be cultured, and that it is technically difficult to conduct bacterial counts during episodes of diarrhoea because the specimens are diluted. In these conditions, it is likely that numbers of obligate anaerobes are under-estimated. There are no studies of the colonic microflora in the course of infectious diarrhoea in humans based on the recognition of 16S ribosomal RNA molecules.

This field remains a major area of investigation for the description and comprehension of pathogenic mechanisms underlying modification of the bacterial ecosystem. By way of example, a study in pigs showed destabilization of the colonic microflora in the course of infectious diarrhoea induced experimentally using *Brachyspira hyodysenteriae* (the etiologic agent of porcine dysentery) [24]. Restriction fragment length polymorphism analysis of the gene encoding the 16S ribosomal RNA molecule showed major fluctuations in restriction profiles in the course of episodes of diarrhoea, contrasting with remarkable stability in profile over time in a control group (not suffering from infectious diarrhoea). Inversely, in conventional mice, experimentally induced rotaviral diarrhoea in the newborn did not modify the establishment of *Lactobacillus spp.* or *Escherichia coli* prior to weaning, development of a barrier effect against *Escherichia coli,* or population of the duodenum by IgA-producing plasma cells after weaning [19]. In humans, destabilization of the microflora warrants better characterization at the scale of phylogenetic groups or molecular species.

Theoretical bases for using probiotics in infectious diarrhoea

Infectious diarrhoea is an international public health problem, representing one of the main causes of neonatal and paediatric mortality in developing countries [25, 26]. The recognition of pathogenic bacteria in the course of bacterial diarrhoea led to the rational use of antibiotics. However, with viral etiologies representing the leading cause of infectious diarrhoea, treatment depends mainly on symptomatic measures aimed at correcting hydro-electrolytic problems. Reducing the intensity and duration of an episode of infectious diarrhoea seems, therefore, to be a justified goal of treatment. Recognition of the barrier effect, i.e., the protective role of the endogenous microflora countering the establishment of a pathogenic microorganism, associated with observed modifications of the commensal colonic microflora in the course of infectious diarrhoea led to the proposition of curative and preventive bacteriotherapy for infectious diarrhoea based on probiotics. In practice, in order to re-establish a balanced commensal microflora, the administration of bacteria ingested live seems an attractive concept. The rational use of probiotics in the course of infectious diarrhoea involves a better understanding of imbalances in the microflora, but also a description of the mechanisms of action of probiotics. A broad field of investigation, both clinical and fundamental, remains open. The use of molecular tools should make it possible, in the coming years, to be able to acquire new information in these areas.

Key points

- The commensal colonic microflora is specific to each individual and remains stable over time, largely by virtue of a protective effect of the microflora itself, referred to as the barrier effect.

- Infectious diarrhoea is an international public health problem, representing one of the main causes of neonatal and paediatric mortality in developing countries.

- Few studies have focused on modifications of the commensal microflora in the course of infectious diarrhoea, and almost all bacterial counts conducted in these studies have been carried out using conventional bacteriological methods.

- Global modifications seem to be similar whichever the etiologic agent causing the diarrhoea: an increase in aerobic bacteria coupled with a decrease in obligate anaerobes.

- Recognition of the barrier effect associated with these modifications of the commensal colonic microflora in the course of infectious diarrhoea has led to the proposal of curative and preventive bacteriotherapy for infectious diarrhoea based on probiotics.

References

1. Suau A, Bonnet R, Sutren M, *et al*. Direct analysis of genes encoding 16S rRNA from complex communities reveals many novel molecular species within the human gut. *Appl Environ Microbiol* 1999 ; 65 : 4799-807.

2. Ducluzeau R. Role of experimental microbial ecology in gastroenterology. In : Bergogner-Berezin E, ed. *Microbial ecology and intestinal infection*. Berlin : Spriger-Verlag, 1988 : 7-26.

3. Marteau P, Pochart P, Doré J, Bera-Maillet C, Bernalier A, Corthier G. Comparative study of bacterial groups within the human cecal and fecal microbiota. *Appl Environ Microbiol* 2001 ; 67 : 4939-42.

4. Wilson KH. The gastrointestinal microflora. In : Yamada T, ed. *Textbook of gastroenterology*. Philadelphia : JB Lippincott, 1991 ; 26 : 532-43.

5. Blaut M, Collins MD, Welling GW, Doré J, van Loo J, de Vos W. Molecular biological methods for studying the gut microbiot : the EU human gut flora project. *Br J Nutr* 2002 ; 87 Suppl 2 : S203-11.

6. Gorbach SL, Nahas L, Lerner PI, Weinstein L. Studies of intestinal microflora. I. Effects of diet, age, and periodic sampling on numbers of fecal microorganisms in man. *Gastroenterology* 1967 ; 53 : 845-55.

7. Seksik P, Rigottier-Gois L, Gramet G, *et al*. Alterations of the dominant faecal bacterial groups in patients with Crohn's disease of the colon. *Gut* 2003 ; 52 : 237-42.

8. Freter R. Factors influencing the microecology of the gut. In : Fuller R, ed. *Probiotics: the scientific basis*. London : Chapman & Hall, 1992 : 11-45.

9. Duncan HE, Edberg SC. Host-microbe interaction in the gastrointestinal tract. Crit Rev Microbiol 1995 ; 21 : 85-100.

10. Duval-Iflah Y, Ouriet MF, Moreau C, Daniel N, Gabilan JC, Raibaud P. Implantation précoce d'une souche d'*Escherichia coli* dans l'intestin de nouvau-né humain : effet de barrière vis-à-vis de souches d'*E. coli* antibiorésistants. *Ann Microbiol* 1982 ; 133 : 393-408.

11. Corthier G, Dubos F, Raibaud P. Modulation of cytotoxin production by *Clostridium difficile* in the intestinal tracts of gnotobiotic mice inoculated with various human intestinal bacteria. *Appl Environ Microbiol* 1985 ; 49 : 250-2.

12. Corthier G, Muller MC. Emergence in gnotobiotic mice of nontoxinogenic clones of *Clostridium difficile* from a toxinogenic one. *Infect Immun* 1988 ; 56 : 1500-4..

13. Schwan A, Sjolin S, Trottestam U, Aronsson B. Relapsing *Clostridium difficile* enterocolitis cured by rectal infusion of normal faeces. *Scand J Infect Dis* 1984 ; 16 : 211-5.

14. Wilson KH, Sheagren JN. Antagonism of toxigenic *Clostridium difficile* by nontoxigenic *C. difficile*. *J Infect Dis* 1983 ; 147 : 733-6.

15. Yurdusev N, Ladire M, Ducluzeau R, Raibaud P. Antagonism exerted by an association of a *Bacteroides thetaiotaomicron* strain and a *Fusobacterium necrogenes* strain against *Clostridium perfringens* in gnotobiotic mice and in fecal suspensions incubated *in vitro*. *Infect Immun* 1989 ; 57 : 724-31.

16. Roussin Bretagne S, Barge J, Boussougant Y, Hagiage M, Devars du Mayne JF, Cerf M. La diarrhée aiguë de l'adulte en région parisienne. Aspects cliniques, bactériologiques, endoscopiques et histologiques. Étude de 52 cas. *Gastroenterol Clin Biol* 1989 ; 13 : 804-10.

17. Beaugerie L, Barbut F, Delas N, *et al*. Caractérisation des colites aiguës de l'adulte immunocompétent : résultats préliminaires d'une série prospective multicentrique de 93 cas. *Gastroenterol Clin Biol* 1998 ; 22 : A15.

18. Schumacher G, Kollberg B, Sandstedt B, *et al*. A prospective study of first attacks of inflammatory bowel disease and non-relapsing colitis. Microbiologic findings. *Scand J Gastroenterol* 1993 ; 28 : 1077-85.

19. Moreau MC, Corthier G, Muller MC, Dubos F, Raibaud P. Relationships between rotavirus diarrhea and intestinal microflora establishment in conventional and gnotobiotic mice. *J Clin Microbiol* 1986 ; 23 : 863-8.

20. Gorbach SL, Banwell JG, Jacobs B, *et al*. Intestinal microflora in Asiatic cholera. I. « Rice-water » stool. *J Infect Dis* 1970 ; 121 : 32-7.

21. Gorbach SL, Banwell JG, Chatterjee BD, Jacobs B, Sack RB. Acute undifferentiated human diarrhea in the tropics. I. Alterations in intestinal micrflora. *J Clin Invest* 1971 ; 50 : 881-9.

22. Fujita K, Kaku M, Yanagase Y, *et al*. Physicochemical characteristics and flora of diarrhoeal and recovery faeces in children with acute gastro-enteritis in Kenya. *Ann Trop Paediatr* 1990 ; 10 : 339-45.

23. Albert MJ, Bhat P, Rajan D, Maiya PP, Pereira SM, Baker SJ. Faecal flora of South Indian infants and young children in health and with acute gastroenteritis. *J Med Microbiol* 1978 ; 11 : 137-43.

24. Leser TD, Lindecrona RH, Jensen TK, Jensen BB, Moller K. Changes in bacterial community structure in the colon of pigs fed different experimental diets and after infection with *Brachyspira hyodysenteriae*. *Appl Environ Microbiol* 2000 ; 66 : 3290-6.

25. Snyder GD, Holmes RW, Bates JN, Van Voorhis BJ. Nitric oxide inhibits aromatase activity: mechanisms of action. *J Steroid Biochem Mol Biol* 1996 ; 58 : 63-9.

26. Ho MS, Glass RI, Pinsky PF, *et al*. Diarrheal deaths in American children. Are they preventable? *JAMA* 1988 ; 260 : 3281-5.

Microflora and Diarrhoea: Antibiotic-Associated Diarrhoea

Yoram Bouhnik

Hépato-Gastro-entérologie
et Assistance Nutritive,
Hôpital Lariboisière,
Paris, France.

Diarrhoea is defined by the WHO as the passing of loose or watery stools more than three times a day. Antibiotic-associated diarrhoea (AAD) is defined as an otherwise unexplained episode of diarrhoea appearing in association with a course of antibiotic treatment.

Somewhat artificially, distinction can be made between three different clinical situations:
- simple diarrhoea, the most common form with many possible underlying mechanisms;
- haemorrhagic colitis, possibly related to the emergence of a toxigenic strain of *Klebsiella oxytoca*;
- pseudomembranous colitis, linked to the emergence of a toxigenic strain of *Clostridium difficile* made possible by compromise of the barrier effect.

In all the pathogenic mechanisms involved, a common and necessary feature is antibiotic-induced changes in the intestinal bacterial ecosystem [1]. Thus, taking an antibiotic belonging to any family can have two types of consequence:
- a change in the composition of the microflora, leading to compromise of the "barrier effect" which is itself due to the presence of dominant, commensal anaerobic bacteria which form a complex, subtle equilibrium and inhibit the proliferation of endogenous or exogenous pathogens;
- modification of bacterial metabolism leading to reduced hydrolysis and fermentation by the colonic microflora causing "metabolic" diarrhoea [2].

As a general rule, the perturbed balance returns to normal soon after the subject has stopped taking the antibiotic, which suggests that the barrier-mediating bacteria of the microflora are only temporarily eradicated, or perhaps more probably that their multiplication is only inhibited while the drug is being taken.

Epidemiology and risk factors for antibiotic-associated diarrhoea

The incidence of AAD varies depending on the antibiotic prescribed. It occurs in 5-10% of patients taking ampicillin, 10-25% of those taking amoxicillin-clavulanic acid, 15-20% of those taking a third generation cephalosporin, and 2-5% of those taking some other antibiotic [1, 3]. The rates reported for AAD and parenterally administered antibiotics (especially those which pass through the enterohepatic cycle) are similar to those observed with oral administration [4]. Only parenterally administered aminoglycosides never cause diarrhoea.

The epidemiology of AAD in a community was recently described in a prospective study which included 266 adults living near Paris taking a course of antibiotic lasting between five and ten days [5]. Moderately intense, self-limited diarrhoea occurred in 17.5% of the subjects—lasting just one day in 66% of them. In a paediatric study of 650 children of between one month and fifteen years of age being treated with an antibiotic, 11% experienced diarrhoea [6]. In this study, diarrhoea was defined as the production of loose or watery stools three or more times a day for at least two days in a row.

The risk factors for AAD are listed in Table I; it should be noted that neither gender nor the dose nor route of administration of the antibiotic are significant risk factors for AAD [7].

Antibiotic-related factors	Host-related factors
• Broad-spectrum antibiotics - Amoxicillin - Amoxicillin-clavulanic acid - 2nd and 3rd generation cephalosporins - Clindamycin	• Extremes of age - < 6 - > 65
• Length of the course of antibiotic - long courses - repeated courses • Number of antibiotics taken	• Predisposing factors - a history of AAD - serious concomitant disease - chronic digestive disease - co-morbidity - immunodeficiency
• Antibiotics which are excreted in the bile	• Hospitalization - long stays - surgery - gastrointestinal procedures - nasogastric alimentation

Table I.
Risk factors for antibiotic-associated diarrhoea
(taken from [7])

"Simple" diarrhoea

So-called "simple" diarrhoea is by the far the most common form. Usually the onset is within a few days of starting the antibiotic although, in some cases, it appears up to six weeks after the end of the course of treatment [8]. "Simple" diarrhoea is usually moderately intense with watery stools, rarely accompanied with abdominal pain or fever. Most episodes resolve when the drug is stopped or its dosage reduced. In an endoscopic examination (which is rarely carried out), no abnormality is seen or, in some cases, non-specific lesions such as oedema, erythema, petechiae or erosions may be detected. It should nevertheless be noted that there is little accurate information about correlations between the endoscopic picture and the causative agent.

Causes of "simple" antibiotic-associated diarrhoea

The pathogenesis of "simple" forms of diarrhoea is debated but a distinction can be made between "infectious", metabolic and other causes.

Infectious causes

A significant proportion of these cases of diarrhoea (10-20%) have been linked with colonization by *Clostridium difficile* [1, 4, 9-11]. In the above-mentioned community-based study [5], stool analyses were carried out before and two weeks after the beginning of the course of antibiotic treatment, including cultures as well as assays to detect *Clostridium difficile*, its toxin, and cytopathogenic activity due to toxin B. *Clostridium difficile* was isolated before and after treatment in one patient who did not experience diarrhoea. Toxin-producing strains of *Clostridium difficile* were isolated in fewer than 3% (7/262) of all subjects but more often in subjects who had diarrhoea than in those who did not (8.7 *versus* 1.4%, p = 0.02). Nevertheless, *Clostridium difficile* is not the main etiologic agent of AAD in outpatients.

AAD can also be caused by other pathogens, namely *Salmonella*, *Clostridium perfringens* type A, *Staphylococcus aureus*, and possibly *Candida albicans*. *Clostridium perfringens* type A produces an enterotoxin known to cause food poisoning; more recently, a different genotype has been implicated in AAD [12]. There is no specific treatment and few medical test laboratories offer any of the diagnostic tests which would be required to identify this pathogen. Multi-drug resistant *Salmonella newport* from infected cows has been blamed for epidemics of diarrhoea in patients taking ampicillin [13].

The detection of *Candida albicans* at densities exceeding 10^6 cells per gram of faeces in a few patients whose condition improved with nystatin treatment suggested that certain strains of this fungus can cause AAD, although this remains controversial [14].

Metabolic causes

Antibiotics can substantially reduce the density of anaerobic bacteria in the colon thereby inhibiting fermentation processes. In these conditions, osmotically active carbohydrates remain in the colonic lumen and may cause osmotic diarrhoea, a well characterized mechanism in subjects taking ampicillin [15]. In parallel, reduced short-chain fatty acid production (the absorption of which promotes that of electrolytes) results in reductions in the colonic absorption rates of sodium, potassium and therefore water, another well characterized mechanism in humans [2]. Finally, a reduction in the rate of the conversion of primary bile acids to secondary forms is sometimes observed, leading to choleretic secretory diarrhoea due to the direct action of primary bile acids on the colonic mucosa.

Other causes

Antibiotics have many effects in the gastrointestinal tract, in some cases quite independent of their antimicrobial activity. For example, erythromycin acts as a "motilin-like" agonist which speeds transit, and clavulanic acid (which is included in amoxicillin-clavulanic acid preparations) seems to enhance motility in the small intestine [16].

Finally, in many cases, another product administered at the same time as an antibiotic can cause diarrhoea which may then be attributed to the antibiotic; this could apply to laxatives, antacids, contrast media, preparations containing lactose or sorbitol, non-steroid anti-inflammatory drugs, anti-arrhythmic drugs and cholinergic drugs [16, 17].

Treatment of "simple" antibiotic-associated diarrhoea

In most cases, the diarrhoea regresses within hours or days of withdrawal of the causative drug.

The efficacy of probiotics *vis-à-vis* the prevention of AAD has been evaluated to date in nine placebo-controlled trials. A recent meta-analysis of all these studies confirmed the efficacy of these products, with an odds ratio of 0.39 in favour of the active treatment ($IC_{95\%}$ 0.25-0.62; $p < 0.001$) for *Saccharomyces boulardii*, and of 0.34 ($IC_{95\%}$ 0.19-0.61; $p < 0.01$) for *Lactobacillus spp.* [18]. These findings were confirmed in a second meta-analysis which also took into account the results of open studies [19].

Haemorrhagic colitis

Pathogenesis

Klebsiella oxytoca probably plays a role in haemorrhagic colitis. This Gram-negative, facultative anaerobe is detected in 30-40% of human faecal microflora. It is naturally resistant to both penicillin and the streptomycins, so testing for it in the faeces after a course of one of these antibiotics is of little value unless perhaps a pure culture of this bacterium is obtained [20]. On the other hand, its detection in colonic biopsies could reveal adhesive and invasive properties which would be strong evidence of pathogenicity. Moreover, a heat-stable toxin has been isolated from the supernatants of cultures of strains of *Klebsiella oxytoca* isolated from patients with post-antibiotic haemorrhagic colitis. Inoculation of this cytotoxin into the ligated intestinal loops of rabbits induced heavy mucosal bleeding with fluid build-up, further evidence that *Klebsiella oxytoca* is involved in the pathogenesis of post-antibiotic haemorrhagic colitis. However, the very low molecular weight and extremely simple chemical structure of this cytotoxin contrasts with the characteristics of other known bacterial cytotoxins [21].

Clinical picture

Digestive manifestations are stereotypical [22, 23]. The characteristic picture combines:
- abdominal pain of sudden onset, e.g. colic and tenesmus (98%), usually intense;

- diarrhoea with more than fifteen watery stools a day, turning bloody within a matter of hours (100%);
- fever absent or of low-level, i.e., below 38.5 °C (90%);
- inflammatory markers in the blood (in one- to two-thirds of cases).

No signs of gravity have been reported to date. Symptoms appear on average 5.3 days (range: 1-17) after the beginning of the course of antibiotic which was prescribed (88%) for an ENT or bronchial infection in the great majority of cases. In some cases, onset has been reported up to six weeks after the end of treatment. In two cases, the drug had been administered by intramuscular route. The sex ratio is close to 1 and, interestingly, more than 60% of the subjects affected are between the ages of twenty and forty [22, 23].

The antibiotics most commonly responsible are penicillin and its derivatives (ampicillin: 20%; amoxicillin: 45%; amoxicillin-clavulanic acid: 20%; first, second and third generation cephalosporins: 5%; streptomycins: 10%) [8, 22, 23]. Less frequently, a quinolone has been blamed [24]. Concomitant drugs, especially anti-inflammatory drugs (both steroidal and non-steroidal), have not been systematically investigated but do not seem to have any adverse effect.

Special examinations

Endoscopy and biopsies

There are lesions in the right colon in three-quarters of cases, in the transverse, sigmoid and left colons in half of all cases, and in the rectum in one-third of cases. The left colon is the only site involved in 15% of cases, the right colon in 36% of cases, and both segments in 48% of cases [22, 23]. In a recent study, simple sigmoidoscopy revealed typical lesions in seven out of nine patients with acute, bloody diarrhoea, and exclusively rectal involvement was observed in only one of the nine [25].

Colonoscopy reveals typical lesions, mainly characterized by mucosal congestion and sometimes associated with multiple erosions over an extended area resulting in bleeding over a broad mucosal surface (Figure 1), with the disease process generally progressing across the entire surface. Burrowing ulcers have not been reported in this condition.

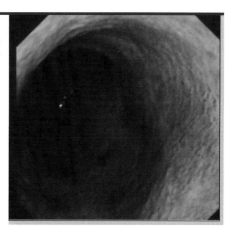

Figure 1.
Typical endoscopic image of haemorragic colitis
due to Klebsiella oxytoca
(photograph: Y. Bouhnik, Hôpital Lariboisière, Paris)

The histology of the lesions is non-specific. Biopsies usually reveal haemorrhagic dissociation of the *lamina propria* which, in this context, becomes all the more significant if it is associated with other signs, such as:
- neutrophilic exocytosis;
- mucosal abrasions and/or erosions;
- inflammation (often mild) of the *lamina propria*, with sparse neutrophils;
- fibrosis of variable severity;
- damage to the crypts with reduced mucus production (Figure 2).

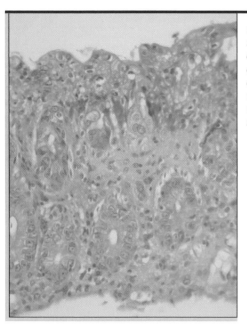

Figure 2.
Right colon biopsy: haemorrhagic dissociation
and low-level inflammation of the lamina propria
as can be seen in haemorragic colitis
due to Klebsiella oxytoca.
(HES. Magnification x 100)
(micrograph: A. Lavergne-Slove, Anatomie pathologique,
Hôpital Lariboisière, Paris)

Bacteriology

Bacteriologic tests include stool cultures and, more importantly, cultures grown from colonic biopsy material. On the basis of a review of the main reports published in the literature which included stool and biopsy cultures, *Klebsiella oxytoca* was isolated from the faeces in one-third of cases and in two-thirds of cases from biopsy cultures. *Clostridium difficile* was present in 10% of the same faecal specimens. In a more recent study, *Klebsiella oxytoca* was isolated from seven out of nine biopsies but not from the faeces in any case [25].

In a recent study, biopsies and colonic fluid samples were collected in the course of colonoscopy on 93 consecutive patients with acute post-antibiotic colitis [26]:
- *Klebsiella oxytoca* was isolated significantly more often from patients with haemorrhagic colitis not associated with the presence of *Clostridium difficile*;
- the strains of *Klebsiella oxytoca* isolated were more often cytotoxic for Hep-2 cells than those isolated from healthy carriers.

Disease course

The lesions generally improve and the clinical symptoms disappear once the antibiotic has been discontinued, within four days in 80% of cases (range: 1-23 days). However, it is important to point out that vancomycin, metronidazole and quinolones are sometimes prescribed on an empirical basis without any real evidence that they are of use.

Whenever follow-up endoscopy was performed, complete normalisation of the mucosa (sometimes in biopsies) was observed, within four to twelve days in 80% of cases [8, 22, 23].

There are no published data on whether resuming the offending antibiotic is followed by reappearance of the symptoms or not, but prudence would rule out ever prescribing that particular drug again.

Pseudomembranous colitis

Epidemiology, risk factors, pathogenesis

The rate of colonization by *Clostridium difficile* in adult subjects in hospital is 20-30%, compared with 3% in outpatients [1, 27] (Figure 3).

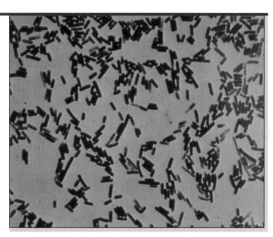

Figure 3.
Optical micrograph of Clostridium difficile (micrograph: Y. Boussougant, Hôpital Louis Mourier, Colombes)

The risk factors for clinical infection are listed in Table I. A Swedish outpatient study showed that *Clostridium difficile* toxin is detected twenty to one hundred times more often in those of over sixty than in those of under twenty [28]. The antibiotics most often involved in *Clostridium difficile*-associated diarrhoea are clindamycin, broad-spectrum penicillins and the cephalosporins [1, 9-11]. However, apart from vancomycin and parenterally administered aminoglycosides, any antibiotic can cause this disease, whatever the length of the course of treatment. Epidemics of pseudomembranous colitis are particularly common in the institutionalised elderly which should lead to conservative antibiotic policies, especially those with a broad-spectrum of activity [11, 19, 29-31]. A few cases of *Clostridium difficile*-associated colitis have been reported following chemotherapy. Recent studies have confirmed that immune status has a role in the expression of *Clostridium difficile* infection.

Clostridium difficile gives rise to intestinal disease mediated by two toxins, A and B: the clinical and pathological characteristics of this disease have been reproduced in an animal model, the hamsters [1].

Our understanding of the mechanism of action of these toxins is constantly expanding. *Clostridium difficile* toxins A and B are responsible for the epithelial lesions, the diarrhoea and the intestinal inflammation seen in the course of infection with this pathogen. These toxins are encoded by two genes, *tox A* and *tox B*, which are close together on the bacterial chromosome. Almost all pathogenic strains produce both toxins whereas non-toxinogenic strains produce neither. A few strains produce only the B toxin. The intestinal effects of the toxins are species-specific: in humans, toxin B is about ten times more potent than toxin A in the colon whereas in the rodent gut, only toxin A induces inflammation or diarrhoea. These differences are probably due to differences between human and rodent receptors. In both humans and rodents, intraluminal exposure of the colon or the ileum to the toxins leads to breakdown of enterocytic actin filaments which increases paracellular permeability. Moreover, chloride ions are actively pumped out of the cell. This is followed by an acute inflammatory reaction in the *lamina propria* which leads to mast cell activation, over-expression of adhesion molecules on leukocytes in the vascular endothelium, and the release of substance P, eicosanoids and chemokines. The result is neutrophil infiltration of the gut wall and the formation of pseudomembranes with secretory and exudative diarrhoea [32].

The clinical spectrum of *Clostridium difficile* infection goes all the way from healthy carriage to fatal colitis. One of the hypotheses to explain this is that humoral immunity (both systemic and the local sIgA response) would be the key determinant. Experiments in animals have shown that passive or active immunisation against toxin A is effective [33]. In humans, the levels of antibodies against *Clostridium difficile* rise following acute infection whereas the levels are low in recurrent infection, in both children [34] and adults [35]. More recently, a prospective study examined the characteristics of *Clostridium difficile* infection in hospitalized patients being treated with antibiotics [36]. Out of 271 patients, 37 (14%) were carrying *Clostridium difficile* on admission, including 18 asymptomatic carriers. Among the 47 patients (17%) who became infected in hospital, 19 remained free of symptoms. The authors noted an association between increased IgG levels against toxin A and asymptomatic *Clostridium difficile* infection. The same researchers also demonstrated that, in a first episode of *Clostridium difficile*-associated diarrhoea, the presence of antibodies in the blood against toxin A was associated with a lower incidence of recurrence [37].

Clinical picture

In 95% of cases, pseudomembranous colitis manifests as severe diarrhoea. The diarrhoea is usually copious with four to ten bowel movements a day and watery, milky or greenish stools. Tenesmus occurs in 70% of cases, and fever exceeding 38.8 °C in 26% of cases. Blood cultures are never positive. Signs of dehydration are seen in 30% of cases, and weight loss corresponding to over 10% of the body weight in 23% of cases. Rectal bleeding is rare (< 5%) and a concomitant cause ought to be considered in patients with this symptom [38]. Testing can reveal leukocytosis and exudative enteropathy, often leading to decreases in the blood levels of cholesterol and/or albumin [39].

Usually the patient is taking or has recently taken an antibiotic, which is the case 95% of the time. The average interval between the beginning of the course of treatment and the onset of symptoms is seven days but it can be as long as several weeks after the end of treatment.

It is important to be aware of atypical pictures in which diarrhoea is absent, e.g. surgical abdomen, toxic megacolon or ileus (especially following surgery). Ascites or pleural effusion may also be observed. Rare locations such as small intestine involvement, an intra-abdominal abscess or even arthritis are possible. Systemic signs are generally severe. This diagnosis must be considered whenever a patient has recently taken an antibiotic [38].

Diagnosis

Endoscopy and biopsies

Endoscopic diagnosis at the florid state (grade II) is easy with lesions of the rectal mucosa observed in 70% of cases. Otherwise, examination of the rectum and sigmoid colon using a flexible sigmoidoscope will be required, or even colonoscopy. The endoscopic picture is pathognomic if it shows yellowish-white, adherent plaques with a diameter of 2-20 millimetres on an erythematous mucosa (Figure 4).

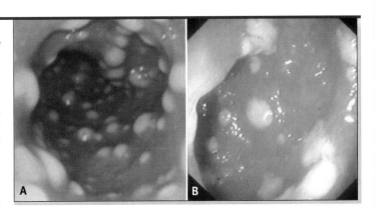

Figure 4.
A : typical endoscopic picture of Clostridium difficile-associated pseudomembranous colitis (photograph: Y. Bouhnik, Hôpital Lariboisière, Paris).
B : rectoscopic picture of false membranes in pseudomembranous colitis (photograph: A. Bitoun, Hôpital Lariboisière, Paris. Traité de Gastro-entérologie, 2000, J.C. Rambaud, ed. Médecine-Sciences Flammarion)

Biopsy analysis reveals superficial necrosis of the mucosa associated with an exudate of leukocytes and fibrin together with tissue debris and mucus (Figure 5). The crypts are distended by copious amounts of mucus and the *lamina propria* is infiltrated with polymorphonuclear cells. This type of colitis is typical of *Clostridium difficile* infection [1, 9-11].

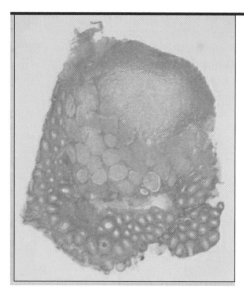

Figure 5.
Colon biopsy: typical histological picture
of pseudomembranous colitis:
the mucosa is coated with a copious
exudate mixed with mucus, and the crypts
are dilated and also filled with mucus
(micrograph: A. Lavergne-Slove,
Anatomie pathologique,
Hôpital Lariboisière, Paris)

Certain forms are more difficult to diagnose, in particular grade I in which pseudomembranes are not seen in an endoscopic examination. Instead, non-specific mucosal damage may be seen or the tissue may appear normal [40]. Biopsies are therefore particularly important. The characteristic abnormality is the apical or "summit" lesion, constituted by focal epithelial necrosis associated with a low-level fibrino-leukocytic exudate. Underneath this lesion, the *lamina propria* may contain fibrin and a few leukocytes but the crypts are normal.

In contrast, in severe forms—grade III—differential diagnosis *vis-à-vis* ischaemic, infectious or inflammatory colitis can prove very difficult. Macroscopic ulcers are due to complete destruction of the mucosa and mucosal muscle tissue, and are covered in a non-specific, mucus-free fibrino-leukocytic exudate. It is important to remember that diagnosis cannot be made on the basis of endoscopic results alone at this stage of the disease. Biopsies are useful for seeking grade II lesions and for trying to rule out other possible causes of ulcerative colitis [40].

Barium contrast enema can reveal a non-specific picture of thumbprinting associated with thickening of the colonic wall. Abdominal CT scanning reveals such thickening in 61% of cases and, less often, an image described as accordion haustration which is considered as more specific for colonic wall thickening [38].

Bacteriology

The isolated presence of *Clostridium difficile* in a stool culture has little value: it is toxin detection which makes diagnosis possible.

The reference diagnostic test is a toxin B assay. This is the most sensitive test [41, 42], capable of detecting just 10 picograms of the toxin, but few laboratories have tissue culture facilities and the result is not usually available in under 24-48 hours. ELISA-based alternatives are now offered by most laboratories [1, 9-11, 34, 37, 41, 43, 44] with good specificity although the sensitivity threshold is of the order of 100-1,000 picograms of toxin A or B: 10-20% of tests give falsely negative results. There are some commercial kits available for detection of toxins A or B [45]. Those which detect both toxins are to be preferred because 1-2% of cases are due to bacterial strains which produce only toxin B [46]. Results are usually available in under 24 hours.

There is no point in testing more than one stool specimen for *Clostridium difficile* toxins: repeating ELISA tests increases the reliability of diagnosis by a factor of 5-10% [47] but the price is increased in parallel, each sample costing about 40 euros.

Treating *Clostridium difficile* infections

Treatment is indicated when *Clostridium difficile* toxin is detected in a patient with any of the following:
- colitis: diarrhoea, fever, leukocytosis and a typical endoscopic picture (warranting the instigation of treatment even before the results of culture and toxin assays are available) or CT scan;
- severe diarrhoea, even in the absence of colitis;
- simple diarrhoea persisting despite discontinuation of the supposedly offending drug;
- a need to continue the antibiotic to treat the original infection.

Various scientific societies have drawn up guidelines for the diagnosis and management of *Clostridium difficile* infections [48]. All recommend metronidazole as the drug of choice, at a dosage of 500 milligrams three times a day or 250 milligrams four times a day. The second-line antibiotic is oral vancomycin at a dosage of 125 milligrams four times a day. Oral metronidazole or vancomycin are successful in over 90% of cases [49, 50]. The usual duration of treatment is ten days. There have been no reports of *Clostridium difficile* resistance to either metronidazole or vancomycin. Given that *Clostridium difficile* colonizes the colonic lumen, the antibiotic is ideally administered by the oral route. If intravenous administration is required, metronidazole (but not vancomycin) is partly effective because it reaches an adequate concentration in the colonic lumen [11].

Metronidazole should be prescribed as the first-line drug because it is less expensive than vancomycin and there is no risk of selecting for resistant enterococci which could exacerbate the problem of nosocomial infection. Indications for oral vancomycin treatment include pregnancy, breast-feeding, intolerance of metronidazole, and the absence of any clinical improvement after three to five days of treatment.

Treatment usually results in disappearance of the fever within 24 hours, and of the diarrhoea in four or five days [11]. If no response is obtained with vancomycin or metronidazole within a reasonable time, it is important to check compliance, consider some other diagnosis (perhaps of a concomitant problem, e.g. inflammatory bowel disease), or seek complications like toxic megacolon or ileus [48]. In the last case, administering high doses of an oral form of vancomycin (500 mg x 4 per day), or the direct instillation of either vancomycin or metronidazole *via* the enteronasal route or as an enema has been proposed. In some cases, the drug has been administered *in situ* into the colon *via* the active channel of an endoscope following exsufflation. Intravenous metronidazole can also be effective [51].

Antimotility drugs ought to be avoided since they promote toxin retention [48]. In severe forms, especially if there is serious dehydration, intensive care measures will be necessary. If there is no rapid response to treatment, subtotal colectomy with temporary ileostomy is indicated.

Recurrent *Clostridium difficile* infection

The main complication of antibiotic treatment is relapse which occurs in 20-25% of cases [9-11, 41, 52, 53]. It is to be suspected if symptoms return anywhere from three days to three weeks after the end of the course of metronidazole or vancomycin. Re-treating a relapse in the same way as the initial episode risks subsequent, serial recurrence which is observed in 40-60% of cases.

Two mechanisms might explain the recurrence of *Clostridium difficile* infection:
- re-infection (exogenous) which can occur after initial eradication if the subject remains exposed to a contaminated environment because clostridial spores can persist in the environment for a matter of months;
- recurrence (endogenous) due to *Clostridium difficile* persisting in the colon because the spores are not killed by antibiotics.

Various strategies proposed for the prevention of relapses of *Clostridium difficile*-associated diarrhoea do not lack originality. The first of these involves administering probiotics or saprophytic bacteria to restore the bacterial balance in the colon:
- administration of *Saccharomyces boulardii* [53, 54];
- administration of *Lactobacillus* GG [37, 50, 52, 55-57];
- rectal infusions of faecal material (which are banned because of the risk of transmitting pathogens) or preferably of mixtures of bacteria [58-60] derived from the faeces.

In a large-scale (124 patients), placebo-controlled trial, *Saccharomyces boulardii* was administered for four weeks—initially combined with standard antibiotics—with a further four-week follow-up period:
- if the episode of diarrhoea had been the first associated with *Clostridium difficile* (64 patients), *Saccharomyces boulardii* brought no significant benefit;
- in patients with a relapse of *Clostridium difficile*-associated diarrhoea (60 patients), *Saccharomyces boulardii* was responsible for a significant reduction in the incidence of further recurrence (35% *versus* 65%; p = 0.04).

Saccharomyces boulardii did not reduce the level of *Clostridium difficile* colonization but was associated with a reduction in the rate of detection of its toxin B. This is consistent with the evidence that proteases released by *Saccharomyces boulardii* inhibit toxins A and B and their receptors without killing the pathogen [53].

After the administration of *Lactobacillus* GG for several days, Gorbach *et al.* observed no recurrence in four out of five patients over a follow-up of at least two months [56]. After a single dose of *Lactobacillus* GG, Bennett *et al.* observed no recurrence in 84% of 32 patients suffering from a recurrent form of *Clostridium difficile* infection over a follow-up period of between one and four years [55].

Attempts have been made to reconstitute the colonic microfloras of patients suffering from recurrent *Clostridium difficile* infection by the rectal infusion of faecal material [58, 59] or mixtures of anaerobic bacteria isolated from healthy volunteers: this strategy yielded promising results in cases which had proved refractory to all other treatment modalities. Rectal infusion of a suspension containing high densities of various bacteria (*Bacteroides, Bifidobacterium* and *Lactobacillus*) eradicated *Clostridium difficile* in five patients [60]. However, no placebo-controlled trial has been published to date and patients tend to be reluctant about this type of treatment. In order to ensure reaching all the lesions (right colon) and perhaps confront this reluctance, it has been proposed that the faecal material could be infused directly using a colonoscope [61].

Another novel approach to the treatment of recurrent *Clostridium difficile* infection is passive immunotherapy by immunoglobulin infusion [31]. Given that experience with this type of modality remains anecdotal, it represents a last resort. Active immunotherapy could also represent a promising avenue [62].

Other preventive measures

Clostridium difficile is a major nosocomial pathogen with a number of hospitals and long-stay units having reported epidemics of clostridial diarrhoea (with or without colitis) of varying duration [35, 36, 40, 44, 45, 47, 63]. Typing the strains of *Clostridium difficile* has been proposed as a way of evaluating epidemics but few laboratories are capable of performing this type of test. Cutting down on the prescription of antibiotics—especially those with a broad-spectrum of activity—has been successful in curtailing some of these epidemics [35, 37]. Most importantly, strict implementation of measures to fight nosocomial infections is a key element in prevention since the transmission of *Clostridium difficile* spores leads to many infections because they spread so widely and persist in the environment for such a long time.

Key points

- Antibiotic-associated diarrhoea complicates 5-20% of courses of treatment (depending on the type of antibiotic prescribed, and the definition of diarrhoea applied).

- "Simple" diarrhoea is the most common form and, in clinical terms, the least severe. However, the underlying mechanisms are complex and etiologies can be infectious (above all *Clostridium difficile*), metabolic (as a result of eradication of bacteria of the dominant anaerobic microflora) or something else (e.g. acceleration of intestinal transit). These forms resolve once the agent responsible has been withdrawn.

- Post-antibiotic haemorrhagic colitis presents a stereotypical picture characterized by the sudden onset of abdominal cramps followed by bloody diarrhoea in a penicillin- or streptogramin-treated patient. The guilty agent woud seem to be *Klebsiella oxytoca* which is most efficiently isolated by the culture of colonic biopsy material. In the great majority of cases, the problem resolves when the antibiotic is withdrawn.

- *Clostridium difficile* causes pseudomembranous colitis. It is now easier to detect as a result of the development of ELISAs for toxins A and B. Metronidazole is the drug of choice in treatment.

- The main complication of antibiotic treatment of *Clostridium difficile* infection is relapse which occurs in 20-25% of cases and is often serial. Among the modalities proposed to prevent multiple recurrence, probiotics—mainly *Saccharomyces boulardii*—occupy a place of choice.

References

1. Bartlett JG. Antibiotic-associated diarrhea. *Clin Infect Dis* 1992 ; 15 : 573-81.

2. Clausen MR, Bonnen H, Tvede M, Mortensen PB. Colonic fermentation to short-chain fatty acids is decreased in antibiotic-associated diarrhea. *Gastroenterology* 1991 ; 101 : 1497-504.

3. Gilbert DN. Aspects of the safety profile of oral antimicrobial agents. *Infect Dis Clin Pract* 1995 ; 4 : Suppl 2 : S103-12.

4. Wistrom J, Norrby SR, Myhre EB, *et al*. Frequency of antibiotic-associated diarrhoea in 2,462 antibiotic-treated hospitalized patients: a prospective study. *J Antimicrob Chemother* 2001 ; 47 : 43-50.

5. Beaugerie L, Flahault A, Barbut F, *et al*., Study Group. Antibiotic-associated diarrhoea and *Clostridium difficile* in the community. *Aliment Pharmacol Ther* 2003 ; 17 : 905-12.

6. Turck D, Bernet JP, Marx J, *et al*. Incidence and risk factors of oral antibiotic-associated diarrhea in an outpatient pediatric population. *J Pediatr Gastroenterol Nutr* 2003 ; 37 : 22-6.

7. McFarland LV. Facteurs de risque de la diarrhée associée aux antibiotiques. Une revue de la littérature. *Ann Med Interne* 1998 ; 149 : 261-6.

8. Caron F, Lerebours E. Effets secondaires gastrointestinaux des antibiotiques. *Gastroenterol Clin Biol* 1991 ; 15(8-9) : 604-12.

9. Kelly CP, Pothoulakis C, LaMont JT. *Clostridium difficile* colitis. *N Engl J Med* 1994 ; 330 : 257-62.

10. Gerding DN. Disease associated with *Clostridium difficile* infection. *Ann Intern Med* 1989 ; 110 : 255-7.

11. Fekety R, Shah AB. Diagnosis and treatment of *Clostridium difficile* colitis. *JAMA* 1993 ; 269 : 71-5.

12. Sparks SG, Carman RJ, Sarker MR, McClane BA. Genotyping of enterotoxigenic *Clostridium perfringens* fecal isolates associated with antibiotic-associated diarrhea and food poisoning in North America. *J Clin Microbiol* 2001 ; 39 : 883-8.

13. Sun M. In search of Salmonella's smoking gun. *Science* 1984 ; 226 : 30-2.

14. Forbes D, Ee L, Camer-Pesci P, Ward PB. Faecal candida and diarrhoea. *Arch Dis Child* 2001 ; 84 : 328-31.

15. Rao SS, Edwards CA, Austen CJ, Bruce C, Read NW. Impaired colonic fermentation of carbohydrate after ampicillin. *Gastroenterology* 1988 ; 94 : 928-32.

16. Chassany O, Michaux A, Bergmann JF. Drug-induced diarrhoea. *Drug Saf* 2000 ; 22 : 53-72.

17. Hogenauer C, Hammer HF, Krejs GJ, Reisinger EC. Mechanisms and management of antibiotic-associated diarrhea. *Clin Infect Dis* 1998 ; 27 : 702-10.

18. D'Souza AL, Rajkumar C, Cooke J, Bulpitt CJ. Probiotics in prevention of antibiotic associated diarrhoea: meta-analysis. *Br Med J* 2002 ; 324 : 1361-7.

19. Cremonini F, Di Caro S, Nista EC, *et al*. Meta-analysis: the effect of probiotic administration on antibiotic-associated diarrhoea. *Aliment Pharmacol Ther* 2002 ; 16 : 1461-7.

20. Wilhelm MP, Lee DT, Rosenblatt JE. Bacterial interference by anaerobic species isolated from human feces. *Eur J Clin Microbiol* 1987 ; 6 : 266-70.

21. Minami J, Katayama S, Matsushita O, *et al*. Enteroxic activity of *K. oxytoca* cytotoxin in rabbit intestinal loops. *Infect Immun* 1994 62 : 172-7.

22. Sakurai Y, Tsuchiya H, Ikegami F, *et al*. Acute right-sided hemorrhagic colitis associated with oral administration of ampicillin. *Dig Dis Sci* 1979 ; 24 : 910-5.

23. Benoit R, Danquechin Dorval E, Loulergue J, *et al*. Diarrhée post-antibiotique : rôle de *Klebsiella oxytoca*. *Gastroenterol Clin Biol* 1992 ; 16 : 860-4.

24. Koga H, Aoyagi K, Yoshimura R, Kimura Y, Iida M, Fujishima M. Can quinolones cause hemorrhagic colitis of late onset? Report of three cases. *Dis Colon Rectum* 1999 ; 42 : 1502-4.

25. Bellaïche G, Le Pennec MP, Choudat L, *et al*. Intérêt de la rectosigmoidoscopie avec cultures bactériologiques de biopsies coliques dans le diagnostic des colites hémorragiques à *Klebsiella oxytoca*. *Gastroenterol Clin Biol* 1997 ; 21 : 764-7.

26. Beaugerie L, Metz M, Barbut F, *et al*., and the Infectious Colitis Study group. *Klebsiella oxytoca* as an agent of antibiotic-associated haemorrhagic colitis. *Clin Gastroenterol Hepatol* : in press.

27. Viscidi R, Willey S, Bartlett JG. Isolation rates and toxigenic potential of *Clostridium difficile* isolates from various patient populations. *Gastroenterology* 1981 ; 81 : 5-9.

28. Karlstrom O, Fryklund B, Tullus K, Burman LG. A prospective nationwide study of *Clostridium difficile*-associated diarrhea in Sweden. *Clin Infect Dis* 1998 ; 26 : 141-5.

29. Gerding DN, Johnson S, Peterson LR, Mulligan ME, Silva J Jr. *Clostridium difficile*-associated diarrhea and colitis. *Infect Control Hosp Epidemiol* 1995 ; 16 : 459-77.

30. Johnson S, Samore MH, Farrow KA, *et al*. Epidemics of diarrhea caused by a clindamycin-resistant strain of *Clostridium difficile* in four hospitals. *N Engl J Med* 1999 ; 341 : 1645-51.

31. Climo MW, Israel DS, Wong ES, Williams D, Coudron P, Markowitz SM. Hospital-wide restriction of clindamycin: effect on the incidence of *Clostridium difficile*-associated diarrhea and cost. *Ann Intern Med* 1998 ; 128 : 989-95.

32. Lamont JT. Recent advances in the structures and function of *Clostridium difficile* toxins. In : Rambaud JC, Lamont JT, eds. *Updates on* Clostridium difficile. Paris : Springer-Verlag, 1996 : 73-82.

33. Kelly CP. Immune response to *Clostridium difficile* infection. *Eur J Gastroenterol* 1996 ; 8 : 1048-53

34. Leung DY, Kelly CP, Boguniewicz M, Pothoulakis C, LaMont JT, Flores A. Treatment with intravenously administered gamma globulin of chronic relapsing colitis induced by *Clostridium difficile* toxin. *J Pediatr* 1991 ; 118 : 633-7.

35. Warny M, Fatimi A, Bostwick EF, *et al*. Bovine immunoglobulin concentrate-*Clostridium difficile* retains *C. difficile* toxin neutralising activity after passage through the human stomach and small intestine. *Gut* 1999 ; 44 : 212-7.

36. Kyne L, Warny M, Qamar A, Kelly CP. Asymptomatic carriage of *Clostridium difficile* and serum levels of IgG antibody against toxin A. *N Engl J Med* 2000 ; 342 : 390-7.

37. Kyne L, Warny M, Qamar A, Kelly CP. Association between antibody response to toxin A and protection against recurrent *Clostridium difficile* diarrhoea. *Lancet* 2001 ; 357 : 189-93.

38. Marteau P, Rambaud JC. Colites pseudomembraneuses et autres manifestations de l'infection à *Clostridium difficile*. In : Rambaud JC, ed. *Traité de gastro-entérologie*. Paris, Flammarion, 2000 : 687-93.

39. Bulusu M, Narayan S, Shetler K, Triadafilopoulos G. Leukocytosis as a harbinger and surrogate marker of *Clostridium difficile* infection in hospitalized patients with diarrhea. *Am J Gastroenterol* 2000 ; 95 : 3137-41.

40. Price AB. Pseudomenbranous colitis. In : Whright R, ed. *Recent advances in gastroenterology*. London : WB Saunders : 15-172.

41. Mylonakis E, Ryan ET, Calderwood SB. *Clostridium difficile*-associated diarrhea: a review. *Arch Intern Med* 2000 ; 161 : 525-5-33.

42. Laughon BE, Viscidi RP, Gdovin SL, Yolken RH, Bartlett JG. Enzyme immunoassays for detection of *Clostridium difficile* toxins A and B in fecal specimens. *J Infect Dis* 1984 ; 149 : 781-8.

43. Barbut F, Kajzer C, Planas N, Petit JC. Comparison of three enzyme immunoassays, a cytotoxicity assay, and toxigenic culture for diagnosis of *Clostridium difficile*-associated diarrhea. *J Clin Microbiol* 1993 ; 31 : 963-7.

44. Merz CS, Kramer C, Forman M, *et al*. Comparison of four commercially available rapid enzyme immunoassays with cytotoxin assay for detection of *Clostridium difficile* toxin(s) from stool specimens. *J Clin Microbiol* 1994 ; 32 : 1142-7.

45. Lozniewski A, Rabaud C, Dotto E, Weber M, Mory F. Laboratory diagnosis of *Clostridium difficile*-associated diarrhea and colitis: usefulness of premier cytoclone A+B enzyme immunoassay for combined detection of stool toxins and toxigenic *C. difficile* strains. *J Clin Microbiol* 2001 ; 39 : 1996-8.

46. Johnson S, Kent SA, O'Leary KJ, *et al*. Fatal pseudomembranous colitis associated with a variant *Clostridium difficile* strain not detected by toxin A immunoassay. *Ann Intern Med* 2001 ; 135 : 434-8.

47. Manabe YC, Vinetz JM, Moore RD, Merz C, Charache P, Bartlett JG. *Clostridium difficile* colitis: an efficient clinical approach to diagnosis. *Ann Intern Med* 1995 ; 123 : 835-40.

48. Guerrant RL. Practice guidelines for the management of infectious diarrhea. *Clin Infect Dis* 2001 ; 32 : 331-51.

49. Teasley DG, Gerding DN, Olson MM, *et al*. Prospective randomised trial of metronidazole *versus* vancomycin for *Clostridium difficile*-associated diarrhoea and colitis. *Lancet* 1983 ; 2 : 1043-6.

50. Wenisch C, Parschalk B, Hasenhundl M, Hirschl AM, Graninger W. Comparison of vancomycin, teicoplanin, metronidazole, and fusidic acid for the treatment of *Clostridium difficile*-associated diarrhea. *Clin Infect Dis* 1996 ; 22 : 813-8. [Erratum, *Clin Infect Dis* 1996 ; 23 : 423.]

51. Friedenberg F, Fernandez A, Kaul V, Niami P, Levine GM. Intravenous metronidazole for the treatment of *Clostridium difficile* colitis. *Dis Colon Rectum* 2001 ; 44 : 1176-80.

52. Bartlett JG. Treatment of *Clostridium difficile* colitis. *Gastroenterology* 1985 ; 89 : 1192-5.

53. McFarland LV, Surawicz CM, Greenberg RN, *et al*. A randomized placebo-controlled trial of *Saccharomyces boulardii* in combination with standard antibiotics for *Clostridium difficile* disease. *JAMA* 1994 ; 271 : 1913-8.

54. Surawicz CM, McFarland LV, Elmer G, Chinn J. Treatment of recurrent *Clostridium difficile* colitis with vancomycin and *Saccharomyces boulardii*. *Am J Gastroenterol* 1989 ; 84 : 1285-7.

55. Gorbach SL, Chang TW, Goldin B. Successful treatment of relapsing *Clostridium difficile* colitis with *Lactobacillus* GG. *Lancet* 1987 ; 2 : 1519.

56. Bennett RG, Gorbach SL. Goldin BR. Treatment of relapsing *Clostridium difficile* diarrhea with *Lactobacillus* GG. *Nutrition Today* 1996 ; 31 (suppl) : 35S-8S.

57. Pochapin M. The effect of probiotics on *Clostridium difficile* diarrhea. *Am J Gastroenterol* 2000 ; 95 : S11-3.

58. Bowden TA Jr, Mansberger AR Jr, Lykins LE. Pseudomembraneous enterocolitis -: mechanism for restoring floral homeostasis. *Am Surg* 1981 ; 47 : 178-83.

59. Schwan A, Sjolin S, Trottestam U, Aronsson B. Relapsing *Clostridium difficile* enterocolitis cured by rectal infusion of normal faeces. *Scand J Infect Dis* 1984 ; 16 : 211-5.

60. Tvede M, Rask-Madsen J. Bacteriotherapy for chronic relapsing *Clostridium difficile* diarrhoea in six patients. *Lancet* 1989 ; 1 (8648) : 1156-60.

61. Persky SE, Brandt LJ. Treatment of recurrent *Clostridium difficile*-associated diarrhea by administration of donated stool directly through a colonoscope. *Am J Gastroenterol* 2000 ; 95 : 3283-5.

62. Kyne L, Kelly C. Prospects for a vaccine for *Clostridium difficile*. *BioDrugs* 1998 ; 10 : 173-81.

63. Fekety R, Kim KH, Brown D, Batts DH, Cudmore M, Silva J Jr. Epidemiology of antibiotic-associated colitis: isolation of *Clostridium difficile* from the hospital environment. *Am J Med* 1981 ; 70 : 906-8.

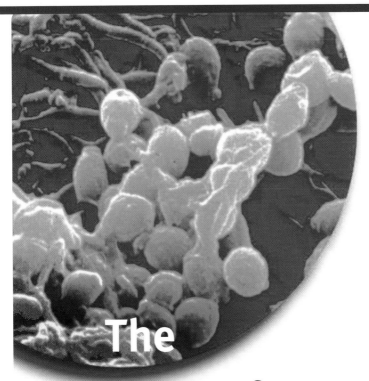

The
Value of
Administering
Live Organisms

Probiotics and Digestive Problems

Thierry Piche[1],
Patrick Rampal[2]

1. Service d'Hépato-
Gastro-entérologie,
CHU de Nice,
Hôpital de l'Archet 2,
Nice, France
2. Service d'Hépato-
Gastro-entérologie,
Centre Hospitalier
Princesse Grace,
Principauté de Monaco,
Monaco

P robiotics are live microorganisms (bacteria or yeasts) which, when administered in adequate amounts, confer a health benefit on the host. A probiotic product must:
- not have any pathogenic activity;
- supply a large number of viable organisms;
- resist gastric, biliary and pancreatic secretions, to survive in the small intestine and the colon;
- confer a health benefit on the host [1].

Probiotics mediate direct effects as they pass through the gastrointestinal tract and can significantly modulate metabolisms of the microflora, thus interacting with the mucosa [2]. Probiotics have been extensively studied leading to nearly 900 articles, some 90% of which were published in the last decade. Many beneficial effects have been documented in digestive and extraintestinal disorders in humans. They have been shown to be effective, especially in the prevention of antibiotic-associated diarrhoea, in decreasing the frequency of recurrent *Clostridium difficile* infection; moreover they have been shown to have preventive and curative activity against acute infectious diarrhoea, inhibitory effects against *Helicobacter pylori* adhesion to the stomach wall, and also a key role in limiting many inflammatory processes. This chapter will review the main digestive and extraintestinal disorders in which probiotics have shown positive effects in controlled studies.

Pharmacology, physiological effects and mechanisms of action

Administering probiotics is a way of delivering active substances (e.g. enzymes, immunomodulatory peptides or antibacterial substances) to a site of action in the digestive tract as well as a means to modulate the endogenous microflora [3]. Pharmacological analysis of probiotics products should result in the identification of active constituents of transiting microorganisms, their pharmacokinetic properties as far as their targets, and their specific beneficial effects. Although the precise nature of many compounds is often uncertain, the capacity of probiotic microorganisms to survive in the digestive tract and their pharmacology have been most fully documented. The density of viable, transiting probiotics varies according to the quantity and nature of the different strains ingested [3]. Some are killed as soon as they arrive in the stomach while others (*Saccharomyces boulardii, Bifidobacterium, Lactobacillus plantarum, Lactobacillus acidophilus*) can reach the colon in large numbers. When they reach their site of action, probiotics mediate direct effects in the lumen and the gut wall (on enterocytes and the immune competent cells of gut-associated lymphoid tissue [GALT]) as well as indirect effects due to modification of the colonic ecosystem (Figure 1).

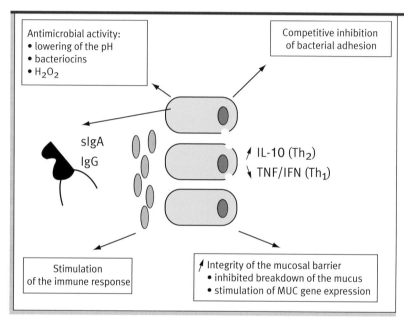

Figure 1.
Molecular effects and mechanisms of action of probiotics in the intestinal or colonic epithelium.
SCFAs: short-chain fatty acids
H_2O_2: hydrogen peroxide
IFN: interferon
TNF: tumour necrosis factor

Although many authors have studied the molecular effects of probiotic microorganisms, the mechanism of action of these agents remains poorly elucidated. The protective effects of certain strains against intestinal infections involve immunomodulatory properties, inhibition of the growth of intracolonic bacteria, the production of antibacterial substances or of the capacity to decrease intracolonic pH [4]. The most fully documented effects are the inhibition of the adhesion of pathogenic bacteria, modulation of macrophage functions, and elimination of toxins (*for a general review, see* [5]). The adhesion of pathogenic bacteria is inhibited by competition of relevant receptors, up-regulation of the expression of mucins RNA messengers (MUC2 and MUC3), the secretion of bacteriocins or even environmental changes such as free radicals, organic acids or hydrogen peroxide productions. The stimulation of macrophage functions by probiotics leads to enhanced phagocytosis of inert particles and, also in certain cases, of live organisms, as it was demonstrated with *Salmonella* cells [6]. Finally, several studies have confirmed that some probiotics can inhibit and sometimes eliminate toxins (e.g. *Clostridium difficile* toxin A in the case of *Saccharomyces boulardii*, and Aflatoxin B1 in the case of bifidobacteria) [7, 8].

Antibiotic-associated diarrhoea

Diarrhoea is a side effect of antibiotics which can sometimes cause patients to discontinue their course of treatment. Changes in stool consistency or full-blown diarrhoea complicate 5-30% of antibiotic treatments, either while the drug is being taken or after the end of the course. The incidence of diarrhoea varies between different antibiotics: it affects 5-10% of those taking ampicillin, 10-20% of those taking a combination of amoxicillin and clavulanic acid, 15-20% of those on cefixime, and finally, 5% of patients receiving other antibiotics such as a quinolone, clarithromycin, erythromycin or tetracycline [9]. The pathogenesis of antibiotic-associated diarrhoea (AAD) is complex and arises from quantitative and qualitative perturbations of the microflora. Two mechanisms underlying AAD have been elucidated, namely the proliferation of pathogenic microbes and reduced fermentative activity on the part of the microflora. The latter can lead to reduced short-chain fatty acids production and an increase in the amount of unabsorbed carbohydrate which can lead to both reduced sodium absorption (which is stimulated by short-chain fatty acids) and osmotic diarrhoea [10]. Clausen *et al.* [11] showed that faecal short-chain fatty acids levels were significantly lower in patients with AAD than in control subjects (with no diarrhoea). In some cases, a course of antibiotics can promote intestinal infection, notably with *Clostridium difficile* and more rarely with *Klebsiella oxytoca* [12, 13]. Probiotics have been demonstrated to be effective in preventing AAD in many studies, the most important of which are shown in Table I.

In two recent meta-analyses, the preventive effects of probiotics against AAD were evaluated. D'Souza *et al.* [14] reviewed nine randomised, placebo-controlled trials covering over one thousand subjects. Five of these trials concerned probiotic bacteria, and four *Saccharomyces boulardii*. The odds ratio in favour of probiotics was 0.37 being more effective than placebo (IC$_{95}$: 0.26 to 0.53; p < 0.001). Another meta-analysis also covering open studies came to the same conclusions [15]. Lactobacilli were the first bacterial probiotics to be evaluated against AAD. Lactobacilli were chosen because the density of this type of bacterium is usually decreased in subjects taking ampicillin. In a recent study, Vanderhoof *et al.* [16] concluded that the GG strain of *Lactobacillus rhamnosus* (*Lactobacillus GG*) effectively prevented diarrhoea in two hundred antibiotic-treated children: 7 children who were administered *Lactobacillus* GG experienced diarrhoea compared with 25 in the placebo group, and the mean duration of the episodes of diarrhoea was significantly reduced (4.7 *versus* 5.8 days). In contrast, Thomas *et al.* [17] did not observe any effect of *Lactobacillus* GG over and above that of placebo in 302 patients treated with *Lactobacillus* GG for fourteen days. In this study, the incidence of diarrhoea in the *Lactobacillus* GG group was 29% compared with 29.9% in the placebo group. Another study showed that *Lactobacillus acidophilus* effectively prevented neomycin-induced diarrhoea whereas *Lactobacillus bulgaricus* had no effect [18]. Gotz *et al.* [19] compared a preparation containing *Lactobacillus acidophilus* and *Lactobacillus bulgaricus* with placebo in patients taking various different antibiotics, and found exactly the same incidence of diarrhoea in both groups. In contrast, if only those cases of diarrhoea associated with ampicillin were considered, no patient being treated with the lactobacilli experienced diarrhoea compared with 14% in the placebo group. Finally, two studies conducted in healthy volunteers suggested that *Bifidobacterium longum* and *Lactobacillus* GG could mitigate side effects attributed to erythromycin, in particular acceleration of intestinal transit [20, 21].

Probiotic	Patients	N	Antibiotic	Duration of the thera-peutic trial	Effect (% diarrhoea)	p	Réf.
Saccharomyces boulardii	Hospitalized patients	180	Various	Variable	9.5% vs 21.8% placebo	= 0.04	[24]
Saccharomyces boulardii	Hospitalized patients	193	β-lactam tetracyclin	Course of treatment + 1 month	7.2% vs 14.6% placebo	= 0.03	[25]
Saccharomyces boulardii	Out-patients	388	β-lactam-tetracyclin	Variable	4.5% vs 17.5% placebo	< 0.01	[26]
Lactobacillus GG	Hospitalized children	202	Various	Variable	2.0% vs 26% placebo	< 0.02	[16]
Lactobacillus GG	Hospitalized patients	302	Various	Variable	29.3% vs 29.9% placebo	NS	[17]

Table I.
Main randomised trials of probiotics in the prevention of antibiotic-associated diarrhoea

Of all the probiotics evaluated in the prevention of AAD, *Saccharomyces boulardii* has been the most extensively studied and has clearly been shown to be effective, cutting down the occurrence of diarrhoea by half. *Saccharomyces boulardii* is a non-pathogenic strain of yeast which is naturally resistant to antibacterial antibiotics, whereas most bacterial probiotics, as a general rule, are highly susceptible to these antibiotics, which makes their viability uncertain and their mechanisms of action imprecise [22, 23]. Surawicz *et al.* [24] evaluated the efficacy of *Saccharomyces boulardii* administered during treatment and continued for two weeks after the end of the course in 180 hospitalized patients receiving antibiotics belonging to various classes. The incidence of diarrhoea was significantly reduced in patients receiving *Saccharomyces boulardii* (9.5% *versus* 21.8% on placebo). The same authors carried out a similar study focusing on β-lactam antibiotics and prolonging the follow-up period out through seven weeks after the drug had been stopped [25]. *Saccharomyces boulardii* (at a dosage of one gram a day) or placebo was administered to 193 patients from the beginning of antibiotic treatment and continued three days after the end of the course. In this study, *Saccharomyces boulardii* mediated a significant preventive effect on the occurrence of diarrhoea (7.2% *versus* 14.6%, p = 0.02). These results have been confirmed by Adam *et al.* [26] in a study of 188 outpatients taking a tetracycline or a β-lactam antibiotic together with *Saccharomyces boulardii* at a dosage of 200 mg/day. Another study, based on the same dosage in hospitalized patients, did not yield any significant results, but the sample size was very small and the subjects were not followed up beyond the end of the course of antibiotic treatment [27].

All these findings suggest that certain probiotics can prevent AAD. This type of modality should be proposed to patients at increased risk of diarrhoea when taking an antibiotic: in a recent outpatient epidemiological survey [28], a high number of bowel movements, a long course of antibiotic and certain antibiotics (amoxicillin/clavulanic acid) were significant risk factors for AAD.

A special case: *Clostridium difficile*

Clostridium difficile is a non-invasive bacillus responsible for the majority of cases of pseudomembranous colitis but also acute, non-pseudomembranous colitis. *Clostridium difficile* is a model of opportunist proliferation of a digestive pathogen after loss of the microflora-mediated barrier effect due to antibiotic therapy. *Clostridium difficile* would be involved in 10-20% of cases of simple AAD in the hospital setting, and in almost all cases of pseudomembranous colitis. The best-documented risk factors for *Clostridium difficile* colitis are, apart from antibiotic consumption, advanced age and hospitalization in an institution. Another risk factor for *Clostridium difficile* colitis is related to immunodeficiency and/or faecal stasis—and therefore perturbation of the colonic ecosystem. After one takes an antibiotic, *Clostridium difficile* may colonize the gut and secretes two exotoxins, A and B which cause diarrhoea. The ability of the bacterium is its capacity to form resistant spores which explains its nosocomial transmission and, in part, the frequency of recurrent infection. All antibiotics can cause *Clostridium difficile*-associated diarrhoea but broad-spectrum penicillins and the cephalosporins are most commonly involved. The standard treatment for *Clostridium difficile* colitis consists of oral metronidazole (500 mg/3 times a day or 250 mg/4 times a day) or vancomycin (125 mg/4 times a day) which has a response rate of 90-97% [29]. Recurrence occurs in 20-25% of cases, on average six days after stopping the initial treatment. In the event of relapse, a new course of the same treatment is most often effective but 40% of patients will experience one or more relapses, with 3-5% of patients presenting more than six relapses. The mechanism underlying recurrence is poorly understood but it may be that *Clostridium difficile* spores can survive in the intestine after withdrawal of the antibiotic. Several open studies have suggested that *Saccharomyces boulardii, Lactobacillus* GG and *Lactobacillus plantarum* LP299v could be beneficial in *Clostridium difficile*-associated diarrhoea [30-32]. In a randomised, placebo-controlled trial, McFarland *et al.* [33] evaluated the effect of *Saccharomyces boulardii* (1 gram a day for 28 days) and placebo as adjunctive therapy to metronidazole or vancomycin in 124 patients. It was a first episode of *Clostridium difficile* infection in 64 cases, and a relapse in 60. In this study, after the administration of *Saccharomyces boulardii*, the authors observed a reduction of about 50% in relapse in patients who had previously experienced a first recurrent *Clostridium difficile* infection. *Saccharomyces boulardii* could mediate its preventive action through proteolysis and inhibition of the binding of *Clostridium difficile* toxin A to its receptor [7, 34].

Infectious diarrhoea

Diarrhoea is a common problem in travellers from a developed country visiting a country with a lower level of hygiene. The incidence of traveller's diarrhoea varies from 20-50% according to the traveler's point of departure as well as destination and also method of transportation. In most cases, it is a mild, short-lived (one to five days) condition although 20% of these digestive problems lead to confinement to bed for few days and, more rarely, hospitalization is necessary. Several infectious agents may be responsible but enterotoxigenic *Escherichia coli* is the most common — as a result of ingestion of contaminated food or water. Prevention mainly depends on observing rules of hygiene as well as improvement of sanitary conditions in developing countries. A cheap treatment modality, free of side effects, would be welcome.

The main studies addressing the administration of probiotics to prevent traveller's diarrhoea are listed in Table II.

Black *et al.* [35] investigated the efficacy of a mixture of probiotics (*Lactobacillus acidophilus, Lactobacillus bulgaricus, Bifidobacterium bifidum* and *Streptococcus thermophilus*) compared with placebo in 94 tourists spending two weeks in Egypt. In the probiotic-treated group, the incidence of diarrhoea was significantly reduced (43% *versus* 71%; p = 0.02). Other authors have shown that *Lactobacillus* GG [36, 37] and *Saccharomyces boulardii* [38] conferred protection against diarrhoea only for those who travel to certain destinations. Different infectious agents could explain the destination-dependent variability in outcome. In the work of Kollaritsch *et al.* conducted in travellers receiving *Saccharomyces boulardii* or placebo, a moderate but statistically significant level of protection against diarrhoea was observed, and the effect was dose-dependent [38]. In contrast, neither Pozo-Olano [39] nor Katelaris [40] observed any protective effect with various lactobacillus-based preparations.

Table II. Main randomised trials of probiotics in the prevention of traveller's diarrhoea	Probiotic	Number of patients	Therapeutic effect	P	Réf.
	Lactobacilli + Bifidobacteria + Streptococci	94	43% vs 71%	= 0.02	[35]
	Lactobacillus GG	756	41% vs 46.5%	NS	[36]
	Lactobacillus GG	245	3.9%/day at risk vs 7.4%	0.05	[37]
	Saccharomyces boulardii	1,016	28.7% vs 39.1%	= 0.005	[38]
	Lactobacillus acidophilus + Lactobacillus bulgaricus	50	35% vs 29%	NS	[39]
	Lactobacillus fermentum strain KLD	282	23.8% vs 23.8%	NS	[40]
	Lactobacillus acidophilus	282	25.7% vs 23.8%	NS	[40]

In children, infectious diarrhoea represents a public health problem and in the Third World, several million children die of dehydration every year. Certain probiotics have been evaluated for their ability to prevent infectious diarrhoea (Table III).

The administration of lactobacilli to healthy volunteers who had ingested an enterotoxigenic strain of *Escherichia coli* had no protective effect against diarrhoea [41]. Oberhelman *et al.* [42] evaluated the efficacy of *Lactobacillus* GG administered for fifteen months to 204 malnourished Peruvian children: a modest but significant effect was observed in children who received *Lactobacillus* GG experiencing fewer episodes of diarrhoea (5.21 *versus* 6.02 episodes per child per year, p = 0.02) than in untreated children. The study of Saavedra *et al.* [43] also showed that administration of a mixture of *Bifidobacterium bifidum* and *Streptococcus thermophilus* to 57 babies in hospital prevented diarrhoea and decreased rotavirus transmission. Similar findings have been shown with *Lactobacillus* GG [44].

Several probiotics have also shown curative efficacy, reducing the severity and duration of episodes of diarrhoea (Table III). Isolauri *et al.* [45] treated 74 children suffering from infectious diarrhoea with either a fermented dairy product supplemented with *Lactobacillus* GG (125 grams twice a day) or placebo. In this study, the authors showed that the duration of the diarrhoea was significantly reduced by *Lactobacillus* GG (1.4 *versus* 2.4 days), and that this effect was more marked when the analysis was confined to children infected with rotavirus. Recently, *Lactobacillus* GG or a placebo were used in a large-scale European trial as an adjunct to rehydration therapy in 283 children with infectious diarrhoea [46]; the duration of the diarrhoea was significantly reduced in those receiving *Lactobacillus* GG, and this effect was again more marked in rotavirus-infected children.

Probiotic	Population studied	Therapeutic effect on the diarrhoea	P	Réf.
Lactobacillus acidophilus, Lactobacillus bulgaricus	Healthy volunteers: challenged with *Escherichia coli* n = 48 Prevention	No benefit	NS	[41]
Lactobacillus GG	Diarrhoea in children n = 204 Prevention	Occurrence reduced (5.21 episodes of diarrhoea/ child/year vs 6.02)	= 0.028	[42]
Bifidobacterium bifidum, Streptococcus thermophilus	Nosocomial diarrhoea in children n = 57 Prevention	Occurrence reduced (7% vs 31%) especially of rotaviral diarrhoea	= 0.035	[43]
Lactobacillus GG	Rotaviral gastroenteritis n = 81 Prevention	Occurrence reduced (2.2% vs 16.7%)	= 0.04	[44]
Lactobacillus GG	Diarrhoea in children (rotavirus in 80 %) n = 74 Treatment	Reduced duration (1 vs 2.4 days)	< 0.001	[45]
Lactobacillus GG	Diarrhoea in children n = 283 Treatment	Reduced duration (58.3 vs 72 hours)	< 0.008	[46]
Saccharomyces boulardii	Diarrhoea in children (n = 130) Treatment	Clinical cure at 96 hours (85% vs 40%)	< 0.01	[47]
Saccharomyces boulardii	Diarrhoea in adult (n = 92) Treatment	Diarrhoea score at 48 hours (number x consistency index) (5.5 vs 6.7)	= 0.035	[48]

Table III.
Main randomised trials of probiotics in infectious diarrhoea

The efficacy of *Saccharomyces boulardii* was evaluated in a double-blind, placebo-controlled study in 130 children between three months and three years of age suffering from acute diarrhoea [47]; the percentage of clinical cure (fewer than four non-watery stools/24 hours) was significantly higher in the *Saccharomyces boulardii* group at both 48 and 96 hours (85% *versus* 40%, p < 0.01). In a double-blind, placebo-controlled trial in 92 adult patients with acute diarrhoea [48], the administration of *Saccharomyces boulardii* significantly reduced the 48-hour diarrhoea score (i.e., the number of bowel movements x the consistency index [1 = normal; 2 = soft; 3 = watery]) (5.5 *versus* 6.7, p = 0.035).

In a recent study, Szajewska *et al*. [49] reviewed all the controlled therapeutic trials addressing the curative or preventive effects of probiotics in acute, paediatric infectious diarrhoea. Analysis of thirteen trials confirmed the therapeutic value of these microorganisms with particularly marked efficacy in rotavirus diarrhoea. Further work will nevertheless be necessary to investigate the usefulness of probiotics in the prevention of gastroenteritis.

Irritable bowel syndrome and dyspepsia

Irritable bowel syndrome (IBS) is defined as chronic gastrointestinal symptoms in the absence of any structural digestive tract abnormality. IBS affects 8-22% of the population as a whole and is more common in women. The etiologies of IBS remains poorly understood. Psychosocial factors, inadequate fibre intake, digestive tract infection, "low grade inflammation", certain forms of food intolerance and impaired gut permeability have all been proposed, but none of these alone can explain the etiology of IBS. Over the last two decades, many studies focused on abnormal motility and then later, on visceral sensitivity. A few studies have shown that the microflora plays an important role in the pathogenesis of IBS with the production of intestinal gas. In a recent study conducted in IBS patients, King *et al*. [50] observed increased colonic fermentation and gas production (methane and hydrogen). In this study, significant improvement in gastrointestinal symptoms and a reduction in excess colonic gas production were observed in patients taking a diet depleted of fermentable substrates. In IBS patients, the faecal microflora often appeared perturbed with increased numbers of certain facultative anaerobes and reduced numbers of lactobacilli and bifidobacteria [51]. However, the efficacy of probiotics on functional symptoms remains debated. In a controlled trial, Maupas *et al*. showed that *Saccharomyces boulardii* could mitigate diarrhoea without any other effect on other functional symptoms [52]. Very recently, Nobaeck *et al*. [53] observed significant improvement in abdominal pain and flatulence in 60 IBS patients who received *Lactobacillus plantarum* for a month.

In contrast, Hentschel *et al*. [54] did not observe any attenuation of symptoms in 126 patients suffering from idiopathic, non-ulcer dyspepsia who were administered a mixture of lactobacilli and *Escherichia coli*.

Inflammatory bowel diseases

Many results indicate that the microflora plays a key role in the pathogenesis of inflammatory bowel diseases (IBD), in particular Crohn's disease (*see chapter entitled* "Influence of the Intestinal Microflora on Host Immunity in Inflammatory Bowel Disease"). Recently, Madsen *et al.* showed that inflammatory lesions caused by certain bacterial components can be attenuated by other organisms, suggesting that probiotics might be useful in the treatment of IBD [55]. These authors studied IL-10 knock-out mice which spontaneously develop colonic ulcers similar to those observed in Crohn's disease. In this study, modification of the microflora was observed two weeks prior to the occurence of the colitis, with increases in both adhesion and bacterial translocation. The concentration of lactobacilli in the lumen decreased, a change which paralleled the development of digestive lesions. Prior administration of lactobacilli *via* the rectal route prevented the colitis. Other authors have obtained similar results by indirectly modulating the density of lactobacilli by administering lactulose, a non absorbed sugar which stimulates the growth of lactobacilli in the colon [56]. Schultz *et al.* [57] also showed that *Lactobacillus plantarum* attenuated the colitis seen in IL-10 knock-out mice. In rats, *Lactobacillus reuteri* R2LC brought about significant improvement in acetic acid-induced colitis whereas *Lactobacillus HLC* had no effect [58]. Wagner *et al.* [59] showed that oral administration of a mixture of four probiotics (*Lactobacillus acidophilus, Lactobacillus* GG, *Lactobacillus reuteri* and *Bifidobacterium animali*) to athymic mice reduced systemic dissemination of *Candida albicans* as well as the rate of mortality due to the infection, suggesting that the product acts on host defence mechanisms against the pathogen. The administration of *Lactobacillus reuteri* R2LC and *Lactobacillus plantarum* DSM 9843 to rats with methotrexate-induced colitis attenuated intestinal permeability, inhibited bacterial translocation and reduced the concentration of endotoxins in the blood [60].

All of these data obtained in animals suggest that the onset of the digestive inflammation that characterizes IBD could be associated with the loss of a protective fraction of the microflora and that therefore, restoring said fraction could be of therapeutic benefit.

In an open study conducted in humans, the administration of *Lactobacillus* GG to 14 children with Crohn's disease increased the number of IgA-producing cells in the gut mucosa, pointing towards interaction between the probiotic and the mucosal immune system [61]. On the other hand, in a recent study, Prantera *et al.* [62] concluded that *Lactobacillus* GG was incapable of preventing clinical and/or endoscopic recurrence in Crohn's disease: the percentage recurrence rate was 16.6% in patients treated with *Lactobacillus* GG and 10.5% in the placebo group (non significant). Of the patients in clinical remission, 60% of those who had received *Lactobacillus* GG presented with an endoscopic relapse compared with 35.2% of those who received the placebo (NS). In a randomised, placebo-controlled trial, Plein & Hotz [63] studied the effect of *Saccharomyces boulardii* on symptoms in patients with stable, relatively inactive Crohn's disease. Twenty patients were given *Saccharomyces boulardii* (or placebo) at a dose of 250 mg/three times a day for seven weeks in addition to conventional modalities to treat IBD. Significant reductions in both the number of bowel movements per day and disease activity index were recorded in those patients who received *Saccharomyces boulardii*. In another recent study, *Saccharomyces boulardii* proved effective at preventing the recurrence of Crohn's disease: relapse was observed in 37.5% of patients treated with mesalazine (3 g/day) compared with 6.25% of patients treated with a combination of mesalazine (2 g/day) and *Saccharomyces boulardii* (1 g/day) [64]. In ulcerative colitis, two studies have compared the efficacy of an oral form of *Escherichia coli* to that of mesalazine on the maintenance of remission [65, 66]: recurrence rates were similar (about 13%) in both the probiotic and mesalazine groups. In patients with ulcerative colitis, the VSL#3 preparation (a combination of several probiotic microorganisms, namely *Lactobacillus* sp., *Bifidobacterium* sp., *Streptococcus salivarius* ssp. *thermophilus*) was recently evaluated in an uncontrolled study [67]; in this study, three-quarters of patients who had been treated for one year remained in remission. In pouchitis too, the VSL#3 preparation has yielded spectacular results. In this condition, there is non-specific inflammation of an ileal reservoir which is made following total colectomy with ileoanal anastomosis performed to manage ulcerative colitis. The cumulative frequency of pouchitis after ten years is about 50%. It may be acute or chronic, with one single episode or recurrence. Its etiology is unknown and is probably multifactorial; nevertheless, the fact that the response to antibiotic treatment is immediate points to the microflora being involved in pathogenesis; pouchitis is associated with a reduction in the ratio of anaerobic to aerobic bacteria as well as decreases in the densities of lactobacilli and bifidobacteria [68]. In a first controlled study, 40 patients with chronic pouchitis in clinical and endoscopic remission following a course of metronidazole were given either VSL#3 or placebo. Over nine months of follow-up, 3 patients on VSL#3 relapsed compared with 100% in the placebo group (p < 0.001). On the active product, the faecal densities of lactobacilli, bifidobacteria and *Streptococcus thermophilus* were significantly higher (p < 0.01) [69]. In a second study, 40 patients with an ileoanal anastomosis for ulcerative colitis were followed up for one year: 2 patients on VSL#3 (10%) developed acute pouchitis compared with 8 (40%) of the placebo patients (p < 0.05) [70].

Helicobacter pylori

In previous work, Bhatia *et al*. [71] suggested that *Lactobacillus acidophilus* could inhibit the growth of *Helicobacter pylori in vitro*.

Canducci *et al.* [72] confirmed this finding in a recent therapeutic trial in which 120 *Helicobacter pylori*-infected patients (Figure 2) were given lyophilised *Lactobacillus acidophilus* or placebo together with conventional treatment modalities (rabeprazole, clarithromycin, amoxicillin).

In this study, the rate of eradication was significantly higher in the *Lactobacillus acidophilus* group than in the placebo group (88% *versus* 72%, p < 0.03). A significant reduction in $^{13}CO_2$ in breath tests with ^{13}C-labelled urea was observed after prolonged daily consumption of *Lactobacillus acidophilus* [73]. However, complete eradication of *Helicobacter pylori* has never been observed with a probiotic alone.

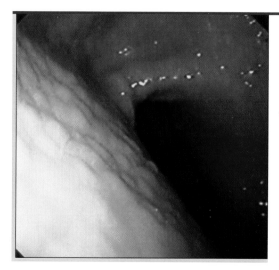

Figure 2.
Helicobacter pylori gastritis:
endoscopic image of nodular antral gastritis
(photograph: A. Bitoun,
Hôpital Lariboisière, Paris.
Traité de Gastro-entérologie, 2000,
J.C. Rambaud, ed. Médecine-Sciences Flammarion)

Colon cancer

The microflora can influence intestinal carcinogenesis (Figure 3) by producing enzymes (glycosidases, β-glucuronidase, azoreductases and nitroreductases) which convert procarcinogenic compounds into active carcinogens. Certain microorganisms of the microflora could have a protective role: in humans, the incidence of colon cancer would be reduced when the microflora is abnormally low in bifidobacteria and rich in anaerobic species such as *Clostridium perfringens* [74]. The beneficial effect of certain probiotics could depend on their capacity to inhibit the bacteria responsible for producing procarcinogenic enzymes and destroy carcinogens such as nitrosamines. Animal studies suggest that certain probiotics could be effective at preventing colon cancer (*for a general review, see* [75]).

In vitro, bifidobacteria inhibit the growth of colonic cell lines. In rats, the ingestion of bifidobacteria reduced the number of colonic tumours induced by dimethylhydrazine or azoxymethane and also inhibited the development of abnormal crypts, cell proliferation and the expression of the oncoprotein p21 encoded by protooncogenes of the *ras* family [76]. In healthy volunteers, Ling *et al.* [77] showed that *Lactobacillus acidophilus* and *Lactobacillus casei* significantly reduced glucuronidase, nitroreductase and azoreductase activities which can convert procarcinogens into carcinogens. In this study, initial enzyme activity was restored ten to thirty days after discontinuation of the probiotics, suggesting that sustained consumption would be required to obtain durable effects. In patients with adenoma of the colon, the ingestion of *Bifidobacterium bifidus* and *Lactobacillus acidophilus* reduces cell proliferation in the upper part of colonic crypts [78]. Interventional studies are now needed to determine the effect of probiotic supplementation on the various stages of colonic carcinogenesis in humans.

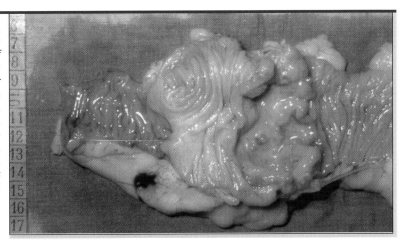

Figure 3.
Ulcerovegetating appearance of anatomical ascending colon cancer (photograph: A. Lavergne-Slove, Hôpital Lariboisière, Paris. Traité de Gastro-entérologie, 2000, J.C. Rambaud, ed. Médecine-Sciences Flammarion)

Disaccharide intolerance

Lactose intolerance is common in people with primary lactase deficiency and in patients who have undergone intestinal resection (secondary deficiency). Many studies have shown that lactase produced by certain lactic bacteria can help digest lactose in the gut, which would explain why the lactose in yogurt is perfectly well digested by lactase-deficient subjects [79, 80]. Arrigoni *et al.* [81] compared the absorption and tolerance of an oral load of 20 grams of lactose administered either in the form of milk or yogurt to patients with short-bowel syndrome. These authors were able to show that the lactose in yogurt is more efficiently absorbed than that in milk. Finally, in young children with congenital saccharase-isomaltase deficiency, it has been shown that tolerance to this disaccharide was enhanced by the regular consumption of *Saccharomyces cerevisiae*, a yeast that produces a saccharase-isomaltase [82].

Microbial overgrowth in the small intestine

Digestive symptoms are often associated with abnormal bacterial proliferation in the small intestine. Therapeutic options are limited to the administration of antibiotics, and responses are often partial and temporary. In a controlled, cross-over study in 10 patients with small intestinal bacterial overgrowth-related diarrhoea, Attar *et al.* [83] showed that norfloxacin (800 mg/day) or amoxicillin (1,500 mg/day) significantly reduced the number of bowel movements per day and the concentration of hydrogen in the breath; no such effect was observed with *Saccharomyces boulardii*. In contrast, Vanderhoof *et al.* [84] showed that both symptoms diarrhoea and bloating in patients with bacterial overgrowth proving refractory to antibiotic treatment could be relieved by administering *Lactobacillus plantarum* and *Lactobacillus* GG, although this was an open study in just 6 children.

Hepatic encephalopathy

The pathogenesis of hepatic encephalopathy remains poorly understood. Neurotoxicity mediated by ammonia produced by gut bacteria is one mechanism proposed. A few old studies showed that the level of urease activity measured in the faeces of subjects with hepatic encephalopathy was lower in patients being treated with a combination of *Lactobacillus acidophilus* and either lactulose or neomycin, compared with those being treated with lactulose or neomycin alone [85, 86]. In these studies, decreased urease activity in the faeces was associated with both a reduction in the blood ammonia concentration and clinical improvement. However, most ammonia comes from the deamination of amino acids.

Preventing allergy

The pathogenesis of food allergy has not been fully elucidated but the gut microflora plays an important role (*see chapter entitled* "Influence of the Intestinal Microflora on Host Immunity: Normal Physiological Conditions"). The commensal microflora mediates mechanisms which protect against allergy: preferential Th1-type responses, the possibility of producing TGF-β which counters the Th2-type responses that predominate in allergic disease and promotes oral tolerance, and finally, sIgA production. At birth, selective colonization of the newborn by an environmental microflora is a major stimulus to establishment of the GALT [87]. The origin of allergy could have its source in complex immune dysfunctions during this period of colonization by the microflora [88]. Probiotics have therefore been evaluated in humans because they are non-toxic, allowing their administration to children and because their immunomodulatory effects have been clearly demonstrated. Majamaa *et al.* [89] evaluated the effect of *Lactobacillus* GG supplementation in young cow's milk intolerant children suffering from atopic dermatitis. In this study, regression of the dermatitis was observed in the children who received *Lactobacillus* GG. More recently, Kalliomäki *et al.* [90] compared the effects of administering *Lactobacillus* GG and placebo to 59 atopic women at the end of pregnancy and then to their neonates for six months: in the newborns, the incidence of atopic dermatitis in the *Lactobacillus* GG group was half that in the placebo group (23% *versus* 46%). The immunomodulatory potential of certain probiotics and their beneficial effects in allergy to animal proteins are supported by the results of very recent randomised, placebo-controlled studies [91, 92].

Conclusion

The great number of articles concerning probiotics reflects the great and increased interest of the medical community to the therapeutic potential of these microorganisms. Over the last ten years, a rigorous scientific methodology for the conduct of therapeutic trials in human subjects has made it possible to show the benefit of certain probiotics in many conditions involving the digestive tract. The best-documented efficacy concerns the use of *Saccharomyces boulardii* to prevent antibiotic-associated diarrhoea and in the treatment of multiply recurrent *Clostridium difficile* infection, and that of the administration of *Lactobacillus* GG or *Bifidobacterium* to decrease the duration of rotaviral gastroenteritis in children. Among therapeutic perspectives, the development of new genetically modified probiotic microorganisms synthetising either cytokines or other therapeutic agents may represent a novel interesting approach for the treatment of IBD [93]. The generation of strains with a targeted biological activity and capable of producing specific compounds makes it possible to imagine new perspectives in the spectrum of activity of probiotics.

Key points

- *Saccharomyces boulardii* is effective in preventing antibiotic-associated diarrhoea and multiple recurrent *Clostridium difficile* infections.

- Certain probiotics can prevent the occurrence of traveller's diarrhoea.

- Probiotic administration in the course of an episode of paediatric rotaviral gastroenteritis reduces duration of the diarrhoea.

- The protective effects of probiotics against intestinal infection are mediated through inhibition of the growth of bacteria in the colon, the production of antibacterial substances, and activation of the gut immune system.

- The beneficial role of probiotics could be applied to many digestive conditions, involving inflammation of the gastrointestinal tract (e.g. IBD and IBS) but also in systemic problems such as allergy and hepatic encephalopathy.

References

1. Collins MD, Gibson GR. Probiotics, prebiotics and symbiotics: approaches for modulating the microbial ecology of the gut. *Am J Clin Nutr* 1999 ; 69 : S1052-7.

2. Bouhnik Y, Pochart P, Marteau P, *et al*. Fecal recovery in man of viable *Bifidobacterium* sp ingested in a fermentable milk. *Gastroenterology* 1992 ;102 : 875-8.

3. Marteau P, Pochart P, Bouhnik Y, *et al*. Fate and effects of some transiting microorganisms in the human gastrointestinal tract. *World Rev Nutr Diet* 1993 ; 74 : 1-21.

4. McFarlane GT, Cummings JH. Probiotics and prebiotics: can regulating the activities of intestinal bacteria benefit health? *Br Med J* 1999 ; 78 : 999-1003.

5. Bengmark S. Pre-, pro- and symbiotics. *Curr Opin Clin Nutr Metab Care* 2001 ; 4 : 571-9.

6. Hatcher GE, Lamprecht RS. Augmentation of macrophage phagocytic activity by cell-free extracts of selected lactic acid-producing bacteria. *J Diary Sci* 1993 ; 76 : 2485-92.

7. Castagliuolo I, LaMont T, Nikulasson ST, *et al*. *Saccharomyces boulardii* protease inhibits *Clostridium difficile* toxin A effects in the rat ileum. *Infect Immun* 1996 ; 64 : 5225-32.

8. Oatley JT, Rarick MD, Ge J, *et al*. Binding of aflatoxin to *Bifidobacteria in vitro*. *J Food Protect* 2000 ; 63 : 1133-6.

9. Bartlett JG. Antibiotic-associated diarrhea. *Clin Infect Dis* 1992 ; 15 : 573-81.

10. McFarland LV, Surawicz CM, Greenberg RN, *et al*. Prevention of beta-lactam associated diarrhea by *Saccharomyces boulardii* compared with placebo. *Am J Gastroenterol* 1995 ; 90 : 439-48.

11. Clausen MR, Bonnen H, Tvede M, *et al*. Colonic fermentation to short chain fatty acids is decreased in antibiotic associated diarrhea. *Gastroenterology* 1991 ; 101 : 1497-504.

12. Benoit R, Dorval D, Loulergue J, *et al*. Post-antibiotic diarrheas: role of *Klebsiella oxytoca*. *Gastroenterol Clin Biol* 1992 ; 16 : 860-4.

13. Soyletir G, Eskiturk A, Kilie G, *et al*. *Clostridium difficile* acquisition rate and its role in nosocomial diarrhoea at a university hospital in Turkey. *Eur J Epidemiol* 1996 ; 12 : 391-4.

14. D'Souza AL, Rajkumar C, Cooke J, *et al*. Probiotics in prevention of antibiotic-associated diarrhoea: meta-analysis. *Br Med J* 2002 ; 324 : 1361-4.

15. Cremonini F, Di Caro S, Nista EC, *et al*. Meta analysis: the effect probiotic administration on antibiotic-associated diarrhoea. *Aliment Pharmacol Ther* 2002 ; 16 : 1461-7.

16. Vanderhoof JA, Whitney DB, Antonson DL, *et al*. *Lactobacillus GG* in the prevention of antibiotic-associated diarrhea in children. *J Pediatr* 1999 ; 135 : 564-8.

17. Thomas MR, Litin SC, Osmon DR, *et al*. Lack of effect of *Lactobacillus GG* on antibiotic-associated diarrhea: a randomised, placebo-controlled trial. *Mayo Clinic Proc* 2001 ; 76 : 883-9.

18. Clements ML, Levine MM, Ristaino PA, *et al*. Exogenous lactobacilli fed to man - their fate and ability to prevent diarrheal disease. *Prog Food Nutr Sci* 1983 ;7 : 29-37.

19. Gotz V, Romankievicz JA, Moss J, *et al*. Prophylaxis against ampicillin-associated diarrhea with a *Lactobacillus* preparation. *Am J Hosp Pharm* 1979 ; 36 : 754-7.

20. Colombel JF, Cortot A, Neut C, *et al*. Yoghurt with *Bifidobacterium longum* reduces erythromycin-induced gastrointestinal effects. *Lancet* 1987 ; 2 : 43.

21. Siitonen S, Vapaatalo H, Salminen S. Effect of *Lactobacillus GG* yoghurt in prevention of antibiotic-associated diarrhoea. *Ann Med* 1990 ; 22 : 57-9.

22. Temmerman R, Pot B, Huys G, *et al*. Identification and antibiotic suceptibility of bacterial isolates from probiotic products. *Int J Food Microbiol* 2000 ; 81 : 1-10.

23. Bergogne-Bérézin E. Place des micro-organismes de substitution dans le contrôle des diarrhées et colites associées aux antibiotiques. *Presse Med* 1995 ; 24 : 145-6.

24. Surawicz CM, Elmer GW, Speelman P, *et al*. Prevention of antibiotic-associated diarrhea by *Saccharomyces boulardii*: a prospective study. *Gastroenterology* 1989 ; 96 : 981-8.

25. McFarland LV, Surawicz CM, Greenberg RN, *et al*. Prevention of beta lactam associated diarrhea by *Saccharomyces boulardii* compared with placebo. *Am J Gastroenterol* 1995 ; 90 : 439-48.

26. Adam J, Barret A, Barret-Bellet C. Essais cliniques contrôlés en double insu de l'Ultralevure lyophilisée : étude multicentrique par 25 médecins de 388 cas. *Méd Chir Dig* 1976 ; 5 : 401-5.

27. Lewis SJ, Potts LF, Barry RE. The lack of therapeutic effect of *Saccharomyces boulardii* in the prevention of antibiotic associated diarrhea. *J Infect* 1998 ; 36 : 171-4.

28. Beaugerie L, Flahault A, Barbut F, *et al*. Antibiotic-associated diarrhoea and *Clostridium difficile* in the community. *Aliment Pharmacol Ther* 2003 ; 17 : 905-12.

29. Wenisch C, Parschalk B, Hasenhundl M, *et al*. Comparison of vancomycin, teicoplanin, metronidazole, and fusidic acid for the treatment of *Clostridium difficile*-associated diarrhea. *Clin Infect Dis* 1996 ; 22 : 813-8.

30. Buts JP, Corthier G, Delmée M. *Saccharomyces boulardii* for *Clostridium difficile* associated enteropathies in infants. *J Pediatr Gastroenterol Nutr* 1993 ; 16 : 419-25.

31. Gorbach SL, Chang TW, Goldin B. Successful treatment of relapsing *Clostridium difficile* colitis with *Lactobacillus GG*. *Lancet* 1987 ; 2 : 1519.

32. Levy J. Experience with live *Lactobacillus plantarum* 299v: a promising adjunct in the management of recurrent *Clostridium difficile* infection. *Gastroenterology* 1997 ; 112 : A379.

33. McFarland LV, Suravwicz CM, Greenberg RN, *et al*. A randomized placebo-controlled trial of *Saccharomyces boulardii* in combination with standard antibiotics for *Clostridium difficile* disease. *J Am Med Assoc* 1994 ; 271 : 1913-8.

34. Czerucka D, Rampal P. Experimental effects of *Saccharomyces boulardii* on diarrheal pathogens. *Microb Infect* 2002 ; 4 : 733-9.

35. Black FT, Anderson PL, Orskov J, *et al*. Prophylactic efficacy of lactobacilli on traveller's diarrhea. *J Travel Med* 1989 ; 7 : 333-5.

36. Oksaken PJ, Salminen S, Saxelin M, *et al*. Prevention of travellers' diarrhoea by *Lactobacillus GG*. *Ann Med* 1990 ; 22 : 53-6.

37. Hilton E, Kolakowski P, Singer C, *et al*. Efficacy of *Lactobacillus* GG as a diarrheal preventive in travelers. *J Travel Med* 1997 ; 4 : 41-3.

38. Kollaritsch H, Holst H, Grobara P, *et al*. Prophylaxe der reisediarrhöe mit *Saccharomyces boulardii*. *Forst Chr Med* 1993 ; 111 : 152-6.

39. Pozo-Olano JD, Warram JH, Gomez RG, *et al*. Effect of a lactobacilli preparation on traveller's diarrhea. A randomized, double blind clinical trial. *Gastroenterology* 1978 ; 74 : 829-30.

40. Katelaris PH, Salam I, Farthing MJ. Lactobacilli to prevent traveller's diarrhea? *N Engl J Med* 1995 ; 333 : 1360-1.

41. Clements ML, Levine MM, Black RE, *et al*. *Lactobacillus* prophylaxis for diarrhea due to enterotoxinogenic *Escherichia coli*. *Antimicrob Agents Chemother* 1981 ; 20 : 104-8.

42. Oberhelman RA, Gilman RH, Sheen P, *et al*. A placebo-controlled trial of *Lactobacillus* GG to prevent diarrhea in undernourished peruvian children. *J Pediatr* 1999 ; 134 : 15-20.

43. Saavedra JM, Bauman NA, Oung I, *et al*. Feeding of *Bifidobacterium bifidum* and *Streptococcus thermophilus* to infants in hospital for prevention of diarrhea and shedding of rotavirus. *Lancet* 1994 ; 344 : 1046-9.

44. Szajewska H, Kotowska M, Mrukowicz JZ, *et al*. Efficacy of *Lactobacillus* GG in prevention of nosocomial diarrhea in infants. *J Pediatr* 2001 ; 138 : 361-5.

45. Isolauri E, Juntunen M, Rautanen T, Sillanaukee P, Kolvula T. A human *Lactobacillus* strain (*Lactobacillus casei* sp GG) promotes recovery from acute diarrhea in children. *Pediatrics* 1991 ; 88 : 90-7.

46. Guandalini S, Pensabene L, Zikri MA, *et al*. *Lactobacillus* GG administered in oral rehydration solution to children with acute diarrhea: a multicenter European study. *J Pediatr Gastr Nutr* 2000 ; 30 : 54-60.

47. Cetina-Sauri G, Sierra Basto G. Évaluation thérapeutique de *Saccharomyces boulardii* chez des enfants souffrant de diarrhée aiguë. *Ann Pediatr* 1994 ; 41 : 397-400.

48. Höchter W, Chase D, Hagenhoff G. *Saccharomyces boulardii* in treatment of acute adult diarrhea. Efficacy and tolerance of treatment. *Münchener Medizinische Wochenschrift* 1990 ; 132(12) : 188-92.

49. Szajewska H, Mrukowicz JZ. Probiotics in the treatment and prevention of acute infectious diarrhea in infants and children: a systematic review of published randomized, double blind, placebo-controlled trials. *J Pediatr Gastroenterol Nutr* 2001 ; 33 : S17-25.

50. King TS, Elia M, Hunter JO. Abnormal colonic fermentation in irritable bowel syndrome. *Lancet* 1998 ; 10 : 1187-9.

51. Hunter JO, Madden JA, Hunter JO. A review of the role of the gut microflora in irritable bowel syndrome and the effects of probiotics. *Br J Nutr* 2002 ; 88 : 67-72.

52. Maupas JL, Champemont P, Delforge M. Traitement des colopathies fonctionnelles. Essai en double aveugle de l'ultra-levure. (Treatment of irritable bowel syndrome with *Saccharomyces boulardii* - a double blind, placebo controlled study.). *Méd Chir Dig* 1983 ; 12 : 77-9.

53. Nobaeck S, Johansson ML, Molin G, *et al*. Alteration of intestinal microflora is associated with reduction in abdominal bloating and pain in patients with irritable bowel syjndrome. *Am J Gastroenterol* 2000 ; 95 : 1231-8.

54. Hentschel C, Bauer J, Dill N. Complementary medicine in non-ulcer dyspepsia: is alternative medicine a real alternative? A randomized placebo-controlled double-blind clinical trial with two probiotic agents-Hylac, and Hylac, forte. *Gastroenterology* 1997 ; 112 : A146.

55. Madsen KL, Doyle JS, Jewell LD, *et al*. *Lactobacillus* species prevents colitis in interleukin 10 gene deficient mice. *Gastroenterology* 1999 ; 116 : 1107-14.

56. Gibson GR, Roberfroid MB. Dietary modulation of the human colonic microbiota: introducing the concept of prebiotics. *J Nutr* 1995 ; 125 : 1401-12.

57. Schultz M, Veltkamp C, Dieleman LA, *et al*. Continuous feeding of *Lactobacillus plantarum* attenuates established colitis in interleukin-10 deficient mice. *Gastroenterology* 1998 ; 114 : A1081.

58. Fabia R, Ar'Rajab A, Johansson ML, *et al*. The effect of exogenous administration of *Lactobacillus reuteri* R2LC and oat fiber on acetic acid-induced colitis in the rat. *Scand J Gastroenterol* 1993 ; 28 : 155-62.

59. Wagner ED, Warner T, Roberts L, *et al*. Colonization of congenitally immunodeficient mice with probiotic bacteria. *Infect Immun* 1997 ; 65 : 3345-51.

60. Mao Y, Nobaeck S, Kasravi B, *et al*. The effects of *Lactobacillus* strains and oat fiber on methotrexate-induced enterocolitis in rats. *Gastroenterology* 1996 ; 111 : 334-44.

61. Malin M, Suolmalainen H, Saxelin M, *et al*. Promotion of IgA immune response in patients with Crohn's disease by oral bacteriotherapy with *Lactobacillus* GG. *Ann Nutr Metab* 1996 ; 40 : 137-45.

62. Prantera C, Scribano ML, Falasco G, *et al*. Ineffectiveness of probiotics in preventing reccurence after curative resction for Crohn's disease: a randomised controlled trial with *Lactobacillus* GG. *Gut* 2002 ; 51 : 405-9.

63. Plein K, Hotz J. Therapeutic effects of *Saccharomyces boulardii* on mild residual symptoms in stable phase of Crohn's disease with special respect to chronic diarrhea - a pilot study. *Z Gastroenterol* 1993 ; 31 : 129-34.

64. Guslandi M, Mezzi G, Sorghi M, *et al*. *Saccharomyces boulardii* in maintenance treatment of Crohn's disease. *Dig Dis Sci* 2000 ; 45 : 1462-4.

65. Kruis W, Schütz E, Fric P, *et al*. Double blind comparison of an oral *Escherishia coli* preparation and mesalazine in maintening remission of ulcerative colitis. *Aliment Pharmacol Ther* 1997 ; 11 : 853-8.

66. Rembacken BJ, Snelling AM, Hawkey PM, *et al*. Non-pathogenic *Escherichia coli versus* mesalazine for the treatment of ulcerative colitis: a randomized trial. *Lancet* 1999 ; 354 : 635-9.

67. Venturi A, Gionchetti P, Rizello F, *et al*. Impact on the composition of the faecal flora by a new probiotic preparation: preliminary data on maintenance treatment of patients with ulcerative colitis. *Aliment Pharmacol Ther* 1999 ; 13 : 1103-8.

68. Ruseler-Van-Embden JGH, Schouten WR, van Lieshaut LMC. Pouchitis: result of microbial imbalance? *Gut* 1994 ; 35 : 658-64.

69. Gionchetti P, Rizello F, Venturi A, *et al*. Oral bacteriotherapy as maintenance treatment in patients with chronic pouchitis: a double blind, placebo-controlled trial. *Gastroenterology* 2000 ; 119 : 305-9.

70. Gionchetti P, Rizello F, Helwig U, *et al*. Prophylaxis of pouchitis ouset with probiotic therapy: a double blind, placebo-controlled trial. *Gastroenterology* 2003 ; 124 : 1202-9.

71. Bhatia SJ, Kochar N, Abraham P. *Lactobacillus acidophilus* inhibits growth of *Campylobacter pylori in vitro*. *J Clin Microbiol* 1989 ; 27 : 2328-30.

72. Canducci F, Armuzzi A, Cremonini F, *et al*. A lyophilised and inactivated culture of *Lactobacillus acidophilus* increases *Helicobacter pylori* eradication rates. *Aliment Pharmacol Ther* 2000 ; 14 : 1625-9.

73. Michetti P, Dorta G, Wiesel PH, *et al*. Effect of whey based culture supernatant of *Lactobacillus acidophilus* (jonsonii) La1 on *Helicobacter pylori* infections in humans. *Digestion* 1999 ; 60 : 203-9.

74. Kubota Y. Fecal intestinal flora in patients with colon adenoma and colon cancer. *Nippon Shoh Gakkai Zasshi* 1990 ; 87 : 771-9.

75. Burns AJ, Rowland IR. Anti-carcinogenicity of probiotics and prebiotics. *Curr Issues Intest Microbiol* 2000 ; 1 : 13-24.

76. Singh J, Rivenson A, Tomita M, *et al*. *Bifidobacterium longum*, a lactic acid-producing intestinal bacterium inhibits colon cancer and modulates the intermediate biomarkers of colon carcinogenesis. *Carcinogenesis* 1997 ;18 : 833-41.

77. Ling WH, Korpela R, Mykkänen H, *et al*. *Lactobacillus* strain GG supplementation decreases colonic hydrolytic reductive enzyme activities in healthy female adults. *J Nutr* 1994 ; 124 : 18-23.

78. Biasco G. Effect of *Lactobacillus acidophilus* and *Bifidobacterium bifidum* on rectal cell kinetics and fecal pH. *Ital J Gastroenterol* 1991 ; 23 : 142-6.

79. Marteau P, Flourié B, Pochart P, *et al*. Effect of the microbial lactase activity in yogurt on the intestinal absorption of lactose: an *in vivo* study in lactase-deficient humans. *Br J Nutr* 1990 ; 64 : 71-9.

80. de Vrese M, Stegelmann A, Richter B, *et al*. Probiotics-compensation for lactase insufficiency. *Am J Clin Nutr* 2001 ; 73 : 421S-9S.

81. Arrigoni E, Marteau P, Briet F, *et al*. Tolerance and absorption of lactose from milk and yogurt during short-bowel syndrome inn humans. *Am J Clin Nutr* 1994 ; 60 : 926-9.

82. Harms HK, Bertele-Harms RM, Bruer-Kleis D. Enzyme substitution therapy with the yeast *Saccharomyces cerevisiae* in congenital sucrase-isomaltase deficiency. *N Engl J Med* 1987 ; 316 : 13-6.

83. Attar A, Flourie B, Rambaud JC, *et al*. Antibiotic efficacy in small intestinal bacterial overgrowth-related chronic diarrhea: a crossover, randomized trial. *Gastroenterology* 1999 ; 117 : 794-7.

84. Vanderhoof JA, Young RJ, Murray N, *et al*. Treatment strategies for small bowel bacterial overgrowth in short bowel syndrome. *J Pediatr Gastroenterol Nutr* 1998 ; 27 : 155-60.

85. Loguercio C, Del Vecchio Blanco C, Coltorti M. *Enterococcus* lactic acid bacteria strain SF68 and lactulose in hepatic encephalopathy: a controlled study. *J Int Med Res* 1987 ; 15 : 335-43.

86. Scevola D, Zambelli A, Concia E, *et al*. Lactitol and neomycin: monotherapy or combined therapy in the prevention and treatment of hepatic encephalopathy. *J Clin Ther* 1989 ; 129 : 105-11.

87. Corthier G, Doré J. La flore intestinale. In : Rampal P, Beaugerie L, Marteau P, Corthier G eds. *Colites infectieuses de l'adulte*. Paris : John Libbey Eurotext, 2000 : 3-25.

88. Lessof M. Food intolerance. *Scand J Gastroenterol* 1985 ; 20 : 117-21.

89. Majamaa H, Isolauri E. Probiotics: a novel approach in the management of food allergy. *J Allergy Clin Immunol* 1997 ; 99 : 179-85.

90. Kalliomäki M, Salminen S, Arvilommi H, *et al*. Probiotics in primary prevention of atopic disease: a randomised placebo-controlled trial. *Lancet* 2001 ; 357 : 1076-9.

91. Pelto L, Isolauri E, Liluis EM, *et al*. Probiotic bacteria down-regulate the milk-induced inflammatory response in milk-hypersensitive subjects but have an immunostimulatory effect in healthy subjects. *Clin Exp Allergy* 1998 ; 28 : 1474-9.

92. Pessi T, Sutas Y, Hurme M, *et al*. Interleukin-10 generation in atopic children following oral *Lactobacillus rhamnosus* GG. *Clin Exp Allergy* 2000 ; 30 : 1804-8.

93. Steidler L, Hans W, Schotte L, *et al*. Treatment of murine colitis by *Lactococcus lactis* secreting interleukin-10. *Science* 2000 ; 289 : 1352-5.

Example of a Medicinal Probiotic: Lyophilised *Saccharomyces boulardii*

Jean-Paul Buts

Université Catholique
de Louvain,
Pédiatrie Générale et
Unité de Gastro-entérologie
Pédiatrique,
Cliniques Universitaires
Saint Luc,
Bruxelles, Belgique

Saccharomyces boulardii is a naturally-occurring yeast which has not been genetically modified. It was first isolated from the skin of lychees grown in Indochina and has an unusually high optimal growth temperature of around 37 °C.

Saccharomyces boulardii is a close but distinct relative of *Saccharomyces cerevisiae*, differing in various taxonomic, metabolic and genetic characteristics [1, 2].

In its lyophilised form, *Saccharomyces boulardii* constitutes the active substance which is available in nearly one hundred countries throughout the world under various brand names and in different presentations and dosages. Lyophilised *Saccharomyces boulardii* is an example of what is referred to as a "probiotic medicinal product":

- "probiotic" because, following oral administration, lyophilised *Saccharomyces boulardii* survives in the digestive tract and "mediates positive effects on the host's health and physiology" [3, 4]. Instead of the word "probiotic", some authors prefer the term "biotherapeutic agent" to distinguish those probiotic microorganisms which are "used to prevent or treat human diseases" [5, 6];

- "medicinal product" because the lyophilised form is prepared, packaged and checked as such, and because the pharmaceutical and clinical files for lyophilised *Saccharomyces boulardii* are subject to the rules pertaining to Marketing Authorization in those countries in which the product is available.

Therefore, lyophilised *Saccharomyces boulardii* is clearly distinct from dietary probiotic products which contain diverse strains of microorganisms and are used in animals to improve zootechnical yields, or in healthy humans (often in the form of yogurt or other dairy products) to strengthen host physiology in the absence of any pathological context.

Presentation and pharmacokinetics

Lyophilised *Saccharomyces boulardii* is produced by freeze-drying in the presence of lactose, a method which preserves the yeast's viability and stability. Analysis of the pharmacodynamic properties of *Saccharomyces boulardii* has shown that its activities are largely dependent upon its ability to survive. As with all yeasts, *Saccharomyces boulardii* is naturally resistant to antibacterial antibiotics: its MIC for almost all antibiotics investigated is very high (over 128 mg/L) [7].

Saccharomyces boulardii is resistant to gastric acidity and to proteolysis, so that it can reach very rapidly high concentrations in the gastrointestinal tract and then persist there at a constant level in viable form [6] (Figure 1).

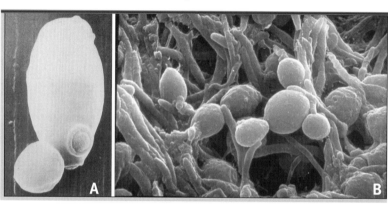

Figure 1.
Saccharomyces boulardii
(micrographs:
M. Bastide, Montpellier).
A: cells visualised
by scanning electron
microscopy
B: murine caecum
three hours after
the administration of
Saccharomyces boulardii

After the administration of a single dose of *Saccharomyces boulardii* to axenic (germ-free) animals, yeast cells establish and persists in the digestive tract at concentrations (5 x 10^7 cells per gram of faeces) which are nevertheless below those of the resident microorganisms of the dominant microflora (10^9-10^{10}), showing that this yeast is able to adapt to the physicochemical conditions of the gut. In contrast, in holoxenic animals (with a normal microflora), *Saccharomyces boulardii* is eliminated rapidly—within a few days. Thus, in the presence of the normal microflora, *Saccharomyces boulardii* fails to establish in the digestive tract [8]. Analysis of the kinetics of the faecal clearance of viable *Saccharomyces boulardii* in healthy adult subjects taking the lyophilisate on a regular basis (± 4 x 10^{10} viable *Saccharomyces boulardii* cells) [9] showed that an equilibrium state of about 10^8 cells per day is reached by the third day of administration. *Saccharomyces boulardii* rapidly disappears from the faeces two to five days after treatment has been stopped. The fraction of ingested cells recovered alive in the faeces has been estimated to be between 0.2-0.4% in both rats [10] and humans [11] with a linear dose/recovery relationship. This ratio is more than doubled when the subjects were concomitantly taking an antibiotic (ampicillin) active against the dominant anaerobic microflora in the colon [11]. A clinical study conducted in patients with multiply recurrent *Clostridium difficile* infection and treated with *Saccharomyces boulardii* at a dose of 1 gram per day showed that the average faecal density of viable yeast cells in patients without any subsequent relapse was higher (1 x 10^6 cells per gram) than that observed in patients who relapsed (2.5 x 10^4/g, p = 0.02). Therefore, there is a significant correlation between the concentration of *Saccharomyces boulardii* in the faeces and the product's therapeutic activity [12].

Pharmacodynamic properties

Table I lists the main mechanisms of action of *Saccharomyces boulardii*. In the course of its transit through the digestive tract, *Saccharomyces boulardii* mediates pharmacodynamic effects which resemble the physiological effects of a balanced gut microflora.

Table I. Mechanisms of action of *Saccharomyces boulardii*	Mechanism	Response
	• Production of antimicrobial substances	Not known
	• Interactions with the microflora	Yes
	• Inactivation of bacterial toxins or their binding sites for receptors	Yes
	• Antisecretory effects	Yes
	• Stimulation of the immune system	Yes
	• Inhibition of the enterotoxin-induced inflammatory response	Yes
	• Trophic effects for the mucosa	Yes

Effects of *Saccharomyces boulardii* in experimental gut infections

The effects of the oral administration of *Saccharomyces boulardii* have been evaluated in several models of intestinal infection and/or intestinal colonization by various microorganisms.

Clostridium difficile

The administration of *Saccharomyces boulardii* significantly reduced mortality due to *Clostridium difficile* colitis in clindamycin-treated hamsters [13] as well as in mice which were given either *Clostridium difficile* [14] or, more directly, the bacterial toxins A and B [15] (Figure 2).

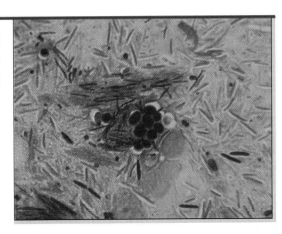

Figure 2.
Gut microflora in a healthy, Saccharomyces boulardii-treated hamster: mucus sampled in the caecum (x 1,000) (micrograph: BCX)

The absence of damage to the intestinal mucosa in animals protected by *Saccharomyces boulardii* was established by both optical [16] and electron [17, 18] microscopy, and was confirmed in an *in vitro* rat intestinal epithelial cell model (IRD 98) [19]. The protective effect against *Clostridium difficile* enterotoxigenicity is more marked if *Saccharomyces boulardii* is taken prophylactically and continuously [13, 14, 20]. It disappears when yeast cells are killed by heating or by treatment with amphotericin B, and is linearly dependent on both the dose administered and the degree of viability of the *Saccharomyces boulardii* [20]. The protective effect is correlated with a drop in the concentration of *Clostridium difficile* in some cases [21], and in all cases with a reduction in the concentration of toxin A and/or toxin B [14, 17, 20, 21]. Moreover, Elmer & Corthier have observed a significant correlation between the rate of survival of *Clostridium difficile*-infected mice and the oral dose of *Saccharomyces boulardii* administered. When the dose of *Saccharomyces boulardii* was increased from 3×10^8 to 3.3×10^{10} cells per millilitre in the drinking water of infected animals, the survival rate rose in a linear fashion from 0 to 85% [20].

The protective action of *Saccharomyces boulardii* against *Clostridium difficile* infection of the gut results from the complementary effects of several different mechanisms (Figure 3):

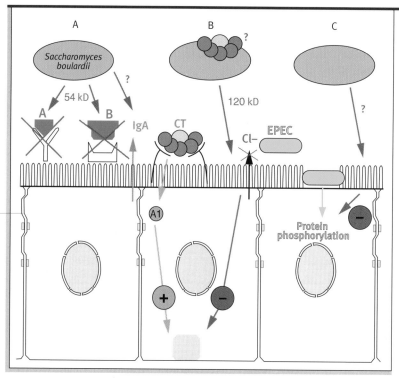

Figure 3.
Saccharomyces boulardii-mediated protective mechanisms against Clostridium difficile, Vibrio cholerae and enteropathogenic Escherichia coli (EPEC) (taken from [22])
A: Saccharomyces boulardii secretes a 54 kD protease which breaks down Clostridium difficile toxins A and B and their receptors.
B: Saccharomyces boulardii secretes a 120 kD protein which mediates effects at the intestinal mucosa, inhibits the stimulation of adenylate cyclase (AC) by cholera toxin (CT), and inhibits chloride secretion.
C: Saccharomyces boulardii mediates activities at the gut mucosa and inhibits EPEC-induced protein phosphorylation. The question mark indicates that the "effector" of this activity (which is released by Saccharomyces boulardii) is as yet unidentified.

- *in vivo*, secretion by the yeast of a 54 kD protease which inhibits the enterotoxic and cytotoxic effects of *Clostridium difficile* toxins A and B. The intestinal receptor for *Clostridium difficile* toxin A is a protease-sensitive, high molecular weight glycoprotein. Pothoulakis *et al.* [23, 24] have shown that, *in vivo*, *Saccharomyces boulardii* produces a protease with a molecular weight of 54 kD which inhibits water and electrolyte secretion in a rabbit isolated loop model. By contrast, this protease has no effect on the cellular lesions induced by *Clostridium difficile* in non-intestinal cell lines such as human lung fibroblasts (IMR-90) or a rat basophilic leukaemia cell line (RBL). This protease inhibits the binding of purified [H^3]-enterotoxin A to the membranes of intestinal villi by a factor of 37%, reduces enterotoxin A-induced water and electrolyte secretion by 55% in rats, and reduces intestinal permeability to mannitol by 93%. Moreover, after oral administration of *Saccharomyces boulardii* to rats for three days, enterotoxin A administered orally no longer had any stimulatory effect on either secretion or intestinal permeability. Castagliuolo *et al.* [24, 25] confirmed that the partially purified protease could directly and specifically attack toxin A and destroy at least part of its binding site on the membranes of intestinal villi, thereby inhibiting the binding of toxins A and B to their receptors (Figure 4);

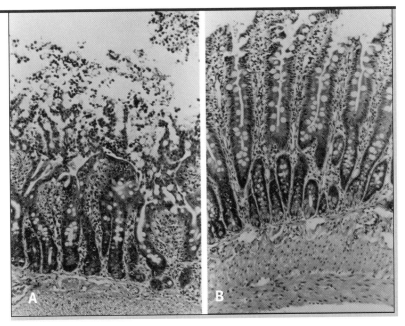

Figure 4.
Inhibition of the enteritis due to Clostridium difficile toxin A by the Saccharomyces boulardii protease. A dose of five milligrams of either toxin A or toxin A that had been pre-treated with the Saccharomyces boulardii protease was injected into rat ileal loops. After four hours of exposure, the animals were sacrificed, the ileal loops were fixed in formaldehyde, and sections were stained using haematoxylin & eosin.
A: in the loop exposed to toxin A, note the presence of necrotic villi and neutrophil infiltration of the lamina propria.
B: in the loop exposed to toxin A that had been pre-treated with the Saccharomyces boulardii protease, note complete absence of lesions [24]

- stimulation of the immune response against toxin A: in mice inoculated orally with a toxoid derived from toxin A, the administration of *Saccharomyces boulardii* induced a strong amplification of the specific immune response as measured by the blood levels of specific secretory IgA and IgM directed against toxin A [26];
- finally, inhibition by *Saccharomyces boulardii* of the adhesion of *Clostridium difficile* to intestinal cells has been demonstrated in an *in vitro* cell culture model [27].

Vibrio cholerae

In an *in vivo* model of ligated jejunal loop in the rat, the administration of *Saccharomyces boulardii* significantly reduced hypersecretion of water and sodium induced by the prior inoculation of cholera toxin [28].

This inhibitory effect was confirmed *in vitro* using models of rat intestinal epithelial cells, such as IRD 98, IEC 17 [29] and IEC 6 [30]. The effect of *Saccharomyces boulardii* was associated with a significant reduction of 50% in the amount of cAMP induced by the cholera toxin. This effect was abolished if the yeast cells had been killed by heating. A culture of supernatant of *Saccharomyces boulardii* (conditioned medium, CM) was able by itself to reduce in a dose-dependent fashion the levels of cAMP induced by cholera toxin in IEC 6 cells; this effect disappeared if the medium was denatured by heat, hydrolysed with trypsin or treated with trichloroacetic acid, pointing to the presence of a proteinic factor; after polyacrylamide gel separation and elution, a signal was identified by autoradiography as a 120 kD protein [30]. In addition, CM did not change the binding of iodinated cholera toxin to its receptor [29] and did not have any proteolytic activity on the cholera toxin [30]. These observations led Czerucka *et al.* [31] to investigate the effects of the CM of *Saccharomyces boulardii* on signal transduction pathways which might be involved in chloride secretion.

The effect of the CM on chloride transport was studied in the cell line T84 which is derived from a human carcinoma. This line has the characteristics of chloride-secreting crypt cells, expressing the Na^+, $K^+ATPase$ pump, the $Na^+/K^+/Cl^-$ co-transporter and the K^+ channel on the basolateral membrane, and the Cl^- channel on the apical membrane. All the exchangers participate to the secretion of chloride induced by agonists which act through cAMP, e.g. forskolin, vasoactive intestinal polypeptide (VIP) and the prostaglandins (PGE)—or through Ca^{2+}, e.g. carbachol [32]. Chloride secretion was measured sixty minutes after exposure of the cells to cholera toxin using the method of Venglarik *et al.* [33].

In the presence of *Saccharomyces boulardii* CM, the increase in chloride secretion and cAMP in T84 cells induced by cholera toxin was reduced to the levels seen in controls. In addition, *Saccharomyces boulardii* CM reduced chloride secretion induced by VIP or PGE_2, but only if the cells had been pretreated for sixty minutes prior to incubation with the agonists: this phenomenon correlates with a reduction in cAMP levels [31].

One hour of pretreatment with *Saccharomyces boulardii* CM was also necessary to reduce carbachol-induced chloride secretion, although this did not affect the intracellular level of inositol-tri-phosphatase. It appears therefore that, in T84 cells, *Saccharomyces boulardii* CM generates a cellular effector which uncouples ion channels from the intracellular Ca^{2+} concentration.

In summary, these studies show that *Saccharomyces boulardii* secretes a 120 kD protein which acts directly on enterocytes and induces a signal transduction pathway involved in regulating Cl^- secretion (Figure 3).

Escherichia coli

In a model of baby mice in which diarrhoea is induced by the heat-stable enterotoxin of enterotoxigenic *Escherichia coli* (ETEC), the simultaneous administration of a suspension of *Saccharomyces boulardii* significantly inhibited intestinal hypersecretion of water and electrolytes [34].

Enteropathogenic *Escherichia coli* (EPEC) is the most common type of bacterium implicated in paediatric diarrhoea, especially in developing countries. Enterohaemorrhagic *Escherichia coli* (EHEC) strains cause food poisoning in industrialized countries (the United States, Canada and Japan), and also hemorrhagic colitis, sometimes associated with a syndrome combining haemolysis and uraemia [35]. These bacteria produce a "Shiga-like toxin" which inhibits protein synthesis in intestinal cells but which does not seem to be involved in EHEC intestinal disease. EPEC and EHEC pathologies begin with attachment of the bacteria to the intestinal mucosa which induces morphological changes in cells of the host, including destruction of the microvilli and formation of so-called "attaching-and-effacing" lesions in which actin filaments build up to form a "pedestal" under the bacterial attachment site [35]. One of the consequences of these changes is the disruption of the tight junctions leading to loss of enterocyte-dependent barrier functions [36]. These infections are associated with migration of polymorphonuclear cells and synthesis of pro-inflammatory cytokines (IL-8) [37]. Some cellular responses to infection have been correlated with an activation through phosphorylation of cellular signalling proteins. For instance, phosphorylation of the myosin light chain (MLC) has been directly implicated in the disruption of tight junctions in EPEC infection [38].

The presence of *Saccharomyces boulardii* during the infection of T84 by an EPEC which produces the "Shiga-like toxin" (strain EDL 931) restores barrier function (measured by transepithelial resistance, diffusion of inulin and immunohistological staining for the ZO-1 protein) (Figure 5). Moreover, study of the cleavage of caspase 32 shows that the yeast is able to delay the process of apoptosis (or programmed cell death) induced by infection of T84 cells by EPEC. The yeast has no effect on the numbers of EPEC or EHEC cells which adhere to the enterocytes, although it inhibits the phosphorylation of certain proteins which are normally phosphorylated in response to infection [39, 40].

Thus, infection of T84 cells by EPEC or EHEC leads to the activation of three intracellular pathways involving MAP (mitogen activating protein) kinases: extra-cellular-regulating protein kinases 1 and 2 (ERK-1 and ERK-2), p38 MAP kinase and JUN-kinase. Activation of these kinases does not seem to be involved in either the "attaching-and-effacing" phenomenon or changes at intercellular tight junctions [41, 42].

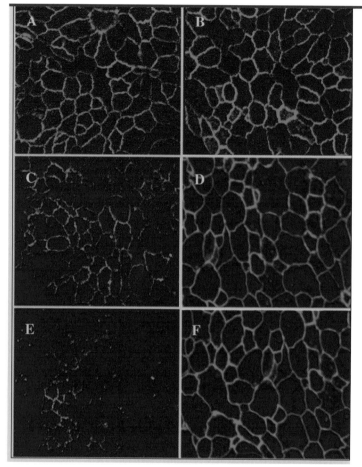

Figure 5.
Immunolocalization of the ZO-1 protein (associated with tight junctions) in T84 cells. Figures A and B show the normal distibution of the ZO-1 protein in uninfected cells (A) and cells exposed to Saccharomyces boulardii (B). The ZO-1 protein disappears in EPEC-infected cells over 6 hours (C) or 9 hours (E). Distribution of the ZO-1 protein is not changed when the EPEC infection is carried out in the presence of Saccharomyces boulardii (D, F) [39]

By contrast, activation of ERK 1,2 is directly linked to bacterial infection. The presence of *Saccharomyces boulardii* reduces the number of infected cells and also modulates phosphorylation of ERK-1 and 2 [41] (Figure 6). Under normal physiological situation, activation of ERK-1 and 2 through a double phosphorylation is involved in the processes of growth and cellular differentiation in response to trophic factors such as insulin and IGF-1.

A double phosphorylation of p38 MAP kinase is involved in the phenomenon of apoptosis. In the course of infection with invasive bacteria such as *Salmonella typhimurium* [43] and *Listeria monocytogenes* [44], it has been suggested that the intracellular MAP kinase signalling pathways are involved in the invasive process and cytokine synthesis. Czerucka *et al.* [41,

42] showed that the MAP kinase pathways stimulated by infection with EPEC and EHEC, as well as the NFκB pathway induced by EHEC, are involved in IL-8 synthesis. *Saccharomyces boulardii* inhibits these pathways as well as the synthesis of IL-8 during infection with these bacteria [40].

In addition, *Saccharomyces boulardii* prevents EHEC-induced apoptosis and inhibits the synthesis of TNFα (Figure 6).

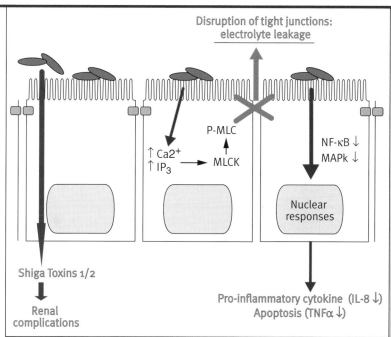

Figure 6. Activities mediated by Saccharomyces boulardii during enterohaemorrhagic Escherichia coli (EHEC) infection.
• *Saccharomyces boulardii inhibits EHEC-dependent phosphorylation of the myosin light chain (MLC), thereby preventing disruption of the tight junctions and reducing electrolyte leakage.*
• *Saccharomyces boulardii inhibits phosphorylation of the MAP kinases (ERK 1/2, p38 and JNK), as well as activation of NFκB, thereby reducing synthesis of the pro-inflammatory cytokine IL-8.*
• *Saccharomyces boulardii inhibits EHEC-induced apoptosis and reduces TNFα synthesis*

Other enteropathogenic bacteria

The administration of a single dose of 10 milligrams of *Saccharomyces boulardii* to gnotoxenic mice inoculated orally with a suspension of *Shigella flexneri* or *Salmonella typhimurium* reduces the mortality (*Shigella flexneri*) or the severity of the intestinal lesions (*Salmonella typhimurium*) induced by these enteropathogenic agents [45]. This protective effect is not linked to a reduction in the degree of intestinal overgrowth of these bacteria.

Effects of *Saccharomyces boulardii* in the intestinal tract

Trophic effects

The oral administration of *Saccharomyces boulardii* to healthy adult volunteers for eight days had no effect on intestinal morphology (conventional histology), neither on the height of villi nor on the depth of crypts. Similarly, electron microscopy of the intestinal epithelial cells of rats treated with *Saccharomyces boulardii* showed no intracellular translocation of the yeast, nor any morphological deterioration of the microvilli, the villi or the crypts [46]. Using a three-dimensional method of microdensification of human biopsies, Jahn *et al.* [47] confirmed that, after oral *Saccharomyces boulardii* treatment, there was no significant difference in the surface of the villi or the depth of the crypts. In a study conducted in humans and rats, Buts *et al.* [46] showed that, compared with baseline observations, biopsies from human volunteers presented significant increases in specific and total activities of sucrase-isomaltase (+82%), lactase (+77%) and maltase (+75%) after eight days of treatment. Similarly, in thirty-day-old rats weaned and treated for fourteen days with *Saccharomyces boulardii*, specific and total activities of sucrase-isomaltase, maltase and lactase were significantly higher than in control, placebo-treated rats.

In a study conducted in healthy adult volunteers, Jahn *et al.* [47] used an *in situ* method to measure enzyme activities in microvilli on frozen sections of intestinal biopsies. After treatment with *Saccharomyces boulardii*, significant increases were observed in the activities of lactase, α-glucosidase and alkaline phosphatase of +22% to +55% over baseline levels as measured before treatment. From these studies, results show that, in both humans and rats, *Saccharomyces boulardii* stimulates the expression of disaccharidases and alkaline phosphatase, microvillous enzymes which are involved in nutrient digestion and which are often perturbed in acute and chronic enteropathies. In the lumen, *Saccharomyces boulardii* secretes a sucrase at such levels that this probiotic is effective in the treatment of congenital sucrase-isomaltase deficiency [48]. A recent study [49] showed that *Saccharomyces boulardii* also releases into the endoluminal medium a leucine aminopeptidase belonging to the zinc-metalloprotease family which enhances the proteolysis of small N-terminal peptides. This mechanism could help to reduce hypersensitisation to dietary proteins, in particular during acute gastroenteritis. Finally, one study [50] showed that the oral administration of *Saccharomyces boulardii* to rats for eight days following 60% proximal enterectomy, not only stimulated disaccharidase activity but also promoted the absorption of D-glucose coupled to Na+ through the glucose/Na+ symport. D-glucose absorption was measured *in vitro* on a preparation of brush border vesicles, as a function of both incubation time and the concentration of glucose in the incubation medium, comparatively to resected but untreated rats and control transected rats. The expression of SGLT-1 (sodium glucose cotransporter-1, 70kD) in the brush border membrane measured by autoradiography was stimulated in rats that had been resected and treated with *Saccharomyces boulardii*. These findings are consistent with those obtained later by Zaouche *et al.* [51].

Saccharomyces boulardii stimulates the production of several glycoproteins in the brush border of microvilli, including hydrolases, transporters, secretory IgA [26, 52] and the receptor for polymeric immunoglobulins [52], whose physiological functions and intracellular synthesis patterns differ profoundly. The mechanism underlying this stimulation has recently been investigated. Because *Saccharomyces boulardii* does not penetrate into enterocytes [46], we evaluated the influence of trophic factors secreted by *Saccharomyces boulardii* during its transit through the intestine. The intestinal functions in both villi and crypts that are stimulated by oral *Saccharomyces boulardii* are shown in Figure 7, together with the enzymatic and trophic factors secreted into the endoluminal medium.

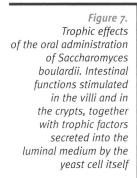

Figure 7.
Trophic effects of the oral administration of Saccharomyces boulardii. Intestinal functions stimulated in the villi and in the crypts, together with trophic factors secreted into the luminal medium by the yeast cell itself

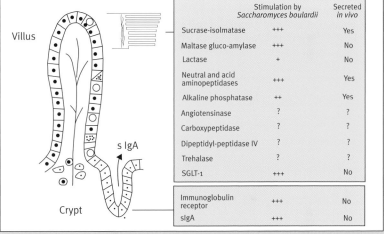

	Stimulation by *Saccharomyces boulardii*	Secreted *in vivo*
Sucrase-isolmatase	+++	Yes
Maltase gluco-amylase	+++	No
Lactase	+	No
Neutral and acid aminopeptidases	+++	Yes
Alkaline phosphatase	++	Yes
Angiotensinase	?	?
Carboxypeptidase	?	?
Dipeptidyl-peptidase IV	?	?
Trehalase	?	?
SGLT-1	+++	No
Immunoglobulin receptor	+++	No
sIgA	+++	No

As shown in Table II, HPLC assays performed on the lyophilised preparation of yeasts reveal significant quantities of polyamines, totaling 679 nanomoles/100 mg of lyophilised preparation, mainly spermidine (55%) and spermine (43%) with a negligible amount of putrescine (1.4%) [53].

In theory, such amounts of polyamines could influence the intestinal expression of brush border membrane glycoproteins (hydrolases, proteases, transport molecules, etc.). In practice, a marked stimulation of disaccharidase and aminopeptidase activities, and of the endoluminal secretion of secretory IgA has been observed in the small intestine of young unweaned rats in response to oral ingestion of spermine and spermidine equivalent to 1,000 nanomoles/day of purified polyamines. When infant rats were given an amount of spermine (500 nanomoles/day) equivalent to the polyamine content of the lyophilised preparation of yeast cells (679 nanomoles/100 mg), similar enzymatic responses were observed, including significant increases in the specific and total activities of both sucrase (x 2.5) and maltase (+24%). In response to 1,000 nanomoles of spermine, the stimulation of enzyme activities was proportionally greater with increased sucrase (x 4.6) and maltase (+70%) activities. Similarly, weaned rats that were treated with either *Saccharomyces boulardii* or equivalent quantities of spermine (500 nanomoles) presented parallel, significant increases in specific sucrase (+157%) and maltase (+47.5%) activities.

	S. boulardii, nanomoles/mg n = 8	S. boulardii, nanomoles/mg protein n = 8	
Putrescine	0.095 ± 0.014	0.28 ± 0.05	*Table II.* *Polyamine concentrations in lyophilised Saccharomyces boulardii preparations*
Spermidine	3.766 ± 0.328	10.9 ± 0.84	
Spermine	2.930 ± 0.268	8.42 ± 0.67	
TOTAL	6.79	19.6	

n = number of individual samples tested
All data are expressed as mean ± SD [53]

Therefore, the oral administration of 100 mg of lyophilised *Saccharomyces boulardii* containing 679 nanomoles of polyamines (compared here to that of 500 nanomoles of purified spermine) to breast-feeding suckling rats or weaned rats, led to similar changes in the enzymatic responses in microvilli. Stimulation of sucrase and maltase activity by the oral administration of spermine is a dose-dependent phenomenon. It is more sensitive than for other enzymes in the microvilli (lactase, aminopeptidase) and becomes detectable at doses of spermine reaching 250 nanomoles/day. Moreover, both *Saccharomyces boulardii* [53] and purified spermine (500 nanomoles/day) can significantly stimulate the intestinal production of the receptor for polymeric immunoglobulins in rats between ten and twenty days after birth.

In parallel to the modulation of enzyme activities, oral *Saccharomyces boulardii* treatment induces parallel modifications in polyamine concentrations, both in the gut mucosa (+21.4%) and the endoluminal fluid (+48% to +316% in the jejunum and +60.8% to +150% in the ileum). The changes in the concentrations of the three polyamines measured in the intestinal mucosa (putrescine: +7%, spermidine: +21.9%, spermine: +21.4%) were proportional to their respective concentrations measured in the lyophilised yeast preparations. In practice, spermine and spermidine, which represent 44% and 55% of all the polyamines released by *Saccharomyces boulardii*, increased by corresponding proportions in the intestinal mucosa of +21.4% and +21.9%.

In accordance with the small quantities of putrescine produced by the yeast (1.4%), the levels of putrescine in the mucosa fluctuated very little and were not affected by the oral treatment.

Experimental data suggest that transepithelial polyamine transport by brush border membrane vesicles is a selective and saturable process which largely depends on their endoluminal concentrations. In samples of jejunal and ileal fluids collected by rinsing the lumen followed by filtration to remove the yeast cells, spermidine and spermine levels were increased by 48% to 316% in *Saccharomyces boulardii*-treated rats compared with controls, whereas putrescine levels were not significantly changed. Since endoluminal polyamines (in particular putrescine) derivate from several sources including some foodstuffs (cheese), intestinal secretions, shed cells and metabolic processes of the bacterial microflora, variations in concentration are far greater in the lumen than in mucosal tissue.

In summary, the data in Table II show that, at the doses used, the lyophilised preparation of *Saccharomyces boulardii* induces trophic effects to the intestinal mucosa (Figure 8) which are probably mediated by the endoluminal release of spermine and spermidine. These polycationic substances could be released by yeast cells during their catabolism rather than being secreted by living cells. In practice, after 96 hours of exponential growth, only traces of putrescine had been detected in media in which yeast have been cultured, while no spermine or spermidine at all could be detected in the conditioned medium.

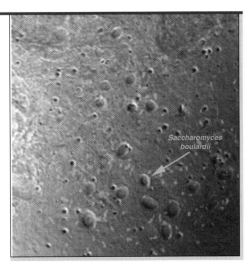

Figure 8.
Confocal microsocopy imaging
of sectioned murine caecum.
Bacteroides vulgatus + antibiotics
+ Saccharomyces boulardii
(micrograph: M.C. Barc, Faculté de Pharmacie,
Université Paris XI)

Because of the well-characterized effects of exogenous polyamines on the maturation of intestinal cells, enzyme expression, transport mechanisms, division of crypt cells, DNA synthesis, and gene expression, the substantial quantity of polyamines brought by *Saccharomyces boulardii* could have major clinical implications. Although the use of *Saccharomyces boulardii* has been well documented in acute gastroenteritis, antibiotic-associated diarrhoea (AAD) and enterocolopathy due to *Clostridium difficile* in children, the possible trophic effects of the yeast for the prevention of persistent chronic diarrhoea, chronic protracted diarrhoea, hypersensitisation to dietary proteins and treatment of congenital enzyme deficiencies (sucrase-isomaltase, trehalase) warrant further investigation.

In addition to the trophic effects mediated by these polyamines, a very promising line of research has been opened by investigation of the effects of *Saccharomyces boulardii* on the short-chain fatty acids (SCFA), i.e., butyrate, acetate and propionate. SCFAs are one of the most important metabolites produced by the anaerobic microflora in the colon: they play a major role in the colonic absorption of water and electrolytes [54]. In an *ex vivo* model of the microbial ecosystem in pigs, the administration of *Saccharomyces boulardii* re-establishes a normal level of SCFA production which had been reduced as a result of clindamycin destruction of the microbial microflora [55]. In a clinical pharmacology study conducted in ten patients receiving total parenteral nutrition, *Saccharomyces boulardii* treatment raised faecal SCFA concentrations (in particular that of butyrate), bringing them back up to levels comparable to those found in normal subjects [56]. This property could explain—at least in part—the antidiarrhoeal effect of *Saccharomyces boulardii* in clinical situations in which SCFAs drop as a result of damage to the colonic microflora, such as those caused by AAD and diarrhoea associated with total parenteral nutrition.

Antisecretory effect

Saccharomyces boulardii decreases the hypersecretion of water (–39%) and permeability to mannitol (–65%) induced by *Clostridium difficile* toxin A in the ileum of rats [23, 25]. In addition, *Saccharomyces boulardii* inhibits chloride secretion induced by the two signal transduction pathways mediated by intracellular cAMP and calcium ions in cells of the intestinal villi [31, 57].

Finally, the prophylactic administration of *Saccharomyces boulardii* exerts a powerful, dose-dependent effect on Castor oil-induced secretory diarrhoea in rats [58]. This effect is significantly reduced by L-arginine, suggesting that the nitrogen oxide (NO) pathway may be involved in this mechanism.

Immunostimulatory effect

In growing rats, *Saccharomyces boulardii* induced a marked increase (+57%) in the concentration of secretory IgA in the intestinal fluid as well as in the concentration of the secretory component (+63%) in crypt cells of the intestinal mucosa [52]. A comparable effect was observed in BALB/c mice which had been orally inoculated with a toxoid derived from *Clostridium difficile* toxin A resulting in large increases in the levels of total secretory IgA (x 1.8) and of specific secretory IgA directed against toxin A (x 4.4) [26].

Anti-inflammatory effect

Experimental models on protective mechanisms mediated by *Saccharomyces boulardii* in EPEC and EHEC infections have shown that *Saccharomyces boulardii* inhibits MAP kinase and NFκB signal transduction pathways, and inhibits secretion of the pro-inflammatory cytokine IL-8 [40].

In addition, Sougioultzis identified a soluble factor secreted by *Saccharomyces boulardii* which also inhibited NFκB-dependent signalling when intestinal cells were exposed to *Clostridium difficile* toxin A [59]. These studies pave the way for clinical trials of *Saccharomyces boulardii* in the treatment of inflammatory bowel diseases (IBD).

In summary, the mechanisms underlying the anti-diarrhoeal activity of *Saccharomyces boulardii* are mainly dependent on two types of pharmacodynamic property:
- inhibition of certain bacterial toxins and/or their pathogenic activities,
- direct effects to the intestinal mucosa involving trophic effects, antisecretory action, stimulation of the mucosal immune system, and anti-inflammatory effects.

Clinical trials

Antibiotic-associated diarrhoea and diarrhoea associated with *Clostridium difficile* enteropathy

Depending on the source, AAD complicates 5-30% of courses of antibiotic treatment. Symptoms range from "simple" diarrhoea (with neither dehydration nor electrolyte or water loss) to severe secretory diarrhoea which can be life-threatening, the extreme cases being colitis or pseudomembranous colitis.

Pathogenesis always includes perturbation of the microecological equilibrium and the barrier microflora due to the elimination of bacteria susceptible to the antibiotic administered. It is generally accepted that *Clostridium difficile* is responsible for 10-30% of cases of AAD and 95% of cases of pseudomembranous colitis [60]. It can also cause refractory enterocolopathy in infants [61]. AAD due to *Clostridium difficile*—above and beyond its potential seriousness—is characterized by frequent recurrence following the initial course of treatment: 20% after the initial episode and up to 60% after a first relapse [62]. The etiology of AAD is not confined to *Clostridium difficile*: a "colonic bacterial insufficiency syndrome" related to a failure to break down carbohydrates on the part of the normal bacterial microflora and/or short-chain fatty acid deficiency have been implicated [63]. In addition, other microorganisms, including *Klebsiella oxytoca* [64], have sometimes been suspected. The risk factors for AAD are now more fully understood. They are related to either the type and duration of the course of antibiotic treatment (long or repeated courses, multiple antibiotics, antibiotics excreted in the bile, antibiotics active against anaerobic species, broad-spectrum antibiotics) or host-related parameters (very young or very old age, severity of the infection being treated, chronic digestive problems, surgery, immunodeficiency, history of AAD and hospitalization) [65]. The existence of one or more of these risk factors can justify selective prevention of AAD. The use in the clinical context of a lyophilised preparation of *Saccharomyces boulardii* has been directly inspired by such epidemiological and pathogenetic considerations.

Prevention of antibiotic-associated diarrhoea

Four prospective, randomised, double-blind, placebo-controlled studies have confirmed the efficacy of *Saccharomyces boulardii* in the prevention of AAD.

In a first study conducted in 180 hospitalized patients [66], *Saccharomyces boulardii* was administered at the dose of 1 gram per day during the course of antibiotic treatment and then for a further two weeks after its end. The percentage of patients who developed AAD was 21.8% in the placebo group compared with 9.5% in the actively treated group (p = 0.038).

In a second study conducted in two centres including 193 patients receiving a β-lactam (with or without other concomitant antibiotics) in a hospital setting [67], *Saccharomyces boulardii* administered at the dose of 1 gram per day (beginning 48 hours after initiation of the antibiotic and continued during three days after the end of the course) reduced the occurrence of diarrhoea in the same proportion: 14.6% in the placebo group *versus* 7.2% in the treated group (p = 0.03).

These results confirm those of a previous study conducted in 388 adult outpatients [68]. Treatment with *Saccharomyces boulardii* at a dose of 200 mg per day throughout the antibiotic course (β-lactams or tetracyclines) reduced the percentage of patients experiencing AAD from 17.5% to 4.5%.

In a recent study, Szajewska *et al.* gave the first demonstration of the efficacy of *Saccharomyces boulardii* in a double-blind, placebo-controlled trial in infants. Two hundred and sixty-nine children were assigned to receive either *Saccharomyces boulardii*, 500 mg/day, or a placebo during the course of the antibiotic treatment. Patients receiving *Saccharomyces boulardii* had a lower prevalence of AAD compared with patients receiving the placebo (3.4% *versus* 17.3%, relative risk: 0.2; 95% confidence interval: 0.07-0.5) [69].

Treatment of recurrent forms of diarrhoea and colitis due to Clostridium difficile

Several clinical trials aimed to evaluate the efficacy of *Saccharomyces boulardii* in the treatment of recurrent colitis and diarrhoea due to *Clostridium difficile* have been conducted.

In a preliminary open study conducted in 13 patients with multiple recurrent *Clostridium difficile*-associated pseudomembranous colitis [70], the administration of *Saccharomyces boulardii* prescribed at a dose of 1 gram per day for one month as an adjunct to standard vancomycin treatment prevented the occurrence of subsequent relapse in eleven of the thirteen patients.

A multicentric, randomised, double-blind, placebo-controlled trial conducted in 124 patients treated with vancomycin or metronidazole for an episode of *Clostridium difficile* colitis or diarrhoea [62] evaluated the effect of *Saccharomyces boulardii* on the occurrence of subsequent relapses. In patients who had already experienced at least one relapse (n = 60), the administration of *Saccharomyces boulardii* significantly reduced the occurrence of subsequent recurrences: 64.7% recurrence in the placebo group *versus* 34.6% in the *Saccharomyces boulardii*-treated group (p = 0.04).

Another multicentric, double-blind, placebo-controlled clinical trial conducted in 170 patients with a recurrent intestinal infection of *Clostridium difficile* treated for ten days by vancomycin, either at a high dosage (2 grams per day) or a low dosage (500 mg), or by metronidazole and by *Saccharomyces boulardii* (1 gram per day) or placebo for four weeks, showed that the "high-dosage vancomycin + *Saccharomyces boulardii*" therapeutic regimen was the association of choice for the management of this disease [71].

Treatment of enterocolopathy due to Clostridium difficile in children

In children, intestinal *Clostridium difficile* infection presents rarely as a pseudomembranous colitis. It causes more commonly an acute diarrhoea or a chronic enterocolopathy. In an open study, 19 infants and children presenting with a clinical picture of chronic diarrhoea and in whom toxigenic *Clostridium difficile* was the only enteropathogen identified by stool culture and sterotyping were evaluated. Most of the patients had been given one or more courses of antibiotic for intestinal infections in the weeks or months preceding admission. Treatment with *Saccharomyces boulardii* at a dosage of 500-1,000 mg per day (depending on age) for 15 days led to a rapid regression of the symptoms in 18 of the children, and clearance of toxin B and *Clostridium difficile* in 16 of them [61].

Acute gastroenteritis

A prospective, randomised study was performed to evaluate the usefulness of *Saccharomyces boulardii* given at a dose of 500 mg per day, as a complement to oral rehydration therapy in moderately severe acute enteritis in infants. Comparison of the treated group (n = 19) and the control group (n = 19) on d1 and d4 revealed significant improvement in four clinical end points, i.e. stool number, weight and consistency of stools, and Carmine Red transit time in the group treated with *Saccharomyces boulardii* [72].

In a double-blind, placebo-controlled clinical trial of 130 children aged between three months and three years of age, the administration of *Saccharomyces boulardii*, at a dose of 200 mg every 8 hours, significantly reduced the frequency of bowel movements as of the 48th hour of treatment. At 48 hours and 96 hours of treatment, the number of patients presenting with normal stools was significantly higher in the treated group than in the control group [73].

In another recent double-blind placebo-controlled study, Kurugöl *et al.* confirmed the efficacy of *Saccharomyces boulardii* when administered to children at a dose of 250 mg/day for 5 days. The duration of diarrhoea was significantly reduced in the *Saccharomyces boulardii* group compared with the placebo group (4.7 *versus* 5.5 days, p = 0.03). The duration of hospital stay was shorter in the *Saccharomyces boulardii* group than in the placebo group (2.9 *versus* 3.9 days, p < 0.001). Four children from the placebo group *versus* only one child from the *Saccharomyces boulardii* group had persisting diarrhoea [74].

In a double-blind, placebo-controlled clinical trial conducted in 92 adults with acute diarrhoea [75], after 48 hours of the administration of *Saccharomyces boulardii,* diarrhoeal symptoms—expressed as a composite score based on stool number and consistency—were significantly reduced (p = 0.035).

Traveller's diarrhoea

Tourists visiting southern countries are exposed to an increased risk of diarrhoea, the most common health problem affecting visitors of tropical and sub-tropical regions.

The efficacy of *Saccharomyces boulardii* in the prevention of traveller's diarrhoea has been demonstrated in many travellers visiting various different parts of the world. A total of 1,016 questionnaires fulfilling the criteria of traveler's diarrhoea were analysed to evaluate the efficacy of *Saccharomyces boulardii*. The treatment was administered five days prior to departure and then throughout the trip.

The patients were divided into three groups: the first took a placebo, the second took *Saccharomyces boulardii* at a dose of 250 mg per day, and the third took *Saccharomyces boulardii* at a dose of 1,000 mg per day.

The incidence of diarrhoea was respectively 39.1%, 34.4% (p = 0.019 *versus* placebo) and 28.7% (p = 0.005 *versus* placebo). Regional differences were observed with the prophylactic effect which was greatest in travellers visiting North Africa [76].

Clinical trials in other conditions

Clinical studies have also been conducted in other conditions which involve perturbation of the balance of the intestinal ecosystem.

Diarrhoea associated with total enteral nutrition

Three randomised, double-blind, placebo-controlled studies have demonstrated the efficacy of *Saccharomyces boulardii* in the prevention of diarrhoea in patients on total enteral nutrition.

In patients treated in an intensive care unit, the oral administration of *Saccharomyces boulardii* at the dose of 500 mg/L of enteral solution reduced the percentage of days of diarrhoea from 16.9% to 8.7% (p < 0.001) [77].

In patients treated in a burn unit, prophylactic *Saccharomyces boulardii* at a dose of 2 grams per day reduced the percentage of days of diarrhoea from 9.1% to 1.5% (p < 0.001) and significantly improved digestive tolerance of continuous enteral nutrition expressed in terms of caloric intake [78].

Finally, a multicentric study (eleven centres) of 128 patients confirmed the efficacy of *Saccharomyces boulardii* administered at a dose of 2 grams per day in the prevention of diarrhoea in subjects on total enteral nutrition in medical and surgical intensive care units [79]. In the *Saccharomyces boulardii*-treated group, there was a significantly lower number of days of diarrhoea (14% *Saccharomyces boulardii versus* 19% placebo, p < 0.01).

Diarrhoea in AIDS

In an open study of 17 patients with AIDS and chronic diarrhoea, *Saccharomyces boulardii* prescribed at the dose of 3 grams per day for 15 days clearly improved the diarrhoea with a reduction in the mean number of daily bowel movements from 9.0 to 2.1 [80]. A double-blind study of 35 patients confirmed these results: after one week of treatment, the diarrhoea had been brought under control in 61% of the patients in the *Saccharomyces boulardii*-treated group compared with 12% in the placebo group (p < 0.002). Significant improvements were recorded in the number, weight and volume of the stools, abdominal pain, body weight and quality of life (according to the Karnofsky index) [81].

Irritable bowel syndrome

A double-blind, placebo-controlled clinical trial including 34 patients suffering from irritable bowel syndrome with predominant diarrhoea showed that *Saccharomyces boulardii* treatment had a significant effect (p < 0.05) on the number and consistency of stools after one month of treatment [82].

Inflammatory bowel diseases

A randomised clinical trial was conducted to evaluate the efficacy of *Saccharomyces boulardii* treatment (1 gram per day) combined with mesalazine (2 grams per day) *versus* mesalazine alone (3 grams per day) in the prevention of relapse in Crohn's disease in remission [83]. At the end of the six months of the study, the recurrence rate was 37.5% in the group treated with mesalazine alone (n = 16) *versus* 6.25% in the group treated with a combination of *Saccharomyces boulardii* and mesalazine (n = 16, p = 0.04).

The results of a recent pilot study have opened interesting perspectives concerning maintenance treatment in moderately to severe forms of ulcerative colitis [84].

Safety

Lyophilised *Saccharomyces boulardii* is a biotherapeutic agent which is well tolerated in usual conditions.

In a few very rare cases, blood cultures positive for *Saccharomyces boulardii* have been recorded and there have been some reports of fungaemia. In the reported cases, all the patients had a central venous catheter installed [85].

Saccharomyces boulardii fungaemia regressed either spontaneously once the product was withdrawn, or responded to antifungal treatment; in some cases, the central venous catheter had to be removed. Contamination of the catheter during the handling of sachets or capsules containing the product would seem to be the most likely source of such infections and in consequence, the administration of lyophilised *Saccharomyces boulardii* is contraindicated in patients with a central venous catheter [85, 86].

Conclusion

Benefiting enormously from progress in our understanding of the physiological role of the intestinal microflora, the mechanisms of action of *Saccharomyces boulardii* have been partly elucidated: release *in vivo* of substances that inhibit certain bacterial toxins and/or their pathogenic effects, trophic effects, antisecretory activity, immunostimulatory and anti-inflammatory effects on the intestinal mucosa.

The efficacy of lyophilised *Saccharomyces boulardii* has been clinically demonstrated in placebo controlled studies for the treatment of various forms of diarrhoea in which the balance of the intestinal microbial ecosystem is disrupted. The efficacy of the product has been especially clearly shown in the prevention of antibiotic-associated diarrhoea, and the treatment of recurrent *Clostridium difficile* intestinal infection.

Key points

- Lyophilised *Saccharomyces boulardii* is an example of a bio-therapeutic agent whose active substance is a live microorganism, designed to treat or prevent various digestive diseases and developed according to the rules governing medicinal products.

- After repeated oral administration, *Saccharomyces boulardii* does not become established in the digestive tract but transits through it in a viable form, reaching a stable concentration by the third day of administration; the yeast disappears from the faeces forty-eight hours after discontinuation of treatment.

- In the course of its passage through the intestine, *Saccharomyces boulardii* mediates pharmacodynamic effects which resemble the protective effects of the normal gut microflora. The mechanisms of action of *Saccharomyces boulardii* mainly depend on the inhibition of certain bacterial toxins and/or their pathogenic effects, antisecretory effects, immunostimulatory activity, and anti-inflammatory effects on the intestinal mucosa.

- The clinical activity of lyophilised *Saccharomyces boulardii* is especially relevant to antibiotic-associated diarrhoea and recurrent *Clostridium difficile* intestinal infection, and also to the prevention and treatment of various other types of diarrhoea.

- Promising research perspectives have been opened in terms of maintenance treatment for inflammatory bowel diseases.

References

1. Hennequin C, Thierry A, Richard GF, *et al*. Microsatellite typing as a new tool for identification of *Saccharomyces cerevisiae* strains. *J Clin Microbiol* 2001 ; 39 : 551-9.

2. Maillié M, Nguyen Van P, Bertout S, Vaillant C, Bastide JM. Genotypic study of *Saccharomyces boulardii* compared to the *Saccharomyces sensu stricto* complex species. *J Mycol Med* 2001 ; 11 : 19-25.

3. Fuller R. Probiotics in human medicine. *Gut* 1991 ; 32 : 439-42.

4. Marteau PR, de Vrese M, Cellier CJ, Schrezenmeir. Protection from gastrointestinal diseases with the use of probiotics. *Am J Clin Nutr* 2001 ; 73 : 4305-65.

5. Elmer GW, Surawicz CM, McFarland LV. Biotherapeutic agents. A neglected modality for the treatment and prevention of selected intestinal and vaginal infections. *JAMA* 1996 ; 275 : 870-6.

6. McFarland LV, Bernasconi P. *Saccharomyces boulardii*: a review of an innovative biotherapeutic agent. *Microbiol Ecology Health Dis* 1993 ; 6 : 57-171.

7. Bergogne-Bérézin E. Impact écologique de l'antibiothérapie. Place des micro-organismes de substitution dans le contrôle des diarrhées et colites associées aux antibiotiques. *Presse Med* 1995 ; 24 : 145-56.

8. Ducluzeau R, Bensaada M. Effet comparé de l'administration unique ou en continu du *Saccharomyces boulardii* sur l'établissement de diverses souches de *Candida* dans le tractus digestif de souris gnotoxéniques. *Ann Microbiol (Paris)* 1982 ; 133 : 491-501.

9. Bléhaut H, Massot J, Elmer GW, Levy RH. Disposition kinetics of *Saccharomyces boulardii* in man and rat. *Biopharm Drug Dispos* 1989 ; 10 : 353-64.

10. Boddy AV, Elmer GW, McFarland LV, Levy RH. Influence of antibiotics on the recovery and kinetics of *Saccharomyces boulardii* in rats. *Pharm Res* 1991 ; 8 : 796-800.

11. Klein SM, Elmer GW, McFarland LV, Surawicz CM, Levy RH. Recovery and elimination of the biotherapeutic agent, *Saccharomyces boulardii*, in healthy human volunteers. *Pharm Res* 1993; 10 : 1615-9.

12. Elmer GW, McFarland LV, Surawicz CM, Dankos L, Greenberg RN. Behavior of *Saccharomyces boulardii* in recurrent *Clostridium difficile* disease patients. *Aliment Pharmacol Ther* 1999 ; 13 : 1663-8.

13. Toothaker RD, Elmer GW. Prevention of Clindamycin-induced mortality in hamster by *Saccharomyces boulardii*. *Antimicrobial Ag Chemother* 1984 ; 26 : 552-6.

14. Corthier G, Dubois F, Ducluzeau R. Prevention of *Clostridium difficile* induced mortality in gnotobiotic mice by *Saccharomyces boulardii*. *Can J Microbiol* 1986 ; 32 : 294-6.

15. Corthier G, Lucas F, Jouvert S, Castex F. Effect of oral *Saccharomyces boulardii* treatment on the activity of *Clostridium difficile* toxins in mouse digestive tract. *Toxicon* 1992 ; 30 : 1583-9.

16. Massot J, Sanchez O, Couchy R, Antoin J, Parodi AL. Bacterio-pharmacological activity of *Saccharomyces boulardii* in Clindamycin induced colitis in the hamster. *Arzn-Forsch/Drug Res* 1984 ; 34 : 794-7.

17. Castex F, Corthier G, Joubert S, Elmer GW, Lucas F, Bastide M. Prevention of *Clostridium difficile*-induced experimental pseudomembranous colitis by *Saccharomyces boulardii*: a scanning electron microscopic and microbiological study. *J Gen Microbiol* 1990 : 136 : 1085-9.

18. Corthier G, Muller MC, Wilkins TD, Lyerly D, L'Haridon R. Protection against pseudomembranous colitis in gnotobiotic mice by use of monoclonal antibodies against *Clostridium difficile* toxin A. *Infect Immun* 1991 ; 59 : 1192-5.

19. Czerucka D, Nano JL, Bernasconi P, Rampal P. Réponse aux toxines A et B de *Clostridium difficile* d'une lignée de cellules épithéliales de rat : IRD 98. Effet de *Saccharomyces boulardii*. *Gastroenterol Clin Biol* 1991 ; 15 : 22-7.

20. Elmer GW, Corthier G. Modulation of *Clostridium difficile* induced mortality as a function of the dose and viability of the *Saccharomyces boulardii* used as a preventative agent in gnotobiotic mice. *Can J Microbiol* 1991 ; 37 : 315-7.

21. Elmer GW, McFarland LV. Suppression by *Saccharomyces boulardii* of toxinogenic *Clostridium difficile* overgrowth after Vancomycin treatment in hamsters. *Antimicrobiol Ag Chemother* 1987 ; 31 : 129-31.

22. Czerucka D, Rampal P. Experimental effects of *Saccharomyces boulardii* on diarrheal pathogens. *Microbes Infect* 2002 ; 4 : 733-9.

23. Pothoulakis C, Kelly CP, Joshi MA, *et al. Saccharomyces boulardii* inhibits *Clostridium difficile* toxin A binding and enterotoxicity in rat ileum. *Gastroenterology* 1993 ; 104 : 1108-15.

24. Castagliuolo I, LaMont JT, Nikulasson ST, Pothoulakis C. *Saccharomyces boulardii* protease inhibits *Clostridium difficile* toxin A effects in the rat ileum. *Infect Immun* 1996 ; 12 : 5225-32.

25. Castagliuolo I, Riegler MF, Valenick L, LaMont JT, Pothoulakis C. *Saccharomyces boulardii* protease mediates *Clostridium difficile* toxin A and B effects in human colonic mucosa. *Infect Immun* 1999 ; 67 : 302-7.

26. Qamar A, Aboudola S, Warny M, *et al. Saccharomyces boulardii* stimulates intestinal immunoglobulin A immune response to *Clostridium difficile* toxin A in mice. *Infect Immun* 2001 ; 69 : 2762-5.

27. Tasteyre A, Barc MC, Karjalainen T, Bourlioux P, Collignon A. Inhibition of *in vivo* cell adherence of *Clostridium difficile* by *Saccharomyces boulardii*. *Microbiol Pathogen* 2002 ; 32 : 219-25.

28. Vidon N, Huchet B, Rambaud JC. Influence de *Saccharomyces boulardii* sur la sécrétion jéjunale induite chez le rat par la toxine cholérique. *Gastroenterol Clin Biol* 1986 ; 10 : 13-6.

29. Czerucka D, Nano JL, Bernasconi P, Rampal P. Réponse à la toxine cholérique de deux lignées de cellules épithéliales intestinales. Effet de *Saccharomyces boulardii*. *Gastroenterol Clin Biol* 1989 ; 13 : 383-7.

30. Czerucka D, Roux I, Rampal P. *Saccharomyces boulardii* inhibits secretagogue-mediated adenosine 3', 5'-cyclic monophosphate induction in intestinal cells. *Gastroenterology* 1994 ; 106 : 65-72.

31. Czerucka D, Rampal P. Effect of *Saccharomyces boulardii* on cAMP-and Ca2+-dependent Cl⁻ secretion in T84 cells. *Dig Dis Sci* 1999 ; 44 : 2359-68.

32. Barrett KE. Positive and negative regulation of chloride secretion. *Am J Physiol* 1993 ; 265 : C859-68.

33. Venglarik CJ, Bridges RJ, Frizel RA. A simple assay for agonist-regulated Cl and K conductances in salt-secreting epithelial cells. *Am J Physiol* 1990 ; 259 : C358-64.

34. Massot J, Desconclois M, Astoin J. Protection par *Saccharomyces boulardii* de la diarrhée à *Escherichia coli* du souriceau. *Annal Pharm Franc* 1982 ; 40 : 445-9.

35. Nataro J, Kaper JB. Diarrheagenic *Escherichia coli*. *Clin Microbiol Rev* 1998 ; 11 : 142-201.

36. Philpott DJ, McKay DM, Sherman PM, Perdue MH. Infection of T84 cells with enteropathogenic *Escherichia coli* alters barrier and transport functions. *Am J Physiol* 1998 ; 33 : G634-45.

37. Savkovic SD, Koutsouris A, Hecht G. Attachment of a non invasive enteric pathogen, enteropathogenic *Escherichia coli*, to cultured human intestinal epithelial monolayers induces transmigration of neutrophils. *Infect Immun* 1996 ; 64 : 4480-7.

38. Yuhan R, Koutsouris A, Savkovic SD, Heicht G. Enteropathogenic *Escherichia coli*-induced myosin light chain phosphorylation alters intestinal epithelial permeability. *Gastroenterology* 1997 ; 113 : 1873-82.

39. Czerucka D, Dahan S, Mograbi B, Rossi B, Rampal P. *Saccharomyces boulardii* preserves the barrier function and modulates the signal transduction pathway induced in enteropathogenic *Escherichia coli*-infected T84 cells. *Infect Immun* 2000 ; 68 : 5998-6004.

40. Dahan S, Dalmasso G, Imbert V, Peyron JF, Rampal P, Czerucka D. *Saccharomyces boulardii* interfers with enterohemorragic *Escherichia coli*-induced signaling pathways in T84 cells. *Infect Immun* 2003 ; 71 : 766-73.

41. Czerucka D, Dahan S, Mograbi B, Rossi B, Rampal P. Implication of mitogen-activated protein kinases in T84 cell responses to enteropathogenic *Escherichia coli* infection. *Infect Immun* 2001 ; 69 : 1298-305.

42. Dahan S, Busutill V, Imbert V, Peyron JF, Rampal P, Czerucka D. Enterohemorragic *Escherichia coli* infection induces interleukin-8 production *via* activation of mitogen-activated protein kinases and the transcription factors NF-kappa B and AP-1 in T84 cells. *Infect Immun* 2002 ; 70 : 2304-10.

43. Hobbies S, Chen LM, Davis RJ, Galan JE. Involvement of mitogen-activated protein kinase pathways in the nuclear responses and cytokine production induced by *Salmonella typhimurium* in cultured intestinal epithelial cells. *J Immunol* 1997 ; 57 : 1290-8.

44. Tang P, Sutherland YA, Gold MR, Finlay BB. *Listeria monocytogenes* invasion of epithelial cells requires the MEK-1/ERK-2 mitogen-activated protein kinase pathway. *Infect Immun* 1998 ; 66 : 1106-12.

45. Rodrigues ACP, Nardi RM, Bambirra EA, Viera EC, Nicoli JR. Effect of *Saccharomyces boulardii* against experimental oral infection with *Salmonella typhimurium* and *Shigella flexneri* conventional and gnotobiotic mice. *J Appl Bacteriol* 1996 ; 91 : 251-6.

46. Buts JP, Bernasconi P, Van Craynest MP, Maldague P, De Meyer R. Response of human and rat small intestinal mucosa to oral administration of *Saccharomyces boulardii*. *Pediatr Res* 1986 ; 20 : 192-6.

47. Jahn HU, Ullrich R, Schneider T, *et al*. Immunology and tropical effects of *Saccharomyces boulardii* on the small intestine in healthy human volunteers. *Digestion* 1996 ; 57 : 95-104.

48. Harms HK, Bertele-Harms RM, Bruer-Kleis D. Enzyme substitution therapy with the yeast *Saccharomyces boulardii* in congenital sucrase isomaltase deficiency. *N Engl J Med* 1987 ; 316 : 1306-9.

49. Buts JP, De Keyser N, Stilmant C, Sokal E, Marandi S. *Saccharomyces boulardii* enhances N-terminal peptide hydrolysis in suckling rat small intestine by endoluminal release of a zinc-binding metalloprotease. *Pediatr Res* 2002 ; 51 : 528-34.

50. Buts JP, De Keyser N, Marandi S, *et al*. *Saccharomyces boulardii* upgrades cellular adaptation after proximal enterectomy in rats. *Gut* 1999 ; 45 : 89-96.

51. Zaouche A, Loukil C, de La Gausie P, *et al*. Effects of oral *Saccharomyces boulardii* on bacterial overgrowth, translocation and intestinal adaptation after small bowel resection in rats. *Scand J Gastroenterol* 2000 ; 35 : 160-5.

52. Buts JP, Bernasconi P, Vaerman JP, Dive C. Stimulation of secretory IgA and secretory component of immunoglobulins in small intestine of rats treated with *Saccharomyces boulardii*. *Dig Dis Sci* 1990 ; 35 : 251-6.

53. Buts JP, De Keyser N, De Raedemaeker L. *Saccharomyces boulardii* enhances rat intestinal enzyme expression by endoluminal release of polyamines. *Pediatr Res* 1994 ; 36 : 522-7.

54. Bowling TF, Raimundo AH, Grimble GK, Silk DB. Reversal by short-chain fatty acids of colonic fluid secretion induced by enteral feeding. *Lancet* 1993 ; 342 : 1266-8.

55. Breves G, Faul K, Schröder B, Holst HF, Caspary W, Stein J. Application of the colon-stimulation technique for studying the effects of *Saccharomyces boulardii* on basic parameters of porcine cecal microbial metabolism disturbed by Clindamycin. *Digestion* 2000 ; 61 : 193-200.

56. Schneider SM, Girard-Pipau F, Filippi J, *et al*. Effects of *Saccharomyces boulardii* on fecal short-chain fatty acids and microflora in patients on long-term total enteral nutrition. *World J Gastroenterol* 2005 ; 11 : 6165-9.

57. Krammer M, Karbach U. Antidiarrheal action of the yeast *Saccharomyces boulardii* in the rat small and large intestine by stimulating chloride absorption. *Z Gastroenterol* 1993 ; 31 : 73-7.

58. Girard P, Pansart Y, Lorette I, Gillardin JM. Dose-response relationship and mechanism of action of *Saccharomyces boulardii* in castor oil-induced diarrhea in rats. *Dig Dis Sci* 2003 ; 48 : 770-4.

59. Sogioultzis, *et al*. *Gastroenterology* 2003 ; 125 : 606 abstract.

60. Kelly CP, Pothoulakis C, LaMont JT. Pseudomembranous colitis. *N Engl J Med* 1994 ; 330 : 257-62.

61. Buts JP, Corthier G, Delmée M. *Saccharomyces boulardii* for *Clostridium difficile*-associated enterocolopathies in infants. *J Pediatr Gastroenterol Nutr* 1993 ; 16 : 419-25.

62. McFarland LV, Surawicz CM, Greenberg RN, *et al*. A randomized placebo-controlled trial of *Saccharomyces boulardii* in combination with standard antibiotics for *Clostridium difficile* disease. *JAMA* 1994 ; 271 : 1913-8.

63. Clausen MR, Bonnen H, Tvede M, Mortensen PB. Colonic fermentation to short-chain fatty acids is decreased in antibiotic-associated diarrhea. *Gastroenterology* 1991 ; 101 : 1497-504.

64. Benoit R, Dorval D, Loulergue J, *et al*. Diarrhée post-antibiotique : rôle de *Klebsiella oxytoca*. *Gastroenterol Clin Biol* 1992 ; 16 : 860-4.

65. McFarland LV. Risk factors for antibiotic-associated diarrhea. A review of the literature. *Ann Med Int* 1998 ; 149 : 261-6.

66. Surawicz CM, Elmer GW, Speelman P, McFarland LV, Chinn J, Van Belle G. Prevention of antibiotic associated diarrhea by *Saccharomyces boulardii*: a prospective study. *Gastroenterology* 1989 ; 96 : 981-8.

67. McFarland LV, Surawicz CM, Greenberg RN, *et al*. Prevention of beta-lactam associated diarrhea by *Saccharomyces boulardii* compared with placebo. *Am J Gastroenterol* 1995 ; 90 : 439-48.

68. Adam J, Barret A, Barret-Bellet C. Essais cliniques contrôlés en double insu de l'Ultra-Levure lyophilisée. Étude multicentrique par 25 médecins de 388 cas. *Med Chir Dig* 1976 ; 5 : 401-5 .

69. Kotowska M, Albrecht P, Szajewska H. *Saccharomyces boulardii* in the prevention of antibiotic-associated diarrhoea in children: a randomized double-blind placebo-controlled trial. *Aliment Pharmacol Ther* 2005 ; 21 : 583-90.

70. Surawicz CM, McFarland LV, Elmer G, Chinn J. Treatment of recurrent *Clostridium difficile* colitis with vancomycin and *Saccharomyces boulardii*. *Am J Gastroenterol* 1989 ; 84 : 1285-7.

71. Surawicz CM, McFarland LV, Greenberg R, *et al*. The search for a better treatment for recurrent *Clostridium difficile* disease: use of high-dose Vancomycin combined with *Saccharomyces boulardii*. *Clin Infect Dis* 2000 ; 31 : 1012-7.

72. Chapoy P. Traitement des diarrhées aiguës infantiles : essai contrôlé de *Saccharomyces boulardii*. *Ann Pediatr* 1985 ; 32 : 561-3.

73. Cetina-Sauri G, Sierra Basto G. Évaluation thérapeutique de *Saccharomyces boulardii* chez des enfants souffrant de diarrhée aiguë. *Ann Pediatr* 1994 ; 41 : 397-400.

74. Kurugol Z, Koturoglu G. Effects of *Saccharomyces boulardii* in children with acute diarrhoea. *Acta Paediatr* 2005 ; 94 : 44-7.

75. Höchter W, Chase D, Hagenhoff G. *Saccharomyces boulardii* in treatment of acute adult diarrhea. Efficacy and tolerance of treatment. *Münch Med Wochen* 1990;132:188-92.

76. Kollaritsch H, Holst H, Grobara P, *et al*. Prophylaxe der reisediarrhöe mit *Saccharomyces boulardii*. *Forst Chr Med* 1993 ; 111 : 152-6.

77. Tempe JD, Steidel AL, Bléhaut H, Hasselmann M, Lutun P, Maurier F. Prévention par *Saccharomyces boulardii* des diarrhées de l'alimentation entérale à débit continu. *Sem Hop (Paris)* 1983 ; 59 : 1409-12.

78. Schlotterer M, Bernasconi P, Lebreton F, Wassermann D. Intérêt de *Saccharomyces boulardii* dans la tolérance digestive de la nutrition entérale à débit continu chez le brûlé. *Nutr Clin Metabol* 1987 ; 1 : 31-4.

79. Bleichner G, Bléhaut H, Mentec H, Moyse D. *Saccharomyces boulardii* prevents diarrhea in critically ill tube-fed patients. A multicenter, randomized, double-blind placebo-controlled trial. *Intensive Care Med* 1997 ; 23 : 517-23.

80. Saint-Marc T, Rossello-Prats L, Touraine JL. Efficacité de *Saccharomyces boulardii* dans le traitement des diarrhées du sida. *Ann Med Int* 1991 ; 142 : 64-5.

81. Saint-Marc T, Bléhaut H, Musial C, Touraine JL. Diarrhées en relation avec le sida. Essai en double aveugle de *Saccharomyces boulardii*. *Sem Hop (Paris)* 1995 ; 71 : 735-41.

82. Maupas JL, Champemont P, Delforge M. Traitement des colopathies fonctionnelles. Essai en double aveugle de l'Ultra-Levure (Treatment of irritable bowel syndrome with *Saccharomyces boulardii*-a double blind, placebo controlled study). *Med Chir Dig* 1983 ;12 : 77-9.

83. Guslandi M, Mezzi G, Sorghi M, Testoni PA. *Saccharomyces boulardii* in maintenance treatment of Crohn's disease. *Dig Dis Sci* 2000 ; 45 : 1462-4.

84. Guslandi M, Giollo P, Testoni PA. A pilot trial of *Saccharomyces boulardii* in ulcerative colitis. *Eur J Gastroenterol Hepatol* 2003 ; 15 : 697-8.

85. Hennequin C, Kauffman-Lacroix C, Jobert A, *et al*. Possible role of catheters in *Saccharomyces boulardii* fungemia. *Eur J Clin Microbiol Infect Dis* 2000 ; 19 : 16-20.

86. Perapoch J, Planes AM, Querol A, *et al*. Fungemia with *Saccharomyces boulardii cerevisiae*, only one of whom had been treated with Ultra-Levure. *Eur J Clin Microbiol Infect Dis* 2000 ; 19 : 468-70.

Index

Proliferation: 22, 42, 49, 97, 107, 110, 112, 113, 115-118, 120, 125, 127, 139, 155, 156, 173, 181, 203, 205, 213, 214

Propionate: 52, 64, 67, 68, 72, 78, 99, 101, 104, 114, 234

Proteases: 61, 71, 72, 164, 193, 216, 224, 225, 231

Pseudomembranous colitis: 181, 187, 189, 190, 205, 235-237

R

Recurrence: 152, 153, 158, 167, 188, 192-194, 205, 206, 210, 211, 235, 236, 239

Reductive acetogenesis: 70

Relapse(s): 192-194, 205, 206, 210, 211, 222, 235, 236, 239

Resident microflora: 21, 22, 32, 38, 40, 141, 160

Ribosomal DNA (rDNA): 7-10, 13, 15, 16, 19, 23, 31, 172

Ribosomal RNA (rRNA): 7-13, 16, 17, 19, 23-25, 172, 177

Risk factor(s): 30, 38, 49, 126, 163, 181, 182, 187, 205, 235, 236

Rome criteria: 102, 103

Rotavirus: 47, 142, 143, 147, 176, 207-209

S

Salmonella: 40, 48, 145, 174, 183, 202, 228, 229

Saprophytic microflora: 171-173, 175-178

Shigella: 174, 176, 229

Short-chain fatty acids (SCFA): 21, 37, 47, 52, 61, 78, 101-103, 105, 107, 120, 153, 183, 202, 203, 234, 235

Stem cells: 107-110, 112

Steroid hormones: 74, 77

Sterol(s): 62, 63, 74, 78

Sucrase: 46, 230, 232, 234

Sulphate-reduction: 69

Survival: 20, 39, 43-45, 110, 155, 224

Symbiosis: 107

Symbiotic: 19, 51, 123, 131

T

TNFα: 48, 133, 136, 155, 156, 158, 163-165, 167, 229

Transit: 21, 55, 71, 82, 85, 86, 89, 90, 92, 99-101, 103, 104, 114, 132, 172, 184, 194, 204, 237

Traveller's diarrhoea: 38, 42, 206, 207, 216, 237, 238

Trophic effect(s): 115, 223, 230, 231, 233-235, 239

U

Ulcerative colitis: 50, 118, 145, 151-153, 156, 158, 159, 161, 162, 185, 186, 190, 211, 239

Ulcers: 49, 151, 152, 185, 190, 209, 210

V

Vancomycin: 49, 51, 187, 191, 192, 205, 206, 236, 237

Vibrio cholerae: 175, 224, 226

Achevé d'imprimer par Corlet, Imprimeur, S.A. - 14110 Condé-sur-Noireau
N° d'Imprimeur : 90964 - Dépôt légal : avril 2006 - *Imprimé en France*